The Evidence for
Plastic Surgery

Edited by Christopher Stone

Foreword by Nicholas Parkhouse

Publisher

tfm Publishing Limited
Castle Hill Barns
Harley
Shrewsbury
SY5 6LX
UK

Tel: +44 (0)1952 510061
Fax: +44 (0)1952 510192
E-mail: nikki@tfmpublishing.com
Web site: www.tfmpublishing.com

Design and layout: Nikki Bramhill
First Edition   © April 2008

ISBN 978 1 903378 50 2

Printed by Gutenberg Press Ltd., Gudja Road, Tarxien, PLA 19, Malta.

Tel: +356 21897037; Fax: +356 21800069.

Contents

Page

Foreword   viii

Introduction   Applying evidence-based medicine to plastic surgery   1
             Christopher Stone

Chapter 1   Timing and method of soft tissue reconstruction in patients with IIIb tibial fractures   3
             Andrew DH Wilson, Christopher Stone

Chapter 2   Vacuum-assisted closure: basic science and clinical practice   15
             J. Alexa Potter, Christopher Stone

Chapter 3   The management of necrotising fasciitis   25
             Rachel Tillett, Tim Ward, Marina Morgan, Christopher Stone

Chapter 4   The relationship between increasing body mass index and complications in plastic surgery   37
             Mark S Lloyd, Peter Budny

Chapter 5   Prophylaxis to prevent venous thrombo-embolic disease in plastic surgery patients   49
             James Seaward, Andrew Watts

Chapter 6   Physiological responses to burn injury and resuscitation protocols for adult major burns   63
             Rob Duncan, Ken Dunn

Chapter 7   Improving outcome in paediatric burns   93
             Siobhán O'Ceallaigh, Mamta Shah

Chapter 8   Biological skin substitutes   103
             Lachlan Currie

Chapter 9   Sentinel lymph node biopsy in melanoma   117
             Gordon J McArthur, Barry W Powell

Chapter 10   Management of inguinal and pelvic nodes in patients with stage III malignant melanoma   127
             Ahmed Ali-Khan, Christopher Stone

Chapter 11   Prognostic indicators in adult soft tissue sarcoma   133
             Paul Wilson, Christopher Stone

Chapter 12   Evidence-based imaging of soft tissue sarcomas   145
             Alun G Davies, David AT Silver

Chapter 13   Hypospadias correction: one or two stages?   159
             Norbert Kang, Marc Pacifico

Chapter 14   Cleft palate closure: the timing and options for surgical repair   171
             Simon van Eeden, Loshan Kangesu, Brian Sommerlad

Chapter 15 Post-traumatic wrist instability   183
          Rob Gilbert, Neil Ashwood

Chapter 16 Wrist arthroscopy: its role in diagnosis and treatment   199
          Cronan Kerin, Neil Ashwood

Chapter 17 The role of small joint arthroplasty in osteoarthritis of the hand   205
          Onur Gilleard, Vikram S Devaraj

Chapter 18 Monitoring of microvascular free tissue transfers   225
          Iain S Whitaker, David W Oliver

Chapter 19 Use of the anterolateral thigh flap for intra-oral reconstruction   235
          Emma Hormbrey, Oliver Cassell

Chapter 20 A comparison of TRAM and DIEP flaps for breast reconstruction   245
          Ashley P Tregaskiss, Robert J Morris

Chapter 21 Immediate versus delayed breast reconstruction   257
          Tom WL Chapman, Robert J Morris

Chapter 22 Strategies for minimising palpable implant rippling in the augmented breast   263
          Jonny Hobman, David T Sharpe

Chapter 23 Gynaecomastia: an algorithmic approach to surgical management   273
          (with special emphasis on liposuction)
          Charles Malata, Devor Kumiponjera, Catherine Lau

Chapter 24 Trends in aesthetic facial surgery: the role of endoscopic brow   287
          and minimal access facial lifts
          Gary L Ross, David J Whitby

Chapter 25 Surgical rejuvenation of the aging neck   299
          Ahid Abood, Charles Malata

Chapter 26 Trends in aesthetic facial surgery: the Hamra lower lid blepharoplasty   311
          Gary L Ross, David J Whitby

Chapter 27 Fibrin sealant in plastic surgery   321
          David W Oliver, Iain S Whitaker

Chapter 28 Ablative and non-ablative techniques for rejuvenation of photo-aged skin   327
          Nick Reynolds, Kay Thomas, John Kenealy

Chapter 29 Hand and facial composite tissue allotransplantation   337
          Iain S Whitaker, John H Barker

Chapter 30 Hyperbaric oxygen therapy in plastic surgery   345
          Christian Mills

Contributors

Ahid Abood MBBS MA MSc MRCS Research Fellow, Plastic Surgery, Addenbrooke's University Hospital, Cambridge University Hospitals NHS Trust, Cambridge, UK

Ahmed Ali-Khan MRCS Specialist Registrar, Plastic Surgery, Royal Devon and Exeter Hospital, Exeter, UK

Neil Ashwood BSc (Hons) MB BS FRCS (Tr & Orth) Consultant Orthopaedic Surgeon, Queen's Hospital, Burton on Trent, UK

John H Barker MD PhD Professor of Surgery, Plastic Surgery Research Laboratory, University of Louisville, Kentucky, USA

Peter Budny MSc (Oxon) FRCS (Plast.) Consultant Plastic Surgeon, Stoke Mandeville Hospital, Aylesbury, UK

Oliver Cassell MB ChB FRCS (Plast.) MS Consultant Plastic and Reconstructive Surgeon, The John Radcliffe Hospital, Oxford, UK

Tom WL Chapman BSc MB ChB MRCS Specialist Registrar, Plastic and Reconstructive Surgery, Frenchay Hospital, Bristol, UK

Lachlan Currie MB BS BSc MD FRCS (Plast.) Fellow in Hand and Microsurgery, The Royal Children's Hospital, Melbourne, Australia

Alun G Davies MA BM BCh MRCS FRCR Specialist Registrar, Radiology, Royal Devon and Exeter Hospital, Exeter, UK

Vikram S Devaraj FRCS (Plast.) Consultant Plastic Surgeon, Royal Devon and Exeter Hospital, Exeter, UK

Rob Duncan MB BCh MRCS (Ed) Burns Research Registrar, Wythenshawe Hospital, Manchester, UK

Ken Dunn BSc FRCS (Plast.) Consultant Burns and Plastic Surgeon, Wythenshawe Hospital, Manchester, UK

Rob Gilbert MB BS BMed Sci (Hons) MRCS (Glasg) Specialist Registrar, Trauma and Orthopaedic Surgery, Queen's Hospital, Burton on Trent, UK

Onur Gilleard MB BS Senior House Officer, Royal Devon and Exeter Hospital, Exeter, UK

Jonny Hobman MB BS MRCS MRCS (Glas) Registrar, Plastic Surgery, Bradford Royal Infirmary, Bradford, UK

Emma Hormbrey BSc MB BS FRCS (Plast.) Fellow in Head and Neck Surgery, The John Radcliffe Hospital, Oxford, UK

Norbert Kang MB BS MD FRCS (Plast.) Consultant Plastic Surgeon, Royal Free Hospital, London, UK and RAFT Institute for Plastic Surgery Research, Mount Vernon Hospital, Northwood, Middlesex, UK

Loshan Kangesu MB BS FRCS (Plast.) Consultant Plastic Surgeon, Great Ormond Street Hospital for Children and St Andrews Centre for Plastic Surgery, Broomfield Hospital, Chelmsford, Essex, UK

John Kenealy FRACS Consultant Plastic Surgeon, Frenchay Hospital, Bristol, UK

Cronan Kerin BSc MRCS (Eng) Specialist Registrar, Trauma and Orthopaedic Surgery, Queen's Hospital, Burton on Trent, UK

Devor Kumiponjera MB BS AFRCS Ed FCS-ECSA Clinical Fellow, Plastic Surgery, Addenbrooke's University Hospital, Cambridge University Hospitals NHS Trust, Cambridge, UK

Catherine Lau MB ChB MRCS Clinical Fellow, Plastic Surgery, Addenbrooke's University Hospital, Cambridge University Hospitals NHS Trust, Cambridge, UK

Mark S Lloyd BM MRCS (Eng) MSc IM&T (Health) MPhil Specialist Registrar, Plastic Surgery, Stoke Mandeville Hospital, Aylesbury, UK

Charles Malata BSc (HB) MB ChB LRCP MRCS FRCS (Glasg) FRCS (Plast.) Consultant Plastic and Reconstructive Surgeon, Addenbrooke's University Hospital, Cambridge University Hospitals NHS Trust, Cambridge, UK

Gordon J McArthur MRCS (Ed) Specialist Registrar, Plastic and Reconstructive Surgery, Melanoma Unit, St George's Hospital, London, UK

Christian Mills MRCS CHT Registrar, Plastic and Reconstructive Surgery, Royal Devon and Exeter Hospital, Exeter, UK and Hyperbaric Medicine Physician, Diving Diseases Research Centre, Plymouth, UK

Marina Morgan MRCPath Consultant Microbiologist, Royal Devon and Exeter Hospital, Exeter, UK

Robert J Morris FRCS (Plast.) Consultant Plastic Surgeon, Derriford Hospital, Plymouth, UK

Siobhán O'Ceallaigh MD AFRCSI Specialist Registrar, Plastic Surgery, Booth Hall Children's Hospital, Manchester, UK

David W Oliver BSc MB ChB FRCS FRCS (Plast.) Consultant Plastic Surgeon, Royal Devon and Exeter Hospital, Exeter, UK

Marc Pacifico BSc MB BS MD MRCS Specialist Registrar, Plastic Surgery, Royal Free Hospital, London, UK and RAFT Institute for Plastic Surgery Research, Mount Vernon Hospital, Northwood, Middlesex, UK

J. Alexa Potter MA MRCS Specialist Registrar, Plastic and Reconstructive Surgery, Royal Devon and Exeter Hospital, Exeter, UK

Barry W Powell MCh MA FRCS (Ed) Consultant, Plastic and Reconstructive Surgery, Melanoma Unit, St George's Hospital, London, UK

Nick Reynolds FRCS Ed Specialist Registrar in Plastic Surgery, Frenchay Hospital, Bristol, UK

Gary L Ross MB ChB MRCS (Ed) MD FRCS (Plast.) Consultant Plastic Surgeon, Christie Hospital NHS Foundation Trust, Manchester, UK

James Seaward MRCS Specialist Registrar, Plastic Surgery, Royal Devon and Exeter Hospital, Exeter, UK

Mamta Shah PhD FRCS (Plast.) Consultant Burns and Plastic Surgeon, Booth Hall Children's Hospital, Manchester, UK

David T Sharpe OBE MA FRCS Consultant Plastic Surgeon, Bradford Royal Infirmary, Bradford, UK

David AT Silver FRCR FRCP Consultant Radiologist, Royal Devon and Exeter Hospital, Exeter, UK

Brian Sommerlad MB BS FRCS (Eng) FRCSEd (Hon) Consultant Plastic Surgeon, Great Ormond Street Hospital for Children and St Andrews Centre for Plastic Surgery, Broomfield Hospital, Chelmsford, Essex, UK

Christopher Stone FRCS (Plast.) Consultant, Plastic and Reconstructive Surgery, Royal Devon and Exeter Hospital, Exeter, UK

Kay Thomas MRCGP Associate Clinical Specialist, Frenchay Hospital, Bristol, UK

Rachel Tillett MRCS MSc Specialist Registrar in Plastic Surgery, Royal Devon and Exeter Hospital, Exeter, UK

Ashley P Tregaskiss MSc MRCS Specialist Registrar, Plastic Surgery, Frenchay Hospital, Bristol, UK

Simon van Eeden BSc MChD FFDRCSI FRCSEd (OMFS) Cleft Fellow, Great Ormond Street Hospital for Children and St Andrews Centre for Plastic Surgery, Broomfield Hospital, Chelmsford, Essex, UK

Tim Ward MRCP FRCR Consultant Radiologist, Musgrove Park Hospital, Taunton, UK

Andrew Watts FRCS (Plast.) Consultant Plastic and Hand Surgeon, Royal Devon and Exeter Hospital, Exeter, UK

Iain S Whitaker BA (Hons) MA MB BChir MRCS Specialist Registrar, Plastic Surgery, The Welsh Centre for Burns and Plastic Surgery, Morriston Hospital, Swansea, UK

David J Whitby MB BS FRCS Consultant Plastic Surgeon, University Hospital of South Manchester NHS Foundation Trust, Manchester, UK

Andrew DH Wilson MRCS Specialist Registrar, Plastic and Reconstructive Surgery, Royal Devon and Exeter Hospital, Exeter, UK

Paul Wilson FRCS (Plast.) Specialist Registrar, Plastic and Reconstructive Surgery, Royal Devon and Exeter Hospital, Exeter, UK

Foreword

The phrase 'evidence-based medicine' has been used increasingly since the early 1990s and is often abused. It has entered the language of health services research and is now part of the currency of health care management.

Christopher Stone has asked the contributors to this book to look systematically at the plastic surgery literature and to review a number of selected topics. The topics chosen reflect important parts of the vast scope of reconstructive and aesthetic plastic surgery. The intention was to come as close as possible to a series of contemporary systematic reviews of the most current evidence-based best practice, with a firm emphasis on evidence rather than opinion.

The Editor and his contributors, many of whom are internationally recognised experts in their field, should be congratulated for taking on this huge task and will be proud to be part of the first book to have successfully, and importantly, set out 'The Evidence for Plastic Surgery'.

Mr Nicholas Parkhouse DM MCh FRCS
Consultant Plastic, Reconstructive and Aesthetic Surgeon
McIndoe Surgical Centre, East Grinstead, UK

The Editor

Christopher Stone MB ChB MSc FRCS (Eng) FRCS (Edin) FRCS (Plast)

Mr Stone was educated in West Sussex before attending medical school at Manchester University in 1985. He subsequently worked as an anatomy tutor at the University before embarking upon a general surgical training in teaching hospitals in the North West, gaining his Fellowship of the Royal Colleges of Surgeons of England (FRCSEng) and Edinburgh (FRCSEdin) in 1994. He was also awarded a Master of Science degree (MSc), with distinction, by the University of London in recognition of scientific research undertaken at University College London between 1995 and 1996.

His plastic surgical training in Manchester, Oxford, Exeter and Plymouth provided experience in all aspects of reconstructive surgery including microsurgery. In 1999 he passed the Intercollegiate Examination in Plastic Surgery - FRCS (Plast.) - and was awarded a Certificate of Completion of Surgical Training in 2001 and accreditation on the General Medical Council's Specialist Register for Plastic Surgery.

Mr Stone was appointed as an NHS Consultant in Reconstructive and Aesthetic Plastic Surgery at the Royal Devon & Exeter Hospital in 2001. As an NHS consultant his work focuses mainly upon the management of malignant melanoma, including sentinel lymph node biopsy, and soft tissue sarcoma. Mr Stone chairs the Peninsula Cancer Network Sarcoma Site Specific Group, which co-ordinates the provision of sarcoma care in the South West, and is a member of the South West Public Health Observatory Sarcoma Panel. Up until December 2007 he also served as regional Training Programme Director for Plastic Surgery with responsibilities for the education of plastic surgeons in training in Bristol, Exeter and Plymouth. He has published extensively in the plastic surgery literature over the past 15 years and has written several textbooks.

Dedication

To Barnaby and Alexander

Introduction

Applying evidence-based medicine to plastic surgery

Christopher Stone FRCS (Plast.)

Consultant, Plastic and Reconstructive Surgery

ROYAL DEVON AND EXETER HOSPITAL, EXETER, UK

Evidence-based practice is now firmly, and correctly, established in the mindset of medical graduates, and its importance to the implementation of modern healthcare is beyond dispute. However, the perspicacious student of evidence-based medicine will point out that not all areas of medical practice, perhaps plastic surgery in particular, can be measured by the precise definitions of evidence levels as cited in this text (Tables 1 and 2). Plastic surgery embodies art within science; it is the fusion of medical principles and a three-dimensional creativity that is difficult to deconstruct by statistical tools alone.

How, for example, can evidence levels be applied to the dilemma facing patients when considering the optimum technique for ameliorating the aging features in the face, or the most appropriate means by which intra-oral lining can be restored following tumour extirpation? Much of what we do defies investigation in a double blind prospectively randomised fashion, so we must make the most insightful conclusions that we can from studies of lesser power. While reliance upon personal series or experiences (level IV evidence) may be an anathema to the most zealous proponents of the evidence level hierarchy, in the quotidian scheme of things we draw our influences more from our trainers and personal mentors than from the meticulous mathematical scrutiny of published material. Evidence levels, therefore, must be cautiously applied to the critical analysis of our results and the true value of personal experience must never be underestimated.

Yet there are many areas of plastic surgery where good data does exist to support currently accepted practice, and where contentious issues arise it is the published evidence to which we inevitably turn for arbitration. Some traditionally well rehearsed debates (one versus two-stage hypospadias repair, TRAM versus DIEP breast reconstruction), along with a number of less easily constrained but educationally invaluable discussions (optimising outcomes in major burns care, timing and method of cleft palate repair), are an important component of this text. Consideration is also given to novel or evolving practice (small joint arthroplasty, artificial skin substitutes, sentinel node biopsy) as well as some of the 'Cinderella' subjects that are too often overlooked (venous thrombo-embolic prophylaxis, management of necrotising fasciitis).

As plastic surgeons we draw upon techniques and knowledge acquired from many other fields of

Table 1. Levels of evidence.

Level	Type of evidence
Ia	Evidence obtained from systematic review of meta-analysis of randomised controlled trials
Ib	Evidence obtained from at least one randomised controlled trial
IIa	Evidence obtained from at least one well-designed controlled study without randomisation
IIb	Evidence obtained from at least one other type of well-designed quasi-experimental study
III	Evidence obtained from well-designed non-experimental descriptive studies, such as comparative studies, correlation studies and case studies
IV	Evidence obtained from expert committee reports or opinions and/or clinical experience of respected authorities

Table 2. Grades of evidence.

Grade of evidence	Evidence
A	At least one randomised controlled trial as part of a body of literature of overall good quality and consistency addressing the specific recommendation (evidence levels Ia and Ib)
B	Well-conducted clinical studies but no randomised clinical trials on the topic of recommendation (evidence levels IIa, IIb, III)
C	Expert committee reports or opinions and/or clinical experience of respected authorities. This grading indicates that directly applicable clinical studies of good quality are absent (evidence level IV)

medicine and we continue to benefit from collaboration with our colleagues in microbiology, radiology, pathology and the many other surgical disciplines in the day to day management of our patients. This diversity is reflected in the wide ranging authorship and subject material presented. As always, it is of paramount importance that the educational baton be shared between trainers and trainees, and the quality of this text is a testament to the diligence and expertise of the contributing authors from both ranks, to whom I remain much indebted.

Ultimately, we are accountable to patients for the appropriateness and efficacy of our work, as well as to those charged with the invidious task of financing healthcare for ensuring that finite resources are not misdirected. How else can we justify the choices that we make on their behalf, if not through an appreciation of the nature of the evidence that underpins those choices?

Chapter 1

Timing and method of soft tissue reconstruction in patients with IIIb tibial fractures

Andrew DH Wilson MRCS

Specialist Registrar, Plastic and Reconstructive Surgery

Christopher Stone FRCS (Plast.)

Consultant, Plastic and Reconstructive Surgery

ROYAL DEVON AND EXETER HOSPITAL, EXETER, UK

Introduction

Lower limb extremity injuries constitute a leading cause of hospital admissions among adolescents and young adults (18-54 years of age), accounting for almost 250,000 hospitalisations each year in the US [1].

For many centuries limb amputation had been the only option for patients disabled by a grossly traumatised or chronically infected lower extremity, with prosthetics providing satisfactory ambulation and support. In this present era when reconstructive options are many and varied, recognising a non-salvageable limb is perhaps the greatest challenge to the orthopaedic and plastic surgeon alike. Advances in fracture management, asepsis and microsurgical techniques have provided the basis for the development of limb salvage procedures and functional reconstruction.

H. Winnett Orr's method of plaster cast immobilisation of open extremity fractures, with wounds covered with dressings under a cast, largely ignored the principles of debridement of devitalised tissues as advocated by Pierre-Joseph Desault (1744-1795). Cases of osteomyelitis were all too frequent, prompting Joseph Trueta to undertake tissue debridement along with secondary wound closure, including the application of skin grafts to granulation tissue. This approach persisted between 1939-1942, but thereafter the importance of restoring the soft tissues over an open fracture within the first week of injury began to be appreciated, as evidenced by the incidence of post-fracture osteomyelitis following World War I (~80%), compared with that following World War II (~25%).

Within the last three decades the inception and development of free tissue transfer techniques for lower limb injuries [2] has revolutionised the management of open fractures and the prevention of osteomyelitis. Whatever the timing and method of reconstruction advocated in the many suggested protocols [3, 4, 5-13], the common aim remains the restoration or maintenance of limb function with expedient bony union and stable soft tissue coverage. More recently, attention has focused upon the additional goal of minimising flap donor-site morbidity [9, 13, 14] and a re-appraisal of the efficacy of free fasciocutaneous flaps as an alternative to muscle flaps for limb reconstruction [5, 6, 8-10, 14].

Methodology

Medline, PubMed and Cochrane databases were used to gather publications on open tibial fractures

Table 1. Gustilo's revised classification of open fractures [15].

Type I	**Open fracture**	
	Clean wound <1cm in length	
Type II	**Open fracture**	
	Laceration >1cm long without extensive soft tissue damage, flaps or avulsions	
Type III	**Open fracture**	
	Extensive soft tissue laceration, damage or loss	
	Open segmental fracture or traumatic amputation	
	High velocity gunshot injuries	
	Open fractures caused by farm injuries	
	Open fractures requiring vascular repair	
	Open fractures older than 8 hours	

Type III subtype (1984)

A	Adequate periosteal cover of a fractured bone despite extensive soft tissue laceration or damage
	High energy trauma irrespective of size of wound
B	Extensive soft tissue loss with periosteal stripping and bone exposure
	Usually associated with massive contamination
C	Associated with arterial injury requiring repair

using the medical subject headings 'tibial fractures', 'open', 'reconstruction', 'lower extremity', 'timing', 'treatment outcome'. Further publications were sourced from cited manuscripts.

Classification of open fractures

As with all classifications, the aim in the classification of open tibial fractures is to guide treatment and predict prognosis. Various systems have been proposed in an attempt to offer useful prognostic indicators and guide the optimal management plan [2, 11, 15, 16]. The most widely used classification is that of Gustilo, first outlined in 1976 [2] and modified in 1984 [15] (Table 1). The revised system divides Type III injuries into subgroups reflecting the state of the periosteum and adequacy of limb perfusion, but it has been criticised for inter-observer discordance [17, 18] and makes no allowance for nerve injury, crucial to treatment planning. Further attempts

at classifying complex limb injuries have resulted in the Mangled Extremity Syndrome Index, Mangled Extremity Severity Score, Predictive Salvage Index and Limb Salvage Index. These indices are complicated and do not always accurately predict outcome [19].

Epidemiology

The annual incidence of open long bone fractures in the UK has been estimated to be around 11.5 per 100,000 population [20], with tibial diaphyseal fractures accounting for approximately 45% of such injuries. In the Edinburgh series of 515 open fractures in 474 patients over a six-year period, Gustilo IIIB fractures were observed in 10% of proximal tibial fractures, 30% of tibial diaphyseal fractures, 27% of distal tibial/pilon fractures and 5% of ankle fractures. Three quarters of tibial diaphyseal fractures occurred in males with a mean age of around 40 years, and 58%

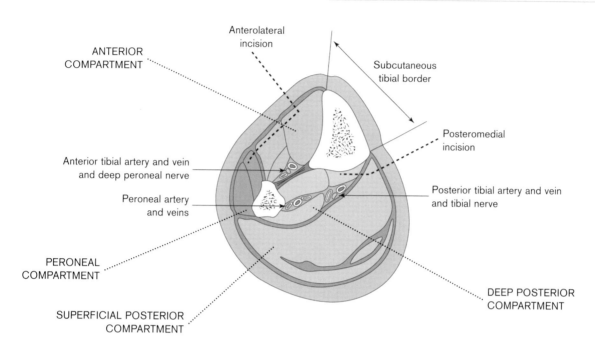

ANTERIOR
COMPARTMENT

Anterolateral
incision

Subcutaneous
tibial border

Posteromedial
incision

Anterior tibial artery and vein
and deep peroneal nerve

Peroneal artery
and veins

Posterior tibial artery and vein
and tibial nerve

PERONEAL
COMPARTMENT

DEEP POSTERIOR
COMPARTMENT

SUPERFICIAL POSTERIOR
COMPARTMENT

Figure 1. Double incision technique. *Reproduced with permission from the BMJ Publishing Group, © 2002. Pearse MF, et al [28].*

of all open fractures were high velocity injuries sustained in road traffic accidents. Similar observations were made in subsequent studies by Gopal et al [8] and Bosse et al [21]. This latter series of 545 patients identified predictors of poor outcome at two years, including readmission for a major complication, low education level, non-white race, poverty, lack of private health care, poor social support, low self-sufficiency, smoking and involvement in disability compensation litigation.

Compartment syndrome in open tibial fractures

The common misconception that open tibial fractures are not accompanied by compartment syndrome, on account of the associated soft tissue damage (automatically decompressing the compartment), does not hold true. A retrospective review of open tibial fractures in 180 patients by Blick et al [22] revealed an incidence of compartment syndrome of 9.1%. Compartment pressure measurements were made in the operating room on the day of admission after reduction and stabilisation of the fracture. Intra-compartmental pressure measurements over 30mmHg were deemed to be pathological and an indication for four-compartment fasciotomies using the double-incision technique described by Mubarak and Owen [23]. Compartment syndrome was found to be directly related to the degree of soft tissue and bony injury, and occurred most often in Gustilo grade III injuries in pedestrians. DeLee and Stiehl [24] observed that 6% of open tibial fractures were accompanied by a compartment syndrome - all Gustilo grade II injuries. In this study, the diagnosis of compartment syndrome was based on clinical findings alone.

Variations exist in the level of intra-compartmental pressure that constitutes a diagnostic value [25]. McQueen et al [26] recommend that decompression should be performed if the differential pressure level (i.e. diastolic pressure minus compartment pressure) drops to under 30 mmHg. When it is less than this, a fasciotomy should be performed unless there is clear evidence that the total tissue pressure is rapidly dropping and the differential pressure is increasing [27].

Pearse et al [28] also recommend the double-incision technique [23] for lower limb decompression (Figure 1), a technique that is endorsed by the Joint Working Committee of the British Association of Plastic Surgeons and the British Orthopaedic Association [27]. The superficial and deep posterior compartments are decompressed via an incision placed 1-2cm posterior to the medial border of the tibia. A second longitudinal incision 2cm lateral to the anterior tibial border decompresses the anterior and peroneal compartments. The medial incision should be anterior to the posterior tibial artery to avoid injury to the perforating vessels that supply the skin used for local fasciocutaneous flaps. When decompressing the deep posterior compartment, care must be taken to avoid damage to the posterior tibial neurovascular bundle which lies just deep to the investing fascia. With the lateral incision, exposure of the fibular periosteum or peroneal tendons is to be avoided as this increases the risk of delayed healing, infection, and ultimately amputation. Muscle viability is then assessed and all non-viable tissue excised.

Timing of soft tissue reconstruction

The optimal timing for the provision of soft tissue cover to open fractures remains controversial. Current evidence indicates that bone infection is more frequently linked with hospital-acquired *Staphylococcus aureus* and aerobic gram-negative bacilli compared with any initial contaminating organisms [16]. Gustilo's landmark review of 1025 open long bone fractures, published in 1976 [3], recommended primary closure of all Type III fractures within five to seven days post-injury for the prevention of non-union and osteomyelitis. Similar recommendations were made in a later report by Russell *et al* [29] in which wound infection, non-union and amputation were all more frequent amongst patients in whom immediate soft tissue closure was achieved, presumably without adequate debridement, compared with those in whom wound closure was delayed but not beyond one week post-injury. Patient numbers were too small to permit statistical comparison. Beyond one week, however, there is clear evidence to demonstrate a worse outcome with regard to wound healing and bone union [3], although arguably the zone of injury is more easily defined following a more protracted period of repeated surgical debridement [10].

A significant contribution to the debate on timing of soft tissue cover emerged from the microsurgical reconstructions undertaken in 532 patients by Godina in Ljubljana in the late '70s and early '80s [6]. The findings of this series are summarised in Table 2. Definitive soft tissue reconstruction within 72 hours of injury translated into fewer failed flaps, a reduction in the incidence of wound infection, a reduced time to bone healing, fewer operations and a shorter hospitalisation time compared with reconstructions undertaken between 72 hours and three months post-injury or beyond three months. Furthermore, there is a measurable increase in wound bacterial count with time after injury and a transition from a contaminated to a colonised wound after day five with a concomitant increase in wound healing complications [4] (Table 3).

Gopal *et al* reported similar findings in their series of 80 Gustilo IIIB or IIIC tibial fractures between 1990 and 1998 [8]. Immediate (within 24 hours of injury) bone and soft tissue debridement and fracture stabilisation was undertaken and, where possible, flap reconstruction was performed in a single stage. Early (up to 72 hours post-injury) or late (beyond 72 hours) flap cover was achieved in the remainder. The series contained 75 free muscle flaps (58 latissimus dorsi, 10 rectus abdominis, 7 gracilis) with a flap failure rate of 3.5%. The observed incidence of deep infection was less following immediate soft tissue replacement (3%), compared with either the early (10%) or late (30%) reconstruction groups, but results lacked statistical significance. The use of external fixator devices was associated with pin tract infections (a proportion of which became chronic), an increased time to bone union, malunion and the practical problems resulting from reduced access for microsurgical anastomosis or even simple skin grafting.

More recently, the Lower Extremity Assessment Project (LEAP) Study Group reported on 601 patients in a prospective multi-centre study of wound-related complications occurring in 190 patients following high energy trauma to the lower extremity, of which 90% were classified as IIIB tibial injuries [30]. Wound-related complications requiring operative intervention were least prevalent when definitive wound closure was achieved between four and seven days post-injury (18%) and greatest when soft tissue reconstruction was undertaken beyond seven days (32%). When

Table 2. How timing of free flap coverage affects outcome in treatment of open fractures. *From Godina* [6].

	Timing of free tissue transfer		
	<72 hours	72 hours-3 months	>3 months
Failure rate (%)	0.75	12	9.5
Infection rate (%)	1.5	17.5	6
Bone healing time (months)	6.8	12.3	29
Hospital time (days)	27	130	256

Table 3. Biological phases of the open fracture wound. *Adapted from Byrd et al* [5].

Category	Time post-injury	Clinical features
Acute	1-5 days	Contaminated but not infected Haemorrhagic and oedematous Ischaemic, devascularised soft tissue and bone Serosanguinous drainage
Subacute	1-6 weeks	Colonised and infected wound Seropurulent drainage Erythema, swollen, cellulitis Exudate
Chronic	>6 weeks	Infection limited to scar and fracture sequestrate Granulating, contracting wound Soft tissues stuck to healthy bone beyond fracture

soft tissue cover was achieved between zero and three days, complications requiring further surgery occurred in 24% of patients (see Table 4).

Overall, there is general agreement that soft tissue closure of IIIB tibial fracture wounds should be undertaken within five to seven days of injury to minimise infection, non-union and flap loss [31]. The level of evidence to support immediate or early wound closure within three days is III/B although at least one prospective study has indicated that this may not be so critical **(III/B)**.

Pre-operative angiography

The role of pre-operative angiography in potential recipients of free flaps remains controversial. Lutz *et al* [32] prospectively examined the indications and limitations of angiography in 36 patients between 1993 and 1998 under a protocol consisting of palpation of the dorsalis pedis and posterior tibial pulses along with pre-operative angiography, to compare findings with intra-operative observations. When at least one of these pulses were palpable, pre-operative angiography was unable to improve upon

Table 4. Studies detailing timing of wound cover for Type III tibial fractures.

Study	Year	Design	Fracture	Timing of closure	Infection rate %	Time to union/ months
Gustilo & Anderson [2]	1976	Retrospective 1961-68	III	Primary	44 (7/16)	
		Prospective 1969-73	III	Delayed (5-7 days)	9 (6/67)	
Cierny [3]	1983	Retrospective	III/IIIa [$]	0-7 days	4 (1/24)	4
				8-30 days	50 (6/12)	6.4
Byrd [5]	1985	Prospective	III [$]	0-5 days	5 (1/21)	5.5
				9-35 days	40 (6/15)	8
Godina [6]	1986	Retrospective	III	<72 hours	1.5	6.8
				72 hours-3months	17.5	12.3
				>3 months	6	29
Francel [7]	1992	Retrospective	IIIB	<15 days		9.1
				>15 days		14.9
Gopal [8]	2000	Retrospective	IIIB IIIC	<24 hours	3 (1/33)	7* 11†
				24-72 hours	10 (3/30)	9* 15†
				>72 hours	30 (6/21) (deep infection)	7.8* 14†
				Wound complication requiring re-operation (%)		
Pollak/ LEAP goup [30]	2000	Prospective	IIIB IIIC	0-3 days	24 (12/49)	
				4-7 days	18 (16/89)	
				>7 days	31 (18/57)	

$ Byrd [5, 11] classification
* internal fixation
† external fixation

the clinical information yielded by simple palpation of foot pulses. Additionally, a normal pre-operative angiography failed to guarantee the suitability of vessels for microsurgical anastomosis. Earlier work by the same group, using osteoseptocutaneous fibula flaps for limb reconstruction following trauma, malunion and osteomyelitis [33], and by Dublin *et al* [34], reached similar conclusions

Where the intended reconstruction is with perforator-based local fasciocutaneous flaps, the role of pre-operative Doppler remains to be fully elucidated and greater emphasis is placed upon the reliability of exploration and direct visualisation of perforators upon which the flap is to be designed. Hallock [35] comments that colour duplex Doppler is superior to conventional Doppler in the identification of perforators and definition of flow characteristics, and so may assist in pre-operative planning. A requirement for pre-operative angiography in these patients usually indicates concern over a significant vascular injury which, in itself, often precludes the use of fasciocutaneous flaps.

A low level of evidence **(III/B)** would seem to exist in the current literature with regard to pre-operative angiography in the context of lower limb trauma. Angiography may only be necessary when pulses are non-palpable or after abnormal Doppler or duplex studies [34-36].

Method of soft tissue cover

There has been a traditional preference for the use of muscle flaps in the reconstruction of lower limb fracture wound sites [2, 8]. *In vivo* studies point to the beneficial effects of the rich vascularity of muscle and its ability to deliver oxygen, antibiotics and leukocytes to the fracture site [37, 38]. Certainly both the medullary blood supply and that derived from the overlying soft tissues are important to fracture healing, as evidenced by animal models [39]. However, clinical studies have demonstrated similarly good outcomes with the use of fasciocutaneous flaps [13, 14] compared with muscle flaps in this setting.

A recent study of the relationship between blood flow and bacterial inoculation at fracture sites beneath musculocutaneous and fasciocutaneous flaps [40] illustrated how blood flow to muscle flaps increases rapidly during the first 24 hours but then plateaus, while blood flow to fascia and subcutaneous tissues is characterised by a gradual and steady increase with time. The most rapid decline in bacterial counts at the undersurface of both muscle and fasciocutaneous flaps occurs within 24 hours, most significantly beneath muscle flaps, and continues to do so beyond 24 hours until there is no significant difference in bacterial count beneath the two types of flap. This suggests a correlation between blood flow and bacterial clearance.

There is some additional evidence from animal studies to indicate that bone segments become re-vascularised faster when contacted by muscle compared with fasciocutaneous flaps [41]. At four weeks, isolated bone segments in a pig model demonstrated superior medullary vascularisation and osteoblastic proliferation when covered by a muscle flap.

There are, however, no prospectively randomised trials comparing muscle with fasciocutaneous flaps for reconstruction of open tibial defects. The largest retrospective series [14] reported on 174 patients with Gustilo IIIB fractures, comparing outcome following reconstructions using both types of flap **(III/B)**. This study failed to demonstrate any significant difference in flap loss, incidence of osteomyelitis, secondary amputations and non-ambulation at two-year follow-up. Free fasciocutaneous flaps were found to be safe and reliable for the closure of distal tibial and ankle defects and offered several advantages over muscle flaps, including easier re-operation, better postoperative monitoring, improved cosmesis and easier thinning. Muscle flaps, however, are able to fill volume defects more easily and so may be better suited to the reconstruction of larger three-dimensional defects as may arise in proximal and middle third tibial fractures [14]. The recipient vessels in the proximal or middle leg are located deep in the muscles, and selected free flaps require a longer pedicle [14, 42]. Choice of reconstruction is generally based on the location of the defect, the size of the wound surface area, the type of deficient tissue components and their volume, the length of the pedicle required and donor site and its morbidity. Subsequent secondary procedures for bone and tendon reconstructions should also be taken into account.

VAC therapy and lower limb trauma

Although not perhaps a method for providing definitive cover for a IIIb tibial fracture, the application of a vacuum-assisted closure (VAC) [43] device may provide a useful adjunct to wound management, particularly between adequate wound excision and preparation for wound cover. The VAC device may aid wound bed preparation whilst minimising dressing changes and wound exposure if further surgery is delayed, for example, while awaiting further investigations or transfer to another hospital.

Several animal studies using VAC to expedite wound healing are presented by Morykwas et al [44]. Using a pig model, studies were undertaken to determine the effect of subatmospheric pressure (125mmHg below ambient) on laser Doppler-measured blood flow in the wound and adjacent tissue, rate of granulation tissue formation and clearance of bacteria from infected wounds. Blood flow levels increased four-fold with VAC, the rate of granulation tissue formation increased significantly and after four days of VAC therapy, bacterial counts significantly decreased to levels below 10^5 organisms per gram of tissue - the traditionally accepted level of organisms for infection.

DeFranzo et al [45] report the successful use of VAC therapy in 71 out of 75 patients with lower extremity wounds with exposed tendon, bone or metal work. The majority (49 out of 75) of these wounds resulted from trauma, but few details are given on the classification of these injuries. The authors report the successful use of VAC following adequate debridement in selected patients with exposed rods and plates, and recommend changing the VAC sponges every 48 hours.

Antibiotics

Studies have shown that approximately 65% of patients with open fractures have wound contamination with micro-organisms [2, 46, 47]. Wound cultures taken at patient presentation or at first operation are of little use as they often fail to identify the organism causing the subsequent infection [48, 49]. Consequently, cultures obtained before wound debridement are no longer recommended [49]. A randomised controlled trial reported that only 3/17 infections (18%) that developed in a series of 171 open fractures were caused by an organism present in the initial cultures [50].

In a double blinded, randomised clinical trial, Patzakis et al reported that the administration of appropriately targeted antibiotics decreased wound infection rate six-fold from 13.9% in the placebo group to 2.3% in the treatment group [46] **(Ia/A)**. In a study on the factors influencing infection rate in open fracture wounds, the single most important factor in reducing the infection rate was the early administration of antibiotics that provide antibacterial activity against both gram-positive and gram-negative micro-organisms. Delay of more than three hours in this study was associated with an increased wound infection risk [47] **(III/B)**.

Smoking-related complications

One retrospective review has been undertaken to determine whether smoking affects fracture healing in open tibial fractures [51], examining time to healing in the context of Type II, IIIA, or IIIB tibia fractures. Smoking correlated with a union rate of 84%, compared with 94% in non-smokers, but this failed to reach statistical significance **(III/B)**.

Outcome studies

Seven-year follow-up results from the Lower Extremity Assessment Project (LEAP) have recently found outcomes following severe lower limb injuries to be poor or average regardless of whether the patient underwent amputation or reconstruction [52] **(III/B)**. The study illustrates wide-ranging variations in outcome following major limb trauma, with a substantial proportion of patients experiencing long-term disability. Patients' economical, social, and personal resources affected outcome more than the initial treatment of the injury - specifically amputation versus reconstruction and level of amputation. These findings concur with those from the earlier LEAP group at two-year follow-up [53]. Factors common amongst those with lower limb injuries that adversely affect outcome included postoperative complications (e.g. infection, malunion), pain, acute stress disorder, post-traumatic stress disorder (PTSD) and depression. The prevalence of PTSD following road traffic accidents is between 24% [54] and 39% [55], with one study suggesting that over 50% of those with PTSD at one-year follow-up were still affected at three years [56]. There is a strong suggestion from the LEAP group that major improvements in functional outcome require intervention in the early post-acute phase of recovery that directly addresses the patient's psychosocial needs **(IV/C)**.

Gopal *et al* [57] could demonstrate no difference in functional outcome between patients treated by limb salvage or by amputation, although Bosse *et al* [21] remain confident that reconstruction provides outcomes equivalent to those of amputation at two-year follow-up. Others report a high proportion of amputees who require retraining and long-term invalidity pensions compared with patients who underwent limb salvage [58, 59] **(III/B)**.

With regard to long-term return to employment, Francel [60] found the re-employment rate for limb salvage patients was improved from 28% to 67% by early soft tissue reconstruction and bone fixation. This equals the re-employment rate amongst traumatic below-knee amputees [7]. Generally, it is unlikely that patients will return to work after two years of unemployment following a severe lower limb injury [7].

The cost-effectiveness of limb salvage versus limb amputation is difficult to determine [61], but expedient free tissue transfer may be less expensive than the combined cost of hospitalisation, prosthetic fitting, rehabilitation and disability payments associated with limb amputation [31, 61].

Conclusions

As with many areas of surgical practice, there is a diversity of opinion regarding the optimum management of patients with IIIb tibial injuries. The evidence, however, points towards a consensus for achieving soft tissue reconstruction within five to seven days of injury. The choice of flap used for soft tissue reconstruction (fasciocutaneous versus muscle) appears to be less important, provided that a timely and adequate debridement is undertaken by appropriately experienced surgeons, preferably with orthopaedic and plastic surgeons working in collaboration. Early antibiotic treatment directed against gram-positive and gram-negative bacteria is advocated. Pre-operative angiography is indicated when distal pulses are absent or after an abnormal Doppler or duplex Doppler study.

Guidelines from the British Orthopaedic Association/ British Association of Plastic, Reconstructive & Aesthetic Surgeons Working Party are currently under review and when published will no doubt provide further evidence for best practice.

Chapter 1

Recommendations	Evidence level
◆ A compartment syndrome may complicate an open tibial fracture in up to 9% of cases.	III/B
◆ Wound-related complications requiring operative intervention are least prevalent when definitive wound closure is achieved within five to seven days post-injury and greatest when soft tissue reconstruction is undertaken beyond seven days.	III/B
◆ The choice of flap for soft tissue reconstruction is less critical than thorough wound debridement and expedient wound closure.	III/B
◆ Pre-operative angiography is necessary when pulses are non-palpable or after an abnormal Doppler or duplex study.	III/B
◆ VAC therapy may be useful in the initial management of IIIB tibial fractures.	III/B
◆ Wound cultures obtained prior to debridement are a poor predictor of infecting organisms and are no longer recommended.	Ib/A
◆ Smoking compromises fracture union and slows wound healing.	III/B
◆ Psychological support and self-management programmes improve the rehabilitation of victims of major limb trauma.	IV/C

References

1. Finkelstein E. Estimates based on Health Care Costs and Utilization Project Inpatient Sample (HCUP-NIS,2003.). http://www.ahcpr.gov/nisoverview.jsp. 2006.

2. Taylor GI, Watson N. One-stage repair of compound leg defects with free, revascularized flaps of groin skin and iliac bone. *Plast Reconstr Surg* 1978; 61(4): 494-506.

3. Gustilo RB, Anderson JT. Prevention of infection in the treatment of one thousand and twenty-five open fractures of long bones: retrospective and prospective analyses. *J Bone Joint Surg Am* 1976; 58(4): 453-8.

4. Cierny G, III, Byrd HS, Jones RE. Primary versus delayed soft tissue coverage for severe open tibial fractures. A comparison of results. *Clin Orthop Relat Res* 1983; 178: 54-63.

5. Byrd HS, Spicer TE, Cierney G, III. Management of open tibial fractures. *Plast Reconstr Surg* 1985; 76(5): 719-30.

6. Godina M. Early microsurgical reconstruction of complex trauma of the extremities. *Plast Reconstr Surg* 1986; 78(3): 285-92.

7. Francel TJ, Vander Kolk CA, Hoopes JE, Manson PN, Yaremchuk MJ. Microvascular soft-tissue transplantation for reconstruction of acute open tibial fractures: timing of coverage and long-term functional results. *Plast Reconstr Surg* 1992; 89(3): 478-87.

8. Gopal S, Majumder S, Batchelor AG, Knight SL, De Boer P, Smith RM. Fix and flap: the radical orthopaedic and plastic treatment of severe open fractures of the tibia. *J Bone Joint Surg Br* 2000; 82(7): 959-66.

9. Guzman-Stein G, Fix RJ, Vasconez LO. Muscle flap coverage for the lower extremity. *Clin Plast Surg* 1991; 18(3): 545-52.

10. Yaremchuk MJ, Brumback RJ, Manson PN, Burgess AR, Poka A, Weiland AJ. Acute and definitive management of traumatic osteocutaneous defects of the lower extremity. *Plast Reconstr Surg* 1987; 80(1): 1-14.

11. Byrd HS, Cierny G, III, Tebbetts JB. The management of open tibial fractures with associated soft-tissue loss: external pin fixation with early flap coverage. *Plast Reconstr Surg* 1981; 68(1): 73-82.

12. Yazar S, Lin CH, Wei FC. One-stage reconstruction of composite bone and soft-tissue defects in traumatic lower extremities. *Plast Reconstr Surg* 2004; 114(6): 1457-66.

13. Erdmann MW, Court-Brown CM, Quaba AA. A five-year review of islanded distally based fasciocutaneous flaps on the lower limb. *Br J Plast Surg* 1997; 50(6): 421-7.

14. Yazar S, Lin CH, Lin YT, Ulusal AE, Wei FC. Outcome comparison between free muscle and free fasciocutaneous flaps for reconstruction of distal third and ankle traumatic open tibial fractures. *Plast Reconstr Surg* 2006; 117(7): 2468-75; Discussion 2476-7.

15. Gustilo RB, Mendoza RM, Williams DN. Problems in the management of type III (severe) open fractures: a new classification of type III open fractures. *J Trauma* 1984; 24(8): 742-6.

16. Templeman DC, Gulli B, Tsukayama DT, Gustilo RB. Update on the management of open fractures of the tibial shaft. *Clin Orthop Relat Res* 1998; 350: 18-25.

17. Brumback RJ, Jones AL. Interobserver agreement in the classification of open fractures of the tibia. The results of a survey of two hundred and forty-five orthopaedic surgeons. *J Bone Joint Surg Am* 1994; 76(8): 1162-6.

18. Horn BD, Rettig ME. Interobserver reliability in the Gustilo and Anderson classification of open fractures. *J Orthop Trauma* 1993; 7(4): 357-60.

19. Bonanni F, Rhodes M, Lucke JF. The futility of predictive scoring of mangled lower extremities. *J Trauma* 1993; 34(1): 99-104.

20. Court-Brown CM, Rimmer S, Prakash U, McQueen MM. The epidemiology of open long bone fractures. *Injury* 1998; 29(7): 529-34.

21. Bosse MJ, MacKenzie EJ, Kellam JF, Burgess AR, Webb LX, Swiontkowski MF, *et al*. An analysis of outcomes of reconstruction or amputation after leg-threatening injuries. *N Engl J Med* 2002; 347(24): 1924-31.

22. Blick SS, Brumback RJ, Poka A, Burgess AR, Ebraheim NA. Compartment syndrome in open tibial fractures. *J Bone Joint Surg Am* 1986; 68(9): 1348-53.

23. Mubarak SJ, Owen CA. Double-incision fasciotomy of the leg for decompression in compartment syndromes. *J Bone Joint Surg Am* 1977; 59(2): 184-7.

24. DeLee JC, Stiehl JB. Open tibia fracture with compartment syndrome. *Clin Orthop Relat Res* 1981; 160: 175-84.

25. Janzing HM, Broos PL. Routine monitoring of compartment pressure in patients with tibial fractures: beware of overtreatment! *Injury* 2001; 32(5): 415-21.

26. McQueen MM, Court-Brown CM. Compartment monitoring in tibial fractures. The pressure threshold for decompression. *J Bone Joint Surg Br* 1996; 78(1): 99-104.

27. A report by the British Orthopaedic Association/British Association of Plastic Surgeons Working Party on the management of open tibial fractures. September 1997. *Br J Plast Surg* 1997; 50(8): 570-83.

28. Pearse MF, Harry L, Nanchahal J. Acute compartment syndrome of the leg. *Br Med J* 2002; 325(7364): 557-8.

29. Russell GG, Henderson R, Arnett G. Primary or delayed closure for open tibial fractures. *J Bone Joint Surg Br* 1990; 72(1): 125-8.

30. Pollak AN, McCarthy ML, Burgess AR. Short-term wound complications after application of flaps for coverage of traumatic soft-tissue defects about the tibia. The Lower Extremity Assessment Project (LEAP) Study Group. *J Bone Joint Surg Am* 2000; 82-A(12): 1681-91.

31. Heller L, Levin LS. Lower extremity microsurgical reconstruction. *Plast Reconstr Surg* 2001; 108(4): 1029-41.

32. Lutz BS, Wei FC, Machens HG, Rhode U, Berger A. Indications and limitations of angiography before free-flap transplantation to the distal lower leg after trauma: prospective study in 36 patients. *J Reconstr Microsurg* 2000; 16(3): 187-91.

Chapter 1

33. Lutz BS, Ng SH, Cabailo R, Lin CH, Wei FC. Value of routine angiography before traumatic lower-limb reconstruction with microvascular free tissue transplantation. *J Trauma* 1998; 44(4): 682-6.

34. Dublin BA, Karp NS, Kasabian AK, Kolker AR, Shah MH. Selective use of preoperative lower extremity arteriography in free flap reconstruction. *Ann Plast Surg* 1997; 38(4): 404-7.

35. Hallock GG. Doppler sonography and color duplex imaging for planning a perforator flap. *Clin Plast Surg* 2003; 30(3): 347-51.

36. Moneta GL, Yeager RA, Antonovic R, Hall LD, Caster JD, Cummings CA, *et al*. Accuracy of lower extremity arterial duplex mapping. *J Vasc Surg* 1992; 15(2): 275-83.

37. Eshima I, Mathes SJ, Paty P. Comparison of the intracellular bacterial killing activity of leukocytes in musculocutaneous and random-pattern flaps. *Plast Reconstr Surg* 1990; 86(3): 541-7.

38. Mathes SJ, Alpert BS, Chang N. Use of the muscle flap in chronic osteomyelitis: experimental and clinical correlation. *Plast Reconstr Surg* 1982; 69(5): 815-29.

39. Holden CE. The role of blood supply to soft tissue in the healing of diaphyseal fractures. An experimental study. *J Bone Joint Surg Am* 1972; 54(5): 993-1000.

40. Gosain A, Chang N, Mathes S, Hunt TK, Vasconez L. A study of the relationship between blood flow and bacterial inoculation in musculocutaneous and fasciocutaneous flaps. *Plast Reconstr Surg* 1990; 86(6): 1152-62.

41. Fisher J, Wood MB. Experimental comparison of bone revascularization by musculocutaneous and cutaneous flaps. *Plast Reconstr Surg* 1987; 79(1): 81-90.

42. Yazar S, Lin CH, Lin YT, Wei FC. Selection of recipient vessels in traumatic lower extremity reconstruction and evaluation of complicated transfers. *Plast Reconstr Surg* 2006; 117(7): 2468-75.

43. Argenta LC, Morykwas MJ. Vacuum-assisted closure: a new method for wound control and treatment: clinical experience. *Ann Plast Surg* 1997; 38(6): 563-76.

44. Morykwas MJ, Argenta LC, Shelton-Brown EI, McGuirt W. Vacuum-assisted closure: a new method for wound control and treatment: animal studies and basic foundation. *Ann Plast Surg* 1997; 38(6): 553-62.

45. DeFranzo AJ, Argenta LC, Marks MW, Molnar JA, David LR, Webb LX, *et al*. The use of vacuum-assisted closure therapy for the treatment of lower-extremity wounds with exposed bone. *Plast Reconstr Surg* 2001; 108(5): 1184-91.

46. Patzakis MJ, Harvey JP, Jr., Ivler D. The role of antibiotics in the management of open fractures. *J Bone Joint Surg Am* 1974; 56(3): 532-41.

47. Patzakis MJ, Wilkins J. Factors influencing infection rate in open fracture wounds. *Clin Orthop Relat Res* 1989; 243: 36-40.

48. Fischer MD, Gustilo RB, Varecka TF. The timing of flap coverage, bone-grafting, and intramedullary nailing in patients who have a fracture of the tibial shaft with extensive soft-tissue injury. *J Bone Joint Surg Am* 1991; 73(9): 1316-22.

49. Lee J. Efficacy of cultures in the management of open fractures. *Clin Orthop Relat Res* 1997; 339: 71-5.

50. Patzakis MJ, Bains RS, Lee J, Shepherd L, Singer G, Ressler R, *et al*. Prospective, randomized, double-blind study comparing single-agent antibiotic therapy, ciprofloxacin, to combination antibiotic therapy in open fracture wounds. *J Orthop Trauma* 2000; 14(8): 529-33.

51. Harvey EJ, Agel J, Selznick HS, Chapman JR, Henley MB. Deleterious effect of smoking on healing of open tibia-shaft fractures. *Am J Orthop* 2002; 31(9): 518-21.

52. MacKenzie EJ, Bosse MJ. Factors influencing outcome following limb-threatening lower limb trauma: lessons learned from the Lower Extremity Assessment Project (LEAP). *J Am Acad Orthop Surg* 2006; 14(10): S205-10.

53. MacKenzie EJ, Bosse MJ, Kellam JF, Burgess AR, Webb LX, Swiontkowski MF, *et al*. Factors influencing the decision to amputate or reconstruct after high-energy lower extremity trauma. *J Trauma* 2002; 52(4): 641-9.

54. Blanchard EB, Hickling EJ, Barton KA, Taylor AE, Loos WR, Jones-Alexander J. One-year prospective follow-up of motor vehicle accident victims. *Behav Res Ther* 1996; 34(10): 775-86.

55. Jeavons S. Long-term needs of motor vehicle accident victims: are they being met? *Aust Health Rev* 2001; 24(1): 128-35.

56. Koren D, Arnon I, Klein E. Acute stress response and posttraumatic stress disorder in traffic accident victims: a one-year prospective, follow-up study. *Am J Psychiatry* 1999; 156(3): 367-73.

57. Gopal S, Giannoudis PV, Murray A, Matthews SJ, Smith RM. The functional outcome of severe, open tibial fractures managed with early fixation and flap coverage. *J Bone Joint Surg Br* 2004; 86(6): 861-7.

58. Arangio GA, Lehr S, Reed JF, III. Reemployment of patients with surgical salvage of open, high-energy tibial fractures: an outcome study. *J Trauma* 1997; 42(5): 942-5.

59. Hertel R, Strebel N, Ganz R. Amputation versus reconstruction in traumatic defects of the leg: outcome and costs. *J Orthop Trauma* 1996; 10(4): 223-9.

60. Francel TJ. Improving reemployment rates after limb salvage of acute severe tibial fractures by microvascular soft-tissue reconstruction. *Plast Reconstr Surg* 1994; 93(5): 1028-34.

61. Heinz TR, Cowper PA, Levin LS. Microsurgery costs and outcome. *Plast Reconstr Surg* 1999; 104(1): 89-96.

Chapter 1

Chapter 1

Chapter 2

Vacuum-assisted closure: basic science and clinical practice

J. Alexa Potter MA MRCS

Specialist Registrar, Plastic and Reconstructive Surgery

Christopher Stone FRCS (Plast.)

Consultant, Plastic and Reconstructive Surgery

ROYAL DEVON AND EXETER HOSPITAL, EXETER, UK

Introduction

Vacuum-assisted closure (VAC®) therapy™ (KCI, USA, San Antonio, TX) is a novel method of wound healing that was initially researched and commercially developed during the 1990s. It is based on surgical principles and observations built up over many years, but the first attempts to analyse its effects scientifically were made by Fleischmann in Germany [1] and Morykwas and Argenta in the US [2]. This led to the development of the commercial system in use today. The VAC system (KCI) consists of a computerised controllable vacuum pump connected to a wound dressing. The dressing consists of an open-cell reticulated foam (either large pore polyurethane or small pore poly-vinyl alcohol), which is inserted into the wound and covered with an air-tight dressing. Suction through the foam dressing applies either continuous or intermittent negative pressure to the wound surface and removes excess wound fluid into a canister.

Since its introduction, much has been written about the use of VAC therapy in various aspects of wound healing, including its role in complex wounds. Accelerated wound healing, as evidenced by increased granulation tissue formation and wound shrinkage, has been demonstrated. However, the physiological basis for the effects of topical negative pressure (TNP) upon wounds has not been fully elucidated and although there are many case studies describing the results seen in clinical practice, few randomised controlled trials have been performed. In addition, there remains some debate as to its cost-effectiveness in a competitive wound healing market.

Methodology

A literature search was performed using Medline and PubMed to obtain published research relating to vacuum-assisted closure therapy. Search terms used included 'vacuum-assisted closure', 'vacuum therapy', 'topical negative pressure therapy', 'suction closure'. Bibliographic linkage was used to further include articles of relevance to the topic.

What is the evidence for the physiological basis of VAC therapy?

Morykwas and Argenta in their seminal paper [2] demonstrated increased wound healing in a pig

Animal studies of specific clinical applications

Animal studies have shown promising results for TNP applied to some specific areas of clinical practice. These include:

- ◆ Increased area of cutaneous flap survival [2].
- ◆ Salvage of muscle flaps up to five hours after ligation of the venous outflow [25].
- ◆ Reduction in ulceration after injection of spider venom [25].
- ◆ Prevention of ulceration after drug extravasation (doxorubicin) [26].
- ◆ Reduction in circulating serum myoglobin after crush injury [27].

There has been one case report of successful VAC use following surgical debridement for toxic beetle bite-induced skin necrosis [28], but there have been no other clinical reports or trials investigating VAC therapy for these other applications **(IV/C)**.

What is the evidence for the use of VAC in clinical practice? (Figures 1-4)

The vast majority of publications regarding the use of VAC therapy are in the form of case reports and small case series [29]. Only a limited number of randomised controlled trials have been performed. Six systematic reviews [30-35] have assessed the evidence available, the most recent and comprehensive of which is the Ontario Health Technology Review (2004) [35]. This summarised randomised controlled trials (RCTs) to August 2004, and discussed the findings of the previous five reviews and health technology assessments. The RCTs analysed are summarised in Table 1 [36-41]. A meta-analysis of the trial data has proven impossible due to the differences in patient populations and outcome measures. Although there may be some evidence that VAC therapy is of benefit to certain wounds, published trials to date have been of small size with significant methodological flaws **(Ia/A)**. This review also included six single-site case series [42-47] and four retrospective analyses **(III/B)** [8, 48-50]. All these studies showed some healing benefit for patients receiving

VAC therapy for a variety of wounds, but as descriptive studies without comparison groups, little conclusion can been drawn as to the true effectiveness of VAC over other wound healing techniques. The Ontario review, like the previous assessments, called for large, well-designed, multi-centred randomised controlled trials to more robustly investigate the efficacy of VAC therapy.

One such trial has been published subsequently [51]. In a multi-centre clinical trial, 162 diabetic patients with trans-metatarsal foot amputations were randomised to receive either VAC therapy or standard wound care. The primary outcome measure was complete closure, with secondary outcome measures including rate of healing and need for further surgery. The results demonstrated a greater proportion of completely healed wounds in the VAC therapy group (p=0.04) and this was achieved in a significantly shorter time (p=0.005). The rate of increase in percentage area of granulation tissue was also calculated to be significantly faster in the VAC treated group (p=0.002). This trial represents the first large study providing evidence for improved healing with VAC therapy over standard therapy in a specific wound type, controlled for comorbid conditions **(Ib/A)**.

Level III evidence

A large case series examining the effect of VAC therapy upon 300 mixed wound types, arbitrarily divided into chronic, subacute and acute wounds, has been reported by Argenta *et al* [52]. In this study, favourable healing in all groups was demonstated, with acute wounds granulating faster than the more chronic or indolent wounds. In particular, healing was achieved in pressure ulcers previously recalcitrant to dressings, and split skin grafting of venous stasis ulcers was facilitated. The length of follow-up was not discussed, however, and it is unclear whether or not these grafts remained stable. Healing was also reported in wounds with exposed bone, orthopaedic metalwork and in thoracic and abdominal wounds (with or without exposed viscera). Wounds either healed directly, or became suitable for direct closure, grafting or flap reconstruction. These results were presented as a first clinical experience with VAC

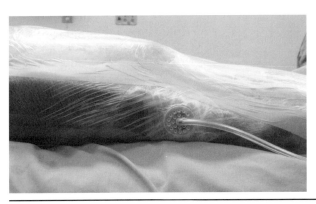
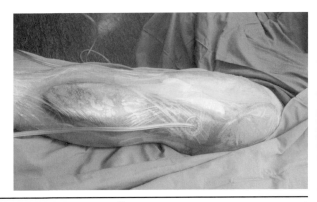

Figure 1. VAC dressings in place prior to attachment of pump. VAC® was used for management of wound exudate before and after skin grafting in this case of upper and lower leg fasciotomy wounds. The photographs show the dressing in place prior to application of the vacuum. The large pore polyurethane foam was cut to the contours of the wound and applied over Adaptic™ as a non-adherent layer. Standard VAC® adhesive dressings have been used, reinforced with Opsite™.

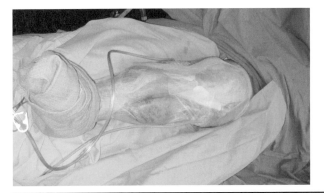
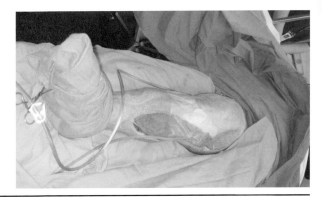

Figure 2. Pre- and post-attachment of pump and application of vacuum (-125mmHg continuous pressure used over meshed graft in this case). The VAC foam shrinks into the wound and should fit exactly within the edges of the wound, without covering any of the surrounding skin, which leads to excoriation.

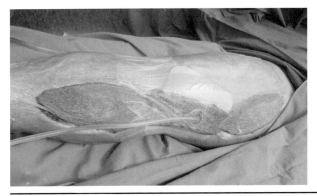
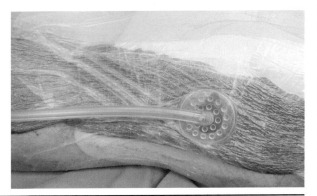

Figure 3. Duoderm™ makes an excellent skin cover to allow a bridge of sponge to connect the upper and lower wounds on each side of the leg, reducing the tubing requirements (two tubes attached via one Y-connector, rather than four tubes).

Table 1. Randomised controlled trials (from Ontario Health Technology Review) [35].

Author/ date	Size/ type of study	Comparison	Length of study	Outcome measurement	Stated result	Comments
Joseph 2000 [36]	24 patients, 36 mixed type chronic wounds	VAC vs saline gauze dressings	6 weeks	Wound volume/ depth assessed by alginate impressions	78% reduction in wound volume with VAC vs 30% with saline gauze at 6 weeks	Methodologically flawed: many potentials for bias
McCallon 2000 [37]	10 patients, diabetic foot ulceration	VAC vs saline gauze dressings	2 weeks + until healed	Wound surface area and time to complete healing	Wound surface area reduced at 2 weeks with VAC, and less time to complete healing	Very small study. No statistics performed
Wanner 2003 [38]	22 paraplegic/ tetraplegic pressure ulcers	VAC vs saline gauze	Until wound reached 50% original volume	Length of time taken for wound to reduce to 50% volume	No difference between VAC and saline gauze	Potential for bias
Ford 2002 [39]	28 patients with 41 pressure ulcers	VAC vs Healthpoint system of gel dressings	6 weeks	Wound volume by plaster impressions*	No significant difference in wound healing	Substantial differences in patient population in the 2 arms of the study
Genecov 1998 [40]	10 patients, 20 SSG donor sites	VAC vs Opsite	Until healed	Rate of healing of SSG donor sites	70% VAC treated wounds re-epithelialised faster than Opsite	Large drop out rate, wide range of patient ages
Moues 2004 [41]	54 patients with chronic or infected wounds awaiting readiness for surgical closure	VAC vs moist gauze (+/- topical anti-microbial ointment)	Until ready for definitive management	i) Readiness for surgery ii) wound surface area	i) No difference between groups ii) larger percentage reduction in wound surface area with VAC	Difference between groups in numbers/types of comorbid conditions (diabetes, vascular disease, etc)

* Other outcome measures also used but not considered robust enough to form part of RCT evidence
SSG = split skin graft

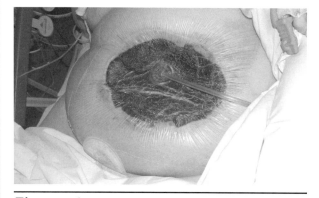

Figure 4. A VAC dressing applied to an abdominal wound.

therapy and further research involving randomised clinical trials was advocated **(III/B)**.

DeFranzo *et al* [53] published a case series of 75 patients with complex open lower limb wounds. Successful wound closure was achieved in 71/75 either with delayed primary closure (12), split skin grafting (58) or a local flap (5). The authors recommended VAC therapy as a good option for patients refusing free tissue transfer or those unfit for surgery. No timescale to healing, or surgical closure was mentioned, but the increased rate of granulation tissue formation and reduced number of dressing changes was thought to reduce the risk of infection where there was exposed bone, tendon and metalwork **(III/B)**.

Sjogren *et al* [54] retrospectively analysed the outcomes of 101 consecutive patients with post-sternotomy mediastinitis. Favourable results were reported with VAC therapy compared with conventional treatment consisting of open dressings, closed irrigation and flap closure. However, the analysis was not contemporaneous, comparing five years of conventional treatment (1994-1998) with five susbsequent years of VAC therapy (1999-2003) **(III/C)**.

TNP therapy has also been reported as a means to secure skin grafts, especially in areas that are difficult to dress or involve complex reconstruction (e.g. uro-genital reconstruction [55, 56]). A series of eight patients in whom VAC therapy was used over Integra™ [57] reported a shorter than expected time to readiness for split skin grafting (seven days compared with 21 days). There are many other individual case reports detailing the use of TNP under a variety of wound conditions, but alone these do not constitute good evidence for its efficacy **(III/ C)**.

Is it safe?

Few complications have been reported with the use of VAC therapy according to the manufacturer's guidelines. However, deaths have been reported due to cardiac rupture [58] secondary to placement of the dressing directly over the heart or cardiac bypass grafts after mediastinitis, and other reports of haemorrhage from erosion of exposed vessels have been published [59] **(III/C)**.

Electrolyte and fluid imbalance has been reported in patients whose wounds produce a high level of exudate [60], and in paediatric patients where smaller fluid losses may be significant. Close monitoring of fluid loss and serum biochemistry (including albumin levels) is advocated in these circumstances **(III/C)**.

Finally, while not a complication of the treatment itself, the lack of a defined endpoint for wound management by TNP therapy can lead to a delay in definitive wound closure [61], emphasising the need to carefully consider its place on the reconstructive ladder **(IV/C)**.

Conclusions

Since its introduction VAC therapy has been used to treat almost every type of wound. The background science originally published has not been reproduced, and the mechanisms underlying its action have not been fully elucidated, although it is likely that a combination of factors is responsible. Numerous case studies report its efficacy in a wide variety of circumstances, but there is little evidence from rigorous studies to support or refute its usefulness. Only one randomised controlled trial provides good evidence for its effectiveness (in diabetic foot wounds [51]). However, the lack of other studies may reflect the difficulty in performing randomised controlled trials for wound treatments. It is largely safe, but the type of wound and the goal of treatment must be carefully considered.

Recommendations	Evidence level
◆ VAC therapy may be used safely on a variety of wounds.	III/C
◆ Care must be taken in its use over exposed vessels, the pericardium, bypass grafts, etc.	III/B
◆ Silicone mesh may be used as an interface dressing without significantly reducing the pressure exerted at the wound surface.	IIb/B
◆ There is a lack of evidence concerning the optimal level of negative pressure or mode of suction (continuous or intermittent).	III/C
◆ Overall, there is little clinical evidence in the form of RCTs to support the use of TNP therapy in the management of the majority of wounds, although good evidence exists for its use in diabetic foot amputations.	Ia/A, Ib/A
◆ TNP therapy should be used as an adjunct to surgical management, and with clear treatment endpoints, in the management of chronic or complex wounds.	IV/C

Chapter 2

References

1. Fleischmann W, Lang E, Kinzl L. Vacuum-assisted wound closure after dermatofasciotomy of the lower extremity. *Unfallchirurg* 1996; 99(4): 283-7.

2. Morykwas MJ, Argenta LC, Shelton-Brown EI, McGuirt W. Vacuum-assisted closure: a new method for wound control and treatment: animal studies and basic foundation. *Ann Plast Surg* 1997; 38(6): 553-62.

3. Wackenfors A, Sjogren J, Gustafsson R, Algotsson L, Ingemansson R, Malmsjo M. Effects of vacuum-assisted closure therapy on inguinal wound edge microvascular blood flow. *Wound Rep Regen* 2004 12(6): 600-6.

4. Wackenfors A, Gustafsson R, Sjogren J, Algotsson L, Ingemansson R, Malmsjo M. Blood flow responses in the peristernal thoracic wall during vacuum-assisted closure therapy. *Ann Thorac Surg* 2005; 79(5): 1724-30; discussion 1730-1.

5. Chen SZ, Li J, Li XY, Xu LS. Effects of vacuum-assisted closure on wound microcirculation: an experimental study. *Asian J Surg* 2005; 28(3): 211-7.

6. Timmers MS, Le Cessie S, Banwell P, Jukema GN. The effects of varying degrees of pressure delivered by negative-pressure wound therapy on skin perfusion. *Ann Plast Surg* 2005; 55(6): 665-71.

7. Moues CM, Vos MC, van de Bemd GJ, Stijnen T, Hovius SE. Bacterial load in relation to vacuum-assisted wound closure therapy: a prospective randomized trial. *Wound Rep Regen* 2004; 12: 11-7.

8. Weed T, Ratliff C, Drake DB. Quantifying bacterial bioburden during negative pressure wound therapy: does the wound VAC enhance bacterial clearance? *Ann Plast Surg* 2004; 52(3): 276-9.

9. Urschel JD, Scott PG, Williams HTG. The effect of mechanical stress on soft and hard tissue repair; a review. *Br J Plast Surg* 1988; 41: 182-6.

10. Saxena V, Hwang CW, Huang S, Eichbaum Q, Ingber D, Orgill DP. Vacuum-assisted closure: microdeformations of wounds and cell proliferation. *Plast Reconstr Surg* 2004; 114(5): 1086-95.

11. Ingber D. Integrins as mechanochemical transducers. *Curr Op Cell Biol* 1991; 3: 841-8.

12. Greene AK, Puder M, Roy R, Arsenault D, Kwei S, Moses MA, Orgill DP. Microdeformational wound therapy: effects on angiogenesis and matrix metalloproteinases in chronic wounds of 3 debilitated patients. *Ann Plast Surg* 2006; 56(4): 418-22.

13. Jones SM, Banwell PE, Shakespeare PG. Advances in wound healing: topical negative pressure therapy. *Postgraduate Medical Journal* 2005; 81: 353-7.

14. Kilpadi DV, Bower CE, Reade CC, Robinson PJ, Sun YS, Zeri R, Nifong LW, Wooden WA. Effect of vacuum-assisted closure therapy on early systemic cytokine levels in a swine model. *Wound Repair Regen* 2006;14(2): 210-5.

15. Labler L, Mica L, Harter L, Trentz O, Keel M. Influence of VAC therapy on cytokines and growth factors in traumatic wounds. *Zentralbl Chir* 2006; 131 Suppl 1: S62-7 [Article in German].

16. Tang SY, Chen SZ, Hu ZH, Song M, Cao DY, Lu XX. Influence of vacuum-assisted closure technique on expression of Bcl-2 and NGF/NGFmRNA during wound healing. *Zhonghua Zheng Xing Wai Ke Za Zhi* 2004; 20(2): 139-42 [Article in Chinese].

17. Kall S, Kilpadi D, Reimers K, Choi CY, Jahn S, Vogt PM. Influence of foam and tubing material of the vacuum-assisted closure device (VAC) on the concentration of transforming growth factor Beta 1 in wound fluid. *Zentralbl Chir* 2004; 129 Suppl 1: S113-5. [Article in German].

18. Banwell PE, Musgrave M. Topical negative pressure therapy: mechanisms and indications. *Int Wound J* 2004; 1(2): 95-106.

19. www.kci1.com.

20. Mokhtari A, Petzina R, Gustafsson L, Sjogren J, Malmsjo M, Ingemansson R. Sternal stability at different negative pressures during vacuum-assisted closure therapy. *Ann Thorac Surg* 2006; 82(3): 1063-7.

21. Fuchs U, Zittermann A, Stuettgen B, Groening A, Minami K, Koerfer R. Clinical outcome of patients with deep sternal wound infection managed by vacuum-assisted closure compared to conventional therapy with open packing: a retrospective analysis. *Ann Thorac Surg* 2005; 79(2): 526-31.

22. Morykwas MJ, Faler BJ, Pearce DJ, Argenta LC. Effects of varying levels of subatmospheric pressure on the rate of granulation tissue formation in experimental wounds in swine. *Ann Plast Surg* 2001; 47(5): 547-51.

23. Banwell PE. Topical negative pressure therapy in wound care. *J Wound Care* 1999; 8: 79.

24. Jones SM, Banwell PE, Shakespeare PG. Interface dressings influence the delivery of topical negative-pressure therapy. *Plast Reconstr Surg* 2005; 116(4): 1023-8.

25. Morykwas MJ, Simpson JBS, Punger KBA, Argenta ABS, Kremers LMD, Argenta JBA. Vacuum-assisted closure: state of basic research and physiologic foundation. *Plast Reconstr Surg, Current Concepts in Wound Healing* 2006; 117(7S) (supplement): 121S-6.

26. Morykwas MJ, Kennedy A, Argenta JP, *et al*. Use of subatmospheric pressure to prevent doxorubicin extravasation ulcers in a swine model. *J Surg Oncol* 1999; 72: 14.

27. Morykwas MJ, Howell H, Bleyer AJ, *et al*. The effect of externally applied subatmospheric pressure on serum myoglobin levels after a prolonged crush/ischemia injury. *J Trauma Injury Inf Crit Care* 2002; 53: 537.

28. von Gossler CM, Horch RE. Rapid aggressive soft-tissue necrosis after beetle bite can be treated by radical necrectomy and vacuum suction-assisted closure. *J Cutan Med Surg* 2004; 4: 219.

29. Pham CT, Middleton PF, Maddern GJ. The safety and efficacy of topical negative pressure in non-healing wounds: a systematic review. *J Wound Care* 2006; 15(6): 240-50.

30. Evans D, Land L. Topical negative pressure for treating chronic wounds. *Cochrane Database of Systematic Reviews* 2004; (2).

31. Higgins S. The effectiveness of vacuum-assisted closure (VAC) in wound healing. Clayton, Victoria: Centre for Clinical Effectiveness (CCE), 2003.

32. Fisher A, Brady B. Vacuum-assisted wound closure therapy. Ottawa: Canadian Coordinating Office for Health Technology Assessment (CCOHTA), 2003.

33. Pham C, Middleton P, Maddern G. Vacuum-assisted closure for the management of wounds: an accelerated systematic review. Australian Safety and Efficacy Register of New Interventional Procedures - Surgical (ASERNIP-S), 2003.

34. Samson DJ, Lefevre F, Aronson Naomi. Wound-healing technologies: low-level laser and vacuum-assisted closure. Evidence report/Technology Assessment No. 111. (Prepared by the Blue Cross and Blue Sheld Association Technology Evaluation Centre Evidenced-based Practice Center, under contract No. 290-02-0026). AHRQ Publication No. 05-E005-

2. Rockville MD: Agency for Healthcare Research and Quality, December 2004.

35. Ontario Ministry of Health and Long-Term Care. Vacuum-assisted closure therapy for wound care. Toronto: Ontario Ministry of Health and Long Term Care, 2004.

36. Joseph E, Hamori C, Bergman S, Roaf E, *et al*. A prospective randomized trial of vacuum-assisted closure versus standard therapy of chronic non-healing wounds. *Wounds* 2000; 12(3): 60-7.

37. McCallon SK, Knight C, Valiulus JP, *et al*. Vacuum-assisted closure versus saline-moistened gauze in the healing of postoperative diabetic foot wounds. *Ostomy Wound Manage* 2000; 46(8): 28-32.

38. Wanner MB, Schwarz F, Strub B, Zaech GA, Pierer G. Vacuum-assisted wound closure for cheaper and more comfortable healing of pressure sores: a prospective study. *Scand J Plast Reconstr Surg Hand Surg* 2003; 37(1): 28-33.

39. Ford CN, Reinhard ER, Yeh D, Syrek D, De las MA, Bergman SB, *et al*. Interim analysis of a prospective, randomized trial of vacuum-assisted closure versus the healthpoint system in the management of pressure ulcers. *Ann Plast Surg* 2002; 49(1): 55-61.

40. Genecov DG, Schneider AM, Morykwas MJ, *et al*. A controlled subatmospheric dressing increases the rate of skin graft donor site reepithelialization. *Ann Plast Surg* 1998; 40(3): 219-25.

41. Moues CM, Vos MC, Van Den BGJ, Stijnen T, Hovius SER. Bacterial load in relation to vacuum-assisted closure wound therapy: a prospective randomized trial. *Wound Repair & Regeneration* 2004; 12(1): 11-7.

42. Isago T, Nozaki M, Kikuchi Y, Honda T, Nakazawa H. Skin graft fixation with negative-pressure dressings. *J Dermatol* 2003; 30(9): 673-8.

43. Isago T, Nozaki M, Kikuchi Y, Honda T, Nakazawa H. Negative-pressure dressings in the treatment of pressure ulcers. *J Dermatol* 2003; 30(4): 299-305.

44. Fleck TM, Fleck M, Moidl R, Czerny M, Koller R, Giovanoli P, *et al*. The vacuum-assisted closure system for the treatment of deep sternal wound infections after cardiac surgery. *Ann Thorac Surg* 2002; 74(5): 1596-600.

45. Wongworawat MD, Schnall SB, Holtom PD, Moon C, Schiller F. Negative pressure dressings as an alternative technique for the treatment of infected wounds. *Clin Orthop Relat Res* 2003; 414: 45-8.

46. Herscovici D, Jr., Sanders RW, Scaduto JM, Infante A, DiPasquale T. Vacuum-assisted wound closure (VAC therapy) for the management of patients with high-energy soft tissue injuries. *J Orthopaedic Trauma* 2003; 17(10): 683-8.

47. Luckraz H, Murphy F, Bryant S, Charman SC, Ritchie AJ. Vacuum-assisted closure as a treatment modality for infections after cardiac surgery. *J Thorac Cardiovasc Surg* 2003; 125(2): 301-5.

48. Carson SN, Overall K, Lee-Jahshan S, Travis E. Vacuum-assisted closure used for healing chronic wounds and skin grafts in the lower extremities. *Ostomy Wound Management* 2004; 50(3): 52-8.

Chapter 2

49. Clare MP, Fitzgibbons TC, McMullen ST, Stice RC, Hayes DF, Henkel L. Experience with the vacuum-assisted closure negative pressure technique in the treatment of non-healing diabetic and dysvascular wounds. *Foot & Ankle International* 2002; 23(10): 896-901.

50. Phillips DE, Rao SJ. Negative pressure therapy in the community: analysis of outcomes. *Wound Care in Canada* 2003; 2(1): 42-5.

51. Armstrong DG, Lavery LA; Diabetic Foot Study Consortium. Negative pressure wound therapy after partial diabetic foot amputation: a multicentre, randomised controlled trial. *Lancet* 2005; 366(9498): 1704-10.

52. Argenta LC, Morykwas MJ. Vacuum-assisted closure: a new method for wound control and treatment: clinical experience. *Ann Plast Surg* 1997; 38(6): 563-76; discussion 577.

53. DeFranzo AJ, Argenta LC, Marks MW, Molnar JA, David LR, Webb LX, Ward WG, Teasdall RG. The use of vacuum-assisted closure therapy for the treatment of lower-extremity wounds with exposed bone. *Plast Reconstr Surg* 2001; 108(5): 1184-91.

54. Sjogren J, Gustafsson R, Nilsson J, Malmsjo M, Ingemansson R. Clinical outcome after poststernotomy mediastinitis: vacuum-assisted closure versus conventional treatment. *Ann Thorac Surg* 2005; 79(6): 2049-55.

55. Hallberg H, Holmstrom H. Vaginal construction with skin grafts and vacuum-assisted closure. *Scand J Plast Reconstr Surg Hand Surg* 2003; 37(2): 97-101.

56. Senchenkov A, Knoetgen J, Chrouser KL, Nehra A. Application of vacuum-assisted closure dressing in penile skin graft reconstruction. *Urology* 2006; 67(2): 416-9.

57. Molnar JA, DeFranzo AJ, Hadaegh A, *et al*. Acceleration of Integra incorporation in complex tissue defects with subatmospheric pressure. *Plast Reconstr Surg* 2004; 133: 1339.

58. Sartipy U, Lockowand U, Gabel J, Jideus L, Dellgren G. *Ann Thor Surg* 2006; 82 (3): 1110-1.

59. White RA, Miki RA, Kazmier P, Anglen JO. Vacuum-assisted closure complicated by erosion and hemorrhage of the anterior tibial artery. *J Orthop Trauma* 2005; 19(1): 56-9.

60. Friedman T, Westreich M, Shalom A. Vacuum-assisted closure treatment complicated by anasarca. *Ann Plast Surg* 2005; 55(4): 420-1.

61. Dieu T, Leung M, Leong J, Morrison W, Cleland H, Archer B, Oppy A. Too much vacuum-assisted closure. *ANZ J Surg* 2003; 73(12): 1057-60.

Chapter 3

The management of necrotising fasciitis

Rachel Tillett MRCS MSc, Specialist Registrar in Plastic Surgery 1
Tim Ward MRCP FRCR, Consultant Radiologist 2
Marina Morgan MRCPath, Consultant Microbiologist 1
Christopher Stone FRCS (Plast.), Consultant, Plastic and Reconstructive Surgery 1

1 ROYAL DEVON AND EXETER HOSPITAL, EXETER, UK
2 MUSGROVE PARK HOSPITAL, TAUNTON, UK

Introduction

Necrotising fasciitis is defined as a deep seated infection of subcutaneous tissue that progressively destroys fascia and fat, but may spare skin and muscle [1]. The condition was first described by Hippocrates in the fifth century BC [2], whilst the first written report, by Claude Pouteau, chief surgeon to the Hôtel Dieu in Lyon, was in 1783 [3]. Meleney (1924) [4], provided the first description of a larger series of 20 Chinese patients and used the term 'haemolytic streptococcal gangrene'. Other historical terms include: hospital gangrene, malignant ulcer, phagedena [3], non-clostridal gas gangrene, necrotising erysipelas and synergistic necrotising cellulitis. More recently, the British media created the incorrect phrase 'flesh-eating virus' to describe severe, invasive streptococcal infections, raising public awareness of the condition. The term 'necrotising fasciitis' was coined by Wilson in 1952 [5], and most accurately describes the key pathological processes involved. Fournier's gangrene is used to describe necrotising fasciitis of the perineum and scrotum and was first reported in 1764 by Bauriene and later described by Jean Alfred Fournier in 1883 [6].

Two broad groups of necrotising fasciitis exist [7]. Type I, or 'synergistic' necrotising fasciitis, is polymicrobial in nature. Different bacterial groups, involving anaerobic bacteria (e.g. gram-positives such as Peptostreptococcus species and gram-negatives such as Bacteroides species) in combination with facultative anaerobic bacteria such as streptococci, staphylococci and Enterobacteriaceae (e.g. *Escherichia coli*, *Klebsiella pneumoniae* and *Proteus mirabilis*) act synergistically to achieve a rapidly progressive infection. Type II necrotising fasciitis is unimicrobial and is usually due to group A, beta-haemolytic streptococci (GAS), occasionally in combination with a staphylococcus. This type of necrotising fasciitis can be complicated by streptococcal toxic shock syndrome (STSS) [8], characterised by hypotension and multi-organ dysfunction. Type I necrotising fasciitis accounts for 70-85% of cases, whilst Type II accounts for the remaining 15-30% [7, 9-11].

Streptococcal toxic shock syndrome was defined in 1993 [12]. The criteria for diagnosis included the isolation of GAS from a usually sterile site (e.g. blood, cerebrospinal fluid) or a non-sterile site such as the throat, vagina, or skin, along with the clinical signs of

Table 1. Case definition of streptococcal toxic shock syndrome.

1.   Isolation of GAS
   a.   From a usually sterile site (e.g. blood, CSF, pleural or peritoneal fluid, tissue biopsy)
   b.   From a non-sterile site (e.g. throat, sputum, vagina, skin lesion)

2.   Clinical signs of severity
   a.   Hypotension: systolic BP ≤90 mmHg in adults or <5th percentile for age in children
   b.   ≥2 of the following:
      i.   Renal impairment
      ii.   Coagulopathy
      iii.   Liver involvement
      iv.   Adult respiratory distress syndrome
      v.   Generalised erythematous macular rash
      vi.   Soft tissue necrosis (NF, myositis, gangrene)

a severe systemic infection (Table 1). Most patients who develop STSS are bacteraemic.

Necrotising fasciitis is known to be rapidly fatal in many patients. McHenry *et al* analysed 29 papers involving a total of 696 cases. The cumulative mortality rate was 34%, ranging from 6-76%[13]. Mortality rates appear to be higher when Type II necrotising fasciitis is complicated by streptococcal toxic shock syndrome (41.4%[14] to 67%[15]).

Methodology

A PubMed search was employed to gather evidence using combinations of the search terms 'necrotising fasciitis', 'synergistic', 'group A streptococcal ± shock', 'epidemiology', 'risk factors', 'aetiology', 'microbiology', 'pathology', 'pathogenesis', 'clinical features', 'imaging', 'ultrasound', 'CT', 'MRI', 'management', 'antibiotics', 'prophylaxis', 'IVIG', 'recombinant protein C', and 'hyperbaric oxygen therapy'.

Epidemiology

The exact incidence of necrotising fasciitis in the UK is unknown because it is not a notifiable disease. However, the Health Protection Agency now performs surveillance of invasive group A streptococcal infection. In 2003, the incidence of invasive infection was 3.8 per 100,000, equivalent to 3000 cases per year [16]. Invasive infection resulted in necrotising fasciitis in 0.19 per 100,000, accounting for 150 cases nationally. If necrotising fasciitis due to group A streptococcus accounts for 15-30% of necrotising fasciitis cases, the likely total number of cases of Type I and II necrotising fasciitis seen in the UK is 0.63-1.26 per 100,000, equivalent to 500-1000 cases per year. In the USA it has been estimated that there are 9600-9700 cases of invasive GAS infections annually, with just under 700 of these demonstrating necrotising fasciitis [14]. This would predict about 3300 cases of necrotising fasciitis of both types per year, with 670-1000 deaths per year.

This estimate concurs with the observed incidence of group A streptococcal necrotising fasciitis in Ontario, Canada of 0.085 per 100,000 in 1991 which rose to 0.4 per 100,000 in 1995 [15]. The 4.7-fold rise in reported cases may be due to increased host susceptibility, increased GAS pathogenicity and increased disease recognition, or a combination of these factors.

In 1994, invasive GAS infections were added to the list of conditions under public health surveillance in the US. The overall incidence of invasive GAS disease reported within five US states was 3.56 per

100,000 in 1999. Necrotising fasciitis accounted for 7.1% of invasive cases, equivalent to 0.5 per 100,000 population [14]. From this it appears that necrotising fasciitis due to GAS may have a higher incidence in North America compared with the UK, or that under-reporting may exist in the UK.

Necrotising fasciitis appears to be more common in the elderly with 69% of affected patients aged 60 years or over in one large series [10]. Similarly, the Canadian experience records incidences of GAS necrotising fasciits as 0.55 per 100,000 in those over 65 years, compared with 0.15 per 100,000 in those under 45 years [15].

With regards to gender and race, there is an unequal sex distribution with males more commonly affected in both types of necrotising fasciitis (ratio of 3:2) [10, 15, 17], while invasive GAS infections (though not necessarily necrotising fasciitis) are more common in black individuals than in other races [14].

Risk factors

Necrotising fasciitis is more common in patients with established comorbidity including diabetes, peripheral vascular disease, malignancy, renal dysfunction, congestive heart failure, chronic lung disease, pancreatitis, cirrhosis and alcoholism, obesity, smoking and intravenous drug abuse [9, 17, 18]. Factors predictive of poor outcome include extremes of age (under one and over 60 years of age), female gender, intravenous drug abuse, past history of cancer, renal failure, congestive cardiac failure and peripheral vascular disease [9, 10].

Amongst adults with invasive GAS infection in one North American series, exposure to children with sore thoats, HIV infection and a history of intravenous drug abuse were significant risk factors, although in the over 45-year age group, an increasing number of persons in the home, diabetes, cardiac disease, cancer, and corticosteroid use were also implicated [19]. The aetiological role of intercurrent illness in the development of Type II necrotising fasciitis (9% [20] - 13.5% [17]) compared with Type I disease (17.3% [14] - 29% [15]) is less well defined.

In the paediatric population, it has been demonstrated that the incidence of invasive GAS infections correlates with the number of children living in the home, reflecting the number of possible streptococcal contacts. This, however, is offset by the number of rooms within the house and the potential for separation of affected children [21]. This crowding phenomenon is also witnessed in adults over 45 years old [19].

In large prospective Canadian suveillance studies, 15% [22] and 25% [23] of children with invasive GAS disease had a history of chicken pox in the month before their illness, possibly as a result of super-infection of chicken pox vesicles. It has been suggested that vaccination against *Varicella zoster* virus could prevent up to a quarter of all paediatric invasive GAS disease.

An association between the use of non-steroidal anti-inflammatory drugs (NSAIDs), which act by reducing the ability of granulocytes to perform chemotaxis, phagocytosis, and bacterial killing [24], and necrotising fasciitis has been highlighted by a recent UK study in which 92% of patients with streptococcal toxic shock syndrome were taking NSAIDs at the time of disease onset [25]. It is not clear, however, whether or not NSAIDs actively participate in the development of the disease or simply delay diagnosis and treatment [26] resulting in a poorer outcome [9, 27].

Aetiology

In many cases of necrotising fasciitis an initiating event, ranging from a minor insult (such as an insect bite) to large, penetrating, injuries can be identified. Iatrogenic cases of necrotising fasciitis, following subcutaneous injections, minor and major operations [13,18], and post partum infections [14] have also been reported along with chronic ulceration, including pressure ulceration [17]. However, in children in particular, there is often no history of antecedent trauma [9].

Microbiology

Type I 'synergistic' necrotising fasciitis, accounts for the majority of cases and is produced by a mixture of bacteria, with a mean value of 4.4 separate pathogens identifiable in any given patient [10]. The most common organisms to be isolated include Bacteroides species, aerobic haemolytic streptococci, staphylococci, enterococci, *Escherichia coli* and other gram-negative rods (*Proteus mirabilis* and klebsiellae). Additionally, clostridial growth is not uncommon [10].

Type II necrotising fasciitis is due to group A beta-haemolytic streptococci as a unique isolate. If a second pathogen is present it is usually a staphylococcus.

Green has proposed that a Type III necrotising fasciitis be added to this classification [28] to account for necrotising fasciitis caused by marine vibrios such as *Vibrio vulnificus* and *Vibrio parahaemolyticus*. *Vibrio vulnificus* appears to be the most virulent of these organisms [29]. Vibrios penetrate the skin via puncture wounds or by surface exposure to minor wounds or abrasions. Systemic infection may be caused by ingestion of contaminated sea food (raw oysters and shellfish).

Vibrio vulnificus multiplies in the warm coastal waters of the Gulf of Mexico, South America, Asia and Australia [29]. If contact with contaminated seawater or raw seafood is suspected an antibiotic protocol of ceftriaxone or ceftazidime combined with doxycycline should be used. These pathogens produce several cytotoxins which can rapidly cause fatal sepsis.

A further type of necrotising fasciitis which is yet to be classified is that due to community-associated methicillin-resistant *Staphylococcus aureus* (MRSA). Historically, *Staphylococcus aureus* has not been a common cause of necrotising fasciitis, but this now appears to be changing [30]. Community-associated MRSA (CA-MRSA) differs from hospital-acquired MRSA (HA-MRSA) in that it is generally far more sensitive to antimicrobials such as cotrimoxazole, ciprofloxacin and clindamycin. In addition, the translation of genes encoding for Panton-Valentine leukocidin (PVL) produces a toxic factor associated with necrotising and recurrent skin and soft tissue infections, and a more serious necrotising pneumonia [31].

Pathology

Necrotising fasciitis is defined by deep seated infection tracking along tissue planes with fascial necrosis and the production of foul-smelling 'dish-water pus' [11, 17].

At a microscopic level, necrosis of fascia, subcutaneous fat, nerves and vessels is seen, often sparing the overlying skin and deeper muscle [9]. Frozen section histopathology can confirm this tissue necrosis [32]. Only when there is extensive necrosis of underlying fat and fascia (liquefactive necrosis) does skin become cyanosed and necrotic [7]. Early in the disease process subcutaneous vessels develop obliterative vasculitis. This is followed by necrosis of subcutaneous tissue and thrombosis of vessels perfusing the skin, the mechanism for producing severe pain. Anaesthesia rapidly supervenes as sensory nerves become critically ischaemic, and the skin undergoes blister formation and ultimately necrosis. Polymorphonuclear leukocytes infiltrate the deep dermis and fascia, and micro-organisms proliferate within the destroyed fascial layer.

Pathogenesis

Although the exact pathogenesis of necrotising fasciitis remains to be fully elucidated, microbial proliferation within fascial planes and the production of bacterial toxins and enzymes (e.g. hyaluronidase) facilitates the extension of the infective process.

Since many cases of GAS necrotising fasciitis follow a flu-like illness, it is presumed that a bacteraemic phase precedes seeding of the organism into an inflamed area of tissue, such as may exist after trauma.

Group A streptococci are gram-positive cocci, occurring as pairs or short to medium length chains in clinical specimens (Figure 1). Although they are extracellular pathogens they have the ability to invade epithelial cells. Group A streptococci are nearly always beta-haemolytic, producing complete lysis of red cells surrounding a colony in culture (Figure 2). The cell surface polysaccharide of GAS [33] accounts for much of the bacteria's virulence, mediating in the

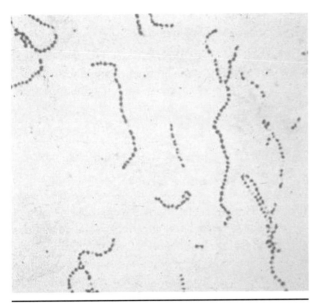

Figure 1. Chains of gram-positive cocci, typical of group A streptococci.

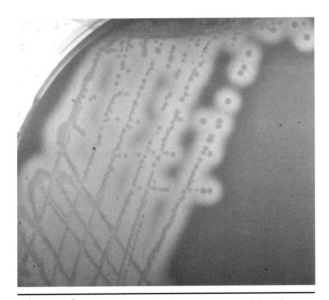

Figure 2. Beta haemolysis seen on a blood agar plate.

are important virulence factors associated with colonisation and resistance to phagocytosis. M proteins bind fibrinogen from serum and block the binding of complement control factors, preventing activation of the alternate complement pathway and protecting the organism from phagocytosis by polymorphonuclear leukocytes. The proteins M1 and M3 are increasingly associated with invasive and fatal infections [34].

Streptococcal 'invasins' lyse eukaryotic cells (including red blood cells and phagocytes) and other host macromolecules resulting in the lysis of ground substance and collagen. Streptococcal toxins include leukocidins (Streptolysin-S and -O, NADase) which damage leukocytes; hyaluronidase which digests host connective tissue; and streptokinase which lyses fibrin. A distinct group of toxins produced by streptococci are the streptococcal pyrogenic exotoxins. These toxins act as superantigens and are able to bypass antigen processing by antigen presenting cells; instead they bind directly in a non-specific manner to the MCH Class II molecule on T-cells. This method of processing leads to the simultaneous activation of up to 3-10% of the T-cell population, compared with only 0.01-0.1% under normal infective conditions [35]. This over-activation leads to the production of large amounts of tumour necrosis factor and interleukins, resulting in hypotension, shock and multi-system organ failure.

Clinical features

The clinical diagnosis of necrotising fasciitis can be difficult as the presenting features are often non-specific, ranging from a relative absence of signs and symptoms to fulminant necrosis associated with hypotension and multi-organ failure (Figures 3 and 4). Failure to make the correct diagnosis at first presentation occurs in up to 15% of patients [36].

The extremities are more often affected than the trunk and perineum [37]. A high index of suspicion should be entertained in patients with a triad of exquisite pain (out of proportion to physical findings), soft tissue swelling or oedema and fever. These clinical features occur independently in 75% to 90% of cases [13, 36]. Blister formation is much less common

avoidance of phagocytosis and host immune responses.

The cell wall of GAS also incorporates a family of M proteins, the hyaluronic acid capsule and fibronectin binding proteins. The M proteins, of which there are more than 50 types associated with GAS,

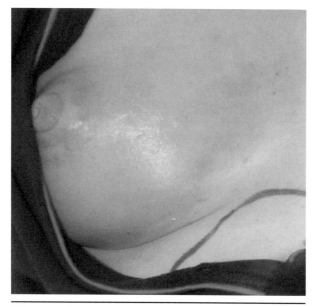

Figure 3. A breast feeding patient presented with pain and swelling of the right breast. The ominous dusky patch on the right breast raised concerns that the patient had a necrotising fasciitis. Debridement and histology confirmed the diagnosis of GAS necrotising fasciitis. *Reproduced with permission from Elsevier, © 2006 [58].*

(16%- 45%) [9, 13, 36, 38] **(III/B)**. Lymphadenopathy and lymphangitis is rarely seen in necrotising fasciitis [28]. Systemic symptoms related to streptococcal TSS, such as nausea, vomiting, diarrhoea and myalgia, should prompt further investigation for a history of GAS contacts (sore throat, flu-like illness, impetigo, scarlet fever).

Laboratory findings

Although necrotising fasciitis is essentially a clinical diagnosis, attempts have been made to distinguish necrotising from non-necrotising conditions on the basis of blood assays [38, 39]. Multivariate analysis showed that a leucocytosis greater than 15.4 x10^9/L, serum sodium less than 135mmol/L, and blood urea of more than 15mg/dL separated patients with necrotising fasciitis from those with non-necrotising infections **(III/B)**. Similarly, ESR [40], C-reactive protein and creatinine kinase [41] levels are significantly elevated in patients with GAS necrotising fasciitis **(III/B)**.

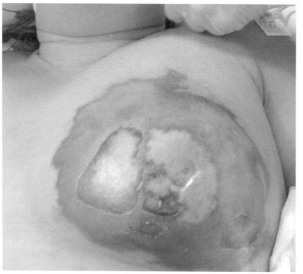

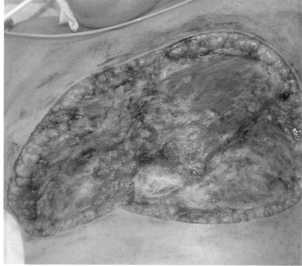

Figure 4. a) This critically ill patient presented to the emergency department. The purple discolouration and blistering are late signs. After a radical debridement, high dose antibiotics, IVIG and treatment in the intensive care unit, she survived. b) The chest wound after debridement.

Imaging

Diagnostic imaging may be of some value in equivocal cases of necrotising fasciitis but should not delay early systemic treatment and surgical debridement [42].

Plain radiography is able to demonstrate the presence of subcutaneous gas; however, this is a late and uncommon sign, seen in only 15% of cases [10] and therefore has limited clinical usefulness.

Computerised tomography (CT) demonstrates asymmetric fascial thickening and fat stranding in up to 80% of patients with necrotising fasciitis, along with fat infiltration, focal fluid collections and soft tissue gas in around 50% [42]. The additional value of CT lies in its ability to accurately demonstrate deep and intra-abdominal collections, and its relative availability, particulary 'out of hours'. However, compared with magnetic resonance (MR) imaging, CT is unable to differentiate between inflamed soft tissue and free fluid tracking along fascial planes. As an imaging modality it provides poor definition of areas of necrosis and fails to demonstrate inflammation of fascial planes. This can lead to both false positive and negative results.

MR may help differentiate cellulitis from necrotising fasciitis on the basis of signal characteristics [43]. Cellulitis typically generates subcutaneous inflammation sometimes accompanied by fluid collections whilst necrotising fasciitis typically generates deep fascial thickening with inflammatory changes, but may also generate free fluid. These water-based changes are best seen on T2-weighted sequences. Muscle necrosis can be identified by the absence of enhancement following intravenous gadolinium on the T1-weighted sequences [44].

T2-weighted sequences have been shown to be 100% sensitive [43] but may not be specific as tissue oedema of any aetiology will be identified. It can not differentiate between infected tissue and adjacent non-infectious inflammation and may overestimate the area of involvement. Thus caution should be exercised when interpreting heavily T2-weighted images (e.g. fast spin echo) which are even more sensitive at identifying free tissue fluid [45].

Tissue-based investigations

Frozen section histopathology may be used to confirm a clinical diagnosis of early necrotising fasciitis [46]. Necrosis of the superficial fascia, a polymorphonuclear inflammatory cell infiltration of deep dermis and fascia, fibrinous thrombosis of vessels passing through the fascia, angiitis with fibrinoid necrosis of arterial and venous walls, the presence of micro-organisms within the destroyed fascia and an absence of muscle involvement are all typical features. Once the disease process is well established, definition between tissue planes is lost and on the basis of histopathology the specimen becomes indistinguishable from other necrotising processes.

Recent progress has been made using trans-cutaneous oximetry as a diagnostic tool for necrotising fasciitis affecting the lower limb, although this technique loses validity in patients with chronic ischaemia or venous hypertension [47].

Treatment

Resuscitation

Systemic fluid and supportive therapy of the shocked patient prior to surgical debridement must be established early, often requiring pre-surgical admission to the Intensive Care Unit. It may be necessary to transfuse blood, fresh frozen plasma and clotting factors to address anaemia or coagulopathy. Occasionally, haemofiltration may also need to be considered.

Antibiotics

Early targeted high dose antibiotic treatment is central to the management of necrotising fasciitis. However, due to the presence of microvascular thrombosis, antimicrobials penetrate infected and necrotic tissue poorly, emphasising the need for expedient surgical debridement. Antibiotic therapy must be effective against gram-positive organisms, anaerobes and gram-negative rods.

Stevens *et al* [48] assessed the efficacy of clindamycin, erythromycin and penicillin in the management of invasive streptococcal infections in a murine model of streptococcal myositis. Penicillin alone was ineffective, unless given at the time of inoculation. Furthermore, if penicillin treatment began two hours after inoculation, survival was no better than in untreated control animals, an observation explained by the 'Eagle effect' [49]. Eagle demonstrated that at a critical mass of bacteria per gram of muscle tissue, streptococci enter a 'stationary phase', effectively protecting the organism from the action of penicillin which depends upon the synthesis of bacterial cell wall penicillin-binding proteins [50].

When mice received erythromycin, survival rates were better than with penicillin-treated and untreated controls; however, therapy had to begin within two hours of inoculation. The survival rates of mice receiving clindamycin were superior, at 100% if treated at zero and two hours, and 70% when treated at 16.5 hours.

Clindamycin is more effective in treating group A streptococci, as it inhibits toxin formation (thereby reducing the inflammatory over-response) and enhances bacterial phagocytosis via down-regulated M protein synthesis [51-53].

Three studies have examined the clinical efficacy of clindamycin in patients with GAS necrotising fasciitis. Kaul *et al* [15] were unable to show improved survival in 77 affected patients **(III/B)**, while more recent studies by Zimbelman *et al* [54] and Mulla *et al* [55] have both demonstrated a clear survival advantage attributable to clindamycin therapy when compared with standard antibiotic regimens **(III/B)**.

The antibiotic protocol for necrotising fasciitis at the Royal Devon & Exeter Hospital, prior to confirmation of the infecting organism, is high-dose intravenous clindamycin (1.2g six-hourly) to combat GAS and other toxin-producing organisms, such as clostridia, combined with intravenous imipenem (500-1000mg six-hourly) to target synergistic organisms. Where MRSA necrotising fasciitis is suspected, intravenous vancomycin or linezolid therapy is indicated.

Other antibiotic regimens have been described in the literature. ß-Lactam/ß-Lactamase combinations,

such as ticarcillin and clavulinic acid, third-generation cephalosporins, including cefotaxime and ceftazidine, with metronidazole or clindamycin, and carbapenems (e.g. imipenem, meropenem) have all been proposed [37] (Young *et al* 2006). However, since none of these prevent toxin production, all patients should receive clindamycin until GAS has been excluded.

Surgical debridement

Expedient surgical debridement is pivotal to reducing mortality rates from necrotising fasciitis. As the time between admission and debridement increases from less than 24 hours to more than 48 hours, mortality rates increase from 6.8% to 24.8% [17], with the mean time to debridement significantly lower for survivors of the disease (25 hours) compared with non-survivors (90 hours)[13] **(IIIb)**.

Early, radical surgical debridement [28] is necessary to remove all non-viable tissue and several returns to the operating theatre are common [17]. A 'second-look' of the wound should be performed 24 hours after the initial debridement, or earlier depending upon the clinical condition of the patient. The large soft tissue defects that are inevitably created are managed in the interim either with simple dressings or by topical negative pressure techniques [56]. A defunctioning colostomy may be required to maintain a clean wound environment for perineal defects.

Wound closure is achieved once the patient has stabilised and the disease process has been eradicated [57]. Reconstructive options include split skin grafts (autologous or cadaveric), full-thickness skin grafts, local, pedicled and free flaps and tissue expansion [58]. Complex reconstructions are, however, best undertaken secondarily.

Adjunctive treatments

Intravenous immunoglobulin

Polyspecific intravenous immunoglobulin (IVIG) has been evaluated in the management of systemic sepsis in several small clinical trials, with varying results. While there are no conclusive data to support the use of IVIG in all cases of sepsis, there is some evidence to demonstrate its efficacy against gram-positive organisms, particularly in the context of streptococcal toxic shock syndrome [59]. The mode of action of IVIG is likely to be three-fold: neutralisation of GAS superantigens, opsonisation of bacteria and modulation of cytokine formation.

An observational cohort study of 21 patients with streptococcal toxic shock syndrome (STSS) treated with a median of 2g of IVIG between 1994-5 and 32 STSS patients treated between 1992-5 who did not receive IVIG [60] demonstrated improved survival amongst STSS patients who received IVIG compared with those in the earlier treatment cohort. This survival advantage was statistically significant with mortality rates of 34% in the IVIG group and 67% in the control group **(III/B)**. However, the patients who had received IVIG were more likely to have received clindamycin and so a multivariate analysis of patients receiving clindamycin was carried out. Those receiving IVIG were still significantly more likely to survive than controls. A reduction in the T-cell production of interleukin-6 and tumour necrosis factor post-IVIG treatment was observed, suggesting a reduced pro-inflammatory response in treated patients.

A later multi-centre European randomised, double-blind placebo-controlled trial assessed the efficacy of IVIG in TSS [61] **(Ib/A)**. This trial terminated prematurely due to the slow recruitment of patients with streptococcal TSS. Results lacked statistical significance but nonetheless illustrated a trend towards a survival benefit conferred by IVIG treatment.

Early recognition of STSS and treatment with high dose IVIG may delay the requirement for, or reduce the extent of, surgical debridement, as evidenced by a recent study by Norrby-Teglund et al [62]. Seven patients with severe GAS sepsis were treated with antimicrobials, IVIG and conservative or even no surgical debridement. All patients survived.

Recombinant protein C

Activated protein C is an endogenous circulating protein that promotes fibrinolysis and inhibits thrombosis and inflammation. Reduced levels of protein C are encountered in patients with severe sepsis and correlate with increased mortality. Although the administration of recombinant human activated protein C (drotrecogin alfa) has been shown to reduce 28-day mortality amongst patients with systemic sepsis [63] **(Ib/A)**, the role of protein C in the management of patients with STSS has not been assessed. Careful consideration should be given to the timing of treatment with protein C as this precludes surgical intervention in the subsequent 12 hours.

Hyperbaric oxygen therapy

Hyperbaric oxygen therapy (HBO) improves oxygen delivery to tissues by increasing dissolved plasma oxygen from 3ml/L at atmospheric pressure to 70ml/L at 3 atmospheres of pressure. An elevated partial pressure of oxygen in the blood enhances leukocyte-mediated bacterial killing. HBO may also reduce tissue oedema, increase angiogenesis and potentiate wound healing [64]. HBO therapy in the management of necrotising fasciitis has not been well evaluated by large prospectively randomised controlled trials. This is partly due to the lack of availability of HBO facilities and the logistic difficulties that arise when transporting critically ill patients.

However, in one prospectively randomised study [65], patients receiving HBO, despite poorer prognosis disease at presentation, had a significantly lower mortality compared with patients in the control group treated by surgical debridement and antibiotic therapy alone (23% vs 66%) **(Ib/A)**. Furthermore, the number of debridements was less in the HBO group. Importantly, HBO should not delay surgical debridement and the potential risks relating to barotrauma, to the middle ear and lungs, and oxygen toxicity of the central nervous system and respiratory tract must be borne in mind.

Secondary cases and prophylactic antibiotics

There have been documented cases of GAS transmission among household contacts and health care workers [66-69]. Air-borne [70] and needlestick [71] transmission of GAS from a single source to health care workers has been reported. It has also been documented in a fire officer following cardiopulmonary resuscitation [72]. Health care workers caring for patients with GAS respiratory infections should wear masks and goggles in addition to the contact precautions (gloves and aprons or gowns) that are required for patients with wounds or skin infections due to GAS [70].

Invasive GAS infection has also been reported in household contacts [66-69, 73]. Although a number of trials have shown successful eradication of GAS from the upper respiratory tract, none have been performed to evaluate the effectiveness of prophylactic antibiotics in preventing invasive GAS disease in household contacts of patients with invasive GAS infection. In the UK, data from surveillance in 2003 have estimated that 2000 contacts would need to be treated to prevent one invasive GAS infection [12].

The current UK guidelines for the management of close community contacts is to offer antibiotic treatment to mother and baby if either develops invasive group A streptococcal infection in the first 28 days of life. Additionally, antibiotics should be administered to close contacts displaying symptoms suggestive of localised GAS infection, e.g. sore throat, fever, skin infection [12]. If contacts have symptoms suggestive of invasive disease (e.g. high fever, severe muscle aches or localised muscle tenderness), then they should be referred immediately to an emergency department.

Conclusions

Necrotising fasciitis is an uncommon condition associated with a high mortality rate. Prompt treatment with intravenous fluid resuscitation, appropriate intravenous antibiotics, intravenous immunoglobulin (where GAS infection is suspected), and urgent surgical debridement is required, followed by supportive treatment in the Intensive Care Unit. Senior intensivist, surgical and microbiology involvement is critical in the diagnosis and emergency management of these patients.

Recommendations	Evidence level
◆ A high index of suspicion of necrotising fasciitis should be held in the presence of exquisite pain, soft tissue swelling or oedema and fever.	III/B
◆ Patients with a leucocytosis of more than 15.4 x10^9/L, serum sodium less than 135mmol/L, and blood urea of more than 15mg/dL are more likely to have a necrotising infection than cellulitis.	III/B
◆ Patients with GAS necrotising fasciitis are more likely to have a raised CRP and CK than patients with cellulitis.	III/B
◆ Antibiotic treatment should consist of high dose intraveous clindamycin in patients where group A streptococcal infection is suspected.	III/B
◆ Urgent surgical debridement, within 24 hours, reduces mortality rates in patients with necrotising fasciitis.	III/B
◆ Intravenous immunoglobulin may reduce mortality rates in patients with STSS.	III/B
◆ Hyperbaric oxygen therapy can reduce mortality rates in patients with necrotising fasciitis but is logistically difficult to obtain.	Ib/A
◆ Regarding chemoprophylaxis for close contacts of patients with GAS necrotising fasciitis, antibiotics should be given to: a) mother and baby if either develops invasive GAS disease in the neonatal period; b) close contacts if they have symptoms suggestive of localised GAS infection.	IV/C

References

1. Stevens DL. Streptococcal toxic syndrome associated with necrotizing fasciitis. *Ann Rev Med* 2000; 51: 271-88.

2. Descamps V, Aitken J, Lee MG. Hippocrates on necrotizing fasciitis. *Lancet* 1994; 344: 566.

3. Loudon I. Necrotizing fasciitis, hospital gangrene, and phagedena. *Lancet* 1994; 344: 1416-9.

4. Meleney FL. Hemolytic streptococcus gangrene. *Arch Surg* 1924; 9: 317-64.

5. Wilson B. Necrotizing fasciitis. *Am J Surg* 1952; 18: 416-31.

6. Eke N. Fournier's gangrene: a review of 1726 cases. *Br J Surg* 2000; 87: 718-28.

7. Giuliano A, Lewis F, Hadley K, Blaisdell FW. Bacteriology of necrotizing fasciitis. *Am J Surg* 1977; 134: 52-7.

8. The working group on severe streptococcal infections. Defining the group A streptococcal toxic shock syndrome. Rationale and consensus definition. *JAMA* 1993; 269 (3): 390-1.

9. Childers BJ, Potyondy LD, Nachreiner R, *et al*. Necrotizing fasciitis: a fourteen-year retrospective study of 163 consecutive patients. *Am Surg* 2002; 68 (2): 109-16.

10. Elliot D, Kufera JA, Myers RAM, *et al*. The microbiology of necrotizing soft tissue infections. *Am J Surg* 2000; 179: 361-6.

11. Nichols RL, Florman S. Clinical presentation of soft-tissue infections and surgical site infections. *Clin Infect Dis* 2001; 33 (Supp 2): S84-93.

12. Health Protection Agency, Group A Streptococcus Working Group. Interim UK guidelines for the management of close community contacts of invasive group A streptococcal disease. *Comm Dis Pub Health* 2004; 7(4): 354-61.

13. McHenry CR, Piotrowski JJ, Petrinic D, Malangoni MA. Determinants of mortality for necrotizing soft-tissue infections. *Ann Surg* 1995; 221 (5): 558-65.

14. O'Brien KL, Beall B, Barrett NL, *et al*. Epidemiology of invasive group A streptococcus disease in the United States, 1995-1999. *Clin Infect Dis* 2002; 35: 268-76.

15. Kaul R, McGeer A, Low DE, *et al*. Population-based surveillance for group A streptococcal necrotizing fasciitis: clinical features, prognostic indicators, and microbiologic analysis of seventy seven cases. *Am J Med* 1997: 103: 18-24.

16. www.strep-euro.lu.se/news_ver3.html.

17. Wong C-H, Chang H-C, Pasupathy S, *et al*. Necrotizing fasciitis: clinical presentation, microbiology and determinants of mortality. *J Bone Joint Surg* Am 2003; 85 (8): 1454-60.

18. Sudarsky LA, Laschinger JC, Coppa GF, Spencer FC. Improved results from a standardised approach in treating patients with necrotising fasciitis. *Ann Surg* 1987; 206: 661-5.

19. Factor SH, Levine OS, Schwartz B, *et al*. Invasive group A streptococcal disease: risk factors for adults. *Emerg Infect Dis* 2003; 9 (8): 970-7.

20. Faucher LD, Morris SE, Edelman LS, *et al*. Burn center management of necrotizing soft-tissue infections in unburned patients. *Am J Surg* 2001; 182: 563-9.

21. Factor SH, Levine OS, Harrison LH, *et al*. Risk factors for pediatric invasive group A streptococcal disease. *Emerg Infect Dis* 2005; 11(7): 1062-6.

22. Laupland KB, Davies HD, Low DE, *et al*. Invasive group A streptococcal disease in children and association with varicella-zoster virus infection. *Pediatrics* 2000; 105 (5): 60-7.

23. Tyrell GJ, Lovgren M, Kress B, *et al*. Invasive group A streptococcal disease in Alberta, Canada (2000 to 2002). *J Clin Microbiol* 2005; 43(4): 1678-83.

24. Stevens DL. Could nonsteroidal anti-inflammatory drugs (NSAIDs) enhance the progression of bacterial infections to toxic shock syndrome? *Clin Infect Dis* 1995; 21 (4): 977-80.

25. Barnham MRD, Weightman NC, Anderson AW, *et al*. Streptococcal toxic shock syndrome: a description of 14 cases from North Yorkshire, UK. *Clin Microbiol Infect* 2002; 8: 174-81.

26. Aronoff DM, Bloch KC. Assessing the relationship between the use of nonsteroidal anti-inflammatory drugs and necrotising fasciitis caused by group A streptococcus. *Medicine* 2003; 82 (4): 225-35.

27. Tillou A, St Hill CR, Brown C, *et al*. Necrotizing soft tissue infections: improved outcomes with modern care. *Am Surg* 2004; 70: 841-4.

28. Green RJ, Dafoe DC, Raffin TA. Necrotizing fasciitis. *Chest* 1996; 110: 219-29.

29. Tsai Y-H, Wen-Wei R, Huang K-C, *et al*. Systemic vibrio infection presenting as necrotizing fasciitis and sepsis. A series of thirteen cases. *J Bone Joint Surg Am* 2004; 86: 2497-502.

30. Miller LG, Perdreau-Remington F, Rieg G, *et al*. Necrotizing fasciitis caused by community-associated methicillin-resistant *Staphylococcus aureus* in Los Angeles. *N Engl J Med* Boston 2005; 352(14): 1445-53.

31. Diep BA, Sensabaugh GF, Somboona NS, *et al*. Widespread skin and soft tissue infections due to two methicillin-resistant *Staphylococcus aureus* strains harbouring the genes for Panton-Valentine leukocidin. *J Clin Microbiol* 2004; 42 (5): 2080-4.

32. Stamenkovic I, Lew PD. Early recognition of potentially fatal necrotizing fasciitis. The use of the frozen section biopsy. *N Engl J Med* 1984; 310 (26): 1690-3.

33. Lancefield RC. Aserological differentiation of human and other groups of haemolytic streptococci. *J Exper Med* 1933; 57: 571-95.

34. Bisno AL, Brito MO, Collins CM. Molecular basis of group A streptococcal virulence. *Lancet Infect Dis* 2003; 3: 191-200.

35. Baracco GJ, Bisno AL. Therapeutic approaches to streptococcal toxic shock syndrome. *Curr Infect Dis Reports* 1999; 1: 230-7.

36. Wong C-H and Wang Y-S. The diagnosis of necrotizing fasciitis. *Curr Opin Infect Dis* 2005; 18: 101-6.

37. Young MH, Engleberg NC, Mulla ZD, *et al*. Therapies for necrotising fasciitis. *Expert Opin Biol Ther* 2006; 6 (2): 155-65.

38. Wall DB, de Virgilio C, Black S, *et al*. Objective criteria may assist in distinguishing necrotizing fasciitis from nonnecrotizing soft tissue infection. *Am J Surg* 2000; 179: 17-21.

39. Wall DB, Klein SR, Black S, *et al*. A simple model to help distinguish necrotizing fasciits from nonnecrotising soft tissue infection. *J Am Coll Surg* 2000; 191: 227-31.

40. Wong CH, Khin LW, Heng KS, *et al*. The LRINEC (Laboratory Risk Indictaor for Necrotising Fasciitis) score: a

tool for distinguishing necrotising fasciitis from other soft tissue infections. *Crit Care Med* 2004; 32: 1535-41.

41. Simonart T, Simonart JM, Derdelinckx I, *et al*. Value of standard laboratory tests for the early recognition of group A beta-haemolytic streptococcal necrotizing fasciitis. *Clin Infect Dis* 2001; 32: e9-12.

42. Wysoki MG, Santora TA, Shah RM, *et al*. Necrotizing fasciitis: CT characteristics. *Radiology* 1997; 203: 859-63.

43. Schmid MR, Kossman T, Duewell S. Differentiation of necrotizing fasciits and cellulitis using MR imaging. *AJR* 1998; 170: 615-20.

44. Brothers TE, Tagge DU, Stutley JE, *et al*. Magnetic resonance imaging differentiates between necrotizing and non-necrotizing fasciitis of the lower extremity. *J Am Coll Surg* 1998; 187 (4): 416-21.

45. Loh N-N, Ch'en IY, Cheung LP, *et al*. Deep fascial hyperintensity in soft tissue abnormalities as revealed by T2-weighted MR Imaging. *Am J Radiol* 1997; 168: 1301-4.

46. Stamenkovic I, Lew PD. Early recognition of potentially fatal necrotizing fasciitis. The use of frozen section biopsy. *N Engl J Med* 1984; 310 (26): 1690-3.

47. Wang TL, Hung CR. Role of tissue oxygen saturation monitoring in diagnosisng necrotising fasciitis of the lower limb. *Ann Emerg Med* 2004; 44: 222-8

48. Stevens DL, Gibbons AE, Bergstrom R, *et al*. The Eagle effect revisited: efficacy of clindamycin, erythromycin and penicillin in the treatment of streptococcal myositis. *J Infect Dis* 1988; 158 (1): 23-8.

49. Eagle H. Experimental approach to the problem of treatment failure with penicillin. Group A streptococcal infection in mice. *Am J Med* 1952; 13: 389-99.

50. Stevens DL. Streptococcal toxic shock syndrome: spectrum of disease, pathogenesis and new concepts in treatment. *Emerg Infect Dis* 1995; 1: 69-78.

51. Coyle EA. Targeting bacterial virulence: the role of protein synthesis inhibitors in severe infections. Insights from the Society of Infectious Diseases Pharmacists. *Pharmacotherapy* 2003; 23 (5): 638-42.

52. Coyle EA, Char R, Rybak MJ. Influences of linezolid, penicillin, and clindamycin, alone and in combination, on streptococcal pyrogenic exotoxin A release. *Antimicrob Agents Chemother* 2003; 47(5): 1752-5.

53. Mulla ZD. Treatment options in the management of necrotising fasciitis casued by group A streptococcus. *Expert Opin Pharmacother* 2004; 5 (8): 1695-700.

54. Zimbelman J, Palmer A, Todd J. Improved outcome of clindamycin compared with beta-lactam antibiotic treatment for invasive *Streptococcus pyogenes* infection. *Pediatr Infect Dis J* 1999; 18: 1096-100.

55. Mulla ZD, Leaverton PE, Wiersma ST. Invasive group A streptococcal infections in Florida. *South Med J* 2003; 96: 968-73.

56. De Geus HRH, van der Klooster JM. Vaccuum-assisted closure in the treatment of large skin defects due to necrotizing fasciitis. *Int Care Med* 2005; 31: 601.

57. Andreasen TJ, Green SD, Childers BJ. Massive soft-tissue injury: diagnosis and management of necrotising fasciitis and purpura fulminans. *Plast Reconstr Surg* 2001; 107 (4): 1025-34.

58. Tillett RL, Saxby PJ, Stone CA, Morgan MS. Group A streptococcal necrotising fasciitis masquerading as mastitis. *Lancet* 2006; 368: 174.

59. Norrby-Teglund A, Ihendayne N, Darenberg J. Intravenous immunoglobulin adjunctive therapy with special emphasis on severe invasive group A streptococcal infections. *Scand J Infect Dis* 2003; 35: 683-9.

60. Kaul R, McGeer A, Norrby-Teglund A, *et al*. Intravenous immunoglobulin therapy for streptococcal toxic shock syndrome - a comparative observational study. *Clin Infect Dis* 1999; 28: 800-7.

61. Darenberg J, Ihendayne N, Sjölin J, *et al*. Intravenous immunoglobulin G therapy in streptococcal toxic shock syndrome: a European randomized, double-blind, placebo-controlled trial. *Clin Infect Dis* 2003; 32: 333-40.

62. Norrby-Teglund A, Muller M, McGeer A, *et al*. Successful management of severe group A streptococcal soft tissue infections using an aggressive medical regimen including intravenous polyspecific immunoglobulin together with a conservative surgical approach. *Scand J Infect Dis* 2005; 37: 166-72.

63. Bernard GR, Vincent J-L, Laterre P-F, *et al*. Efficacy and safety of recombinant human activated protein C for severe sepsis. *N Engl J Med* 2001; 344 (10): 699-709.

64. Jallali N, Withey S, Butler PE. Hyperbaric oxygen as adjuvant therapy in the management of necrotizing fasciitis. *Am J Surg* 2005; 189: 426-66.

65. Riseman JA, Zamboni WA, Curtis A, *et al*. Hyperbaric oxygen therapy for necrotising fasciitis reduces mortality and the need for debridement. *Surgery* 1990; 108: 847-50.

66. DiPersio JR, File TM Jr, Stevens DL, *et al*. Spread of serious disease-producing M3 clones of group A streptococcus among family members and health care workers. *Clin Infect Dis* 1996; 22(3): 490-5.

67. Gamba MA, Martinelli M, Schaad HJ, *et al*. Familial transmission of a serious disease-producing group A streptococcus clone: case reports and review. *Clin Infect Dis* 1997; 24: 1118-21.

68. Ichiyama S, Nakashima K, Shimokata K, *et al*. Transmission of *Streptococcus pyogenes* causing toxic shock-like syndrome among family members and confirmation by DNA macrorestriction analysis. *J Infect Dis* 1997; 175: 723-6.

69. Robinson KA, Rothrock G, Phan Q, *et al*. Risk for severe group A streptococcal disease among patients' household contacts. *Emerg Infect Dis* 2003; 9(4): 443-7.

70. Kakis A, Gibbs L, Eguia J, *et al*. An outbreak of group A streptococcal infection among health care workers. *Clin Infect Dis* 2002; 35:1353-9.

71. Hagberg C, Radulescu A, Rex JH. Necrotizing fasciitis due to group A streptococcus after an accidental needle-stick injury. *N Engl J Med* 1997; 337(23): 1699.

72. Valenzuela TD, Hooton TM, Kaplan EL, *et al*. Transmission of 'toxic strep' syndrome from an infected child to a firefighter during CPR. *Ann Emerg Med* 1991; 20(1): 90-2.

73. The prevention of invasive group A streptococcal infections workshop participants. Prevention of invasive group A streptococcal disease among household contacts of case patients and among postpartum and postsurgical patients: recommendations from the centers for disease control and prevention. *Clin Infect Dis* 2002; 35: 950-9.

Chapter 3

Chapter 4

The relationship between increasing body mass index and complications in plastic surgery

Mark S Lloyd BM MRCS (Eng) MSc IM&T (Health) MPhil
Specialist Registrar, Plastic Surgery
Peter Budny MSc (Oxon) FRCS (Plast.)
Consultant Plastic Surgeon

STOKE MANDEVILLE HOSPITAL, AYLESBURY, UK

Introduction

There is a war on obesity being fought in the UK and USA. The Centres for Disease Control Report stated that 64% of Americans (193 million) are overweight. Of these, 30% are obese (58,000,000) and 4% morbidly obese [1]. These incredible statistics are similar for the UK, which now leads the European Union in having the highest percentage of obese people compared with other European countries.

The overweight and obese are at risk of ischaemic heart disease, cerebrovascular disease, cholelithiasis, respiratory problems, poor female reproductive health, bladder control problems, psychological disorders and complications from pregnancy. These comorbidities have placed an increased workload on health professionals and an increased financial burden on the health economy.

Body mass index (BMI) is calculated using a mathematical formula in which body weight (in kilograms) is divided by the square of the height (in metres). A BMI between 18 and $25kg/m^2$ is regarded as normal. A BMI of $25kg/m^2$ but less than $30kg/m^2$ is considered overweight. A BMI of $30kg/m^2$ is considered obese and over $40kg/m^2$ is morbidly obese.

Surgery undertaken to treat obesity has been named bariatric surgery. The rate of bariatric surgical procedures performed in the USA increased 500% between 1993 and 2003 [1].

Plastic surgeons worldwide will face more overweight and obese patients requesting procedures in the future. With this in mind, plastic surgeons must know whether an increase in complication rate is associated with an increase in BMI. With this knowledge it should be possible to counsel the patient appropriately and manage them safely peri-operatively. The following topics have been reviewed in relation to BMI and associated complications: bilateral reduction mammaplasty, abdominoplasty, panniculectomy, and anaesthetic complications.

Methodology

For each topic, a literature search was performed using MEDLINE, EMBASE, DARE, HTA, CINAHL and internet search engines. Once a paper was found, the abstract was screened for relevance and the methodology scored using the Newcastle-Ottawa Scale to be given a mark out of seven [2]. For each paper studied, the characteristics of the population, technique of the chosen operation, together with the outcome measures, were tabulated and analysed.

The difficulty when trying to extract information on BMI-related complications from these studies was the number of independent variables influencing outcome (Table 1). Once the data were tabulated for each paper, the odds ratios were calculated to weight the study and a meta-analysis performed using a random-effects model with an intention-to-treat protocol together with a sensitivity analysis for heterogeneity. Forest plots were used to display the graphical outputs of meta-analysis.

Table 1. Study characteristics for meta-analysis.

Population	Mean age (years)
	Age range (years)
	BMI (kg/m^2)
	Range of BMI (kg/m^2)
	BMI chosen as overweight (kg/m^2)
	Number of patients below selected BMI
	Number of patients above selected BMI
	Comorbidities
	Number of smokers
	Number of patients who dropped out of study
Reduction mammaplasty	Same/different surgeon
	Grade of surgeon
	Type of pedicle
	Use of adrenaline infiltration
Outcomes	Definition of complication
	Mean follow-up time (years)
	Mean weight of tissue resected in patients below selected BMI
	Mean weight of tissue resected in patients above selected BMI
	Number of patients with complications below selected BMI
	Number of patients with complications above selected BMI
	% complications for total patient sample
	Delayed healing (weeks)
	Wound breakdown
	Fat necrosis
	Nipple loss
	Haematoma
	Deep vein thrombosis
	Infection
	% complications for patients below selected BMI
	% complications for patients above selected BMI
	Appropriate statistical analysis
	Are findings justified?

Chapter 4

Bilateral reduction mammaplasty and BMI

The evidence for an increasing BMI leading to an increase in complications was first stated by Strombeck in 1964 [3] **(III/B)**. He analysed the relationship between various risk factors and complications in reduction mammaplasty. This was a retrospective study of 1042 reductions and he concluded that patients who were more than 10kg over their ideal weight or who had resections greater than 500g were at increased risk of complications. Strombeck stated that the rate of complications in the non-obese population was 4.4% and in the obese population it was 13.5%. This study may have been the start of why plastic surgeons regard BMI as such an important index in the selection of patients for reduction mammaplasty. In the UK, the information for Commissioners of Plastic Surgery Services requires that National Health Service (NHS) patients undergoing reduction mammaplasty should have a BMI less than 30kg/m^2 [4].

Is the BMI the best anthropometric measure for reduction mammaplasty?

A comparison of BMI with other anthropometric measures (such as bra and cup size, weight, height, and triceps fold thickness) as a predictor of complications following reduction mammaplasty and abdominoplasty was studied by Lahiri [5] **(III/B)**. This was a prospective case-controlled trial. The height, weight, waist, percentage body fat and BMI were obtained pre-operatively from 60 patients undergoing body-contouring surgery. To measure the percentage body fat, bioelectrical impedance analysis was used. BMI and waist circumference correlated with the actual body fat content as measured by bioelectrical impedance analysis. This study found that the BMI was still the most robust index of nutritional status and could easily be measured in the clinic.

What proportion of breast tissue is fat?

The study by Cruz-Korchin determined the ratio of fat to glandular tissue in macromastia specimens from 25 patients [6] **(IIa/B)**. The BMI was calculated for each patient together with the amount of fat in breast tissue taken from the central, lateral and pre-axillary areas of the breast, but not from the medial part of the breast. It was found that there was a significant increase in the amount of central fatty breast tissue with increasing BMI. This study did not try and correlate an increase in BMI with an increase in the complication rate but provided evidence that the breasts of a patient requesting reduction mammaplasty seem to have more fat than glandular tissue in the central part of the breast. Lejour studied breast tissue excised post-vertical scar reduction mammaplasty [7] **(IIa/B)**. In order to evaluate the fat content of the breast, 33 unselected specimens removed during breast reductions (20 with liposuction and 13 without liposuction) were subjected to melting in a microwave oven. The fat separated from the residue was weighed. This confirmed that pure glandular breasts were uncommon and that breast fat varied largely from one patient to another, with extremes of 2% and 78% and a mean value of 48%. The Lejour study showed that breast fat increased with age, body mass, and total volume of the breast.

The relationship between BMI and postoperative complications

In order to determine the relationship between BMI and postoperative complications, a systematic review of the literature and meta-analysis of the available data was undertaken. There have been no previous studies of this kind documented in the literature.

For each paper studied, the characteristics of the population, technique of reduction mammaplasty and outcome measures were tabulated and analysed (Tables 2 and 3).

A randomised controlled trial was not a viable study design to answer the question of whether increasing BMI was predictive of increased complications. The only paper with a randomised component was by Platt *et al*, but this was to select patients for adrenaline infiltration [8] **(Ib/A)**. All papers analysed were comparative retrospective case note studies. The numbers of patients with complications were

Table 2. Population and intervention characteristics for meta-analysis. (Studies in italics were excluded).

Author	Year	Quality score	Sample no	μAge/ years	μBMI (kg/m^2)	BMI range (kg/m^2)	BMI used as cut-off	Pedicle	Same surgeon
Budny [10]	1996	*****	101	31	28	20-46	25	Various	No
Blomqvist [9]	1996	******	291	35	23.7	22-26	22	Various	No
Zubowski [12]	2000	*******	267	37.9	25.8	23-32	25	Inferior	No
Wagner [11]	2001	*****	186	37	30	24-36	26	Inferior	Yes
Platt [8]	2003	****	30	33	26.3	21-31	26	Inferior	No
Lahiri [5]	2006	******	43	38.4	28	21.4-36.3	25	Inferior	No
Dabbah [41]	*1995*	*Zero*	*285*	*40*	*-*	*-*	*27*	*-*	*No*
Maxwell-Davis	*1994*	****	*780*	*35.6*	*28*	*-*	*-*	*Inferior*	*No*

Table 3. Outcome data for meta-analysis. (Studies in italics were excluded).

Author	Year	Sample no	μ tissue resection weight per breast (g)	No. patients with complication ≤ BMI/ sample no. (% complication rate)	No. patients with complication ≥ BMI/ sample no. (% complication rate)	Attrition rate (%)
Budny	1996	101	525.0	33 (32.7)	81 (80.2)	16.8
Blomqvist	1996	291	-	17 (5.8)	10 (3.4)	1.0
Zubowski	2000	267	618.2	19 (7.1)	30 (11.2)	2.0
Wagner	2001	186	1013	17 (9.1)	54 (29)	0
Platt	2003	30	635.0	3 (10)	10 (33)	0
Lahiri	2006	43	-	15 (34.9)	23 (53.4)	0
Dabbah	*1995*	*-*	*855.0*	*-*	*-*	*35*
Maxwell-Davis	*1994*	*-*	*676.0*	*-*	*-*	*52*

compared for each group (normal BMI versus overweight/obese BMI) as a proportion of the total number of patients in that group:

$$\frac{\text{Patients with complications}}{\text{Total number of patients with below cut-off BMI}} \quad \textit{Versus} \quad \frac{\text{Patients with complications}}{\text{Total number of patients above cut-off BMI}}$$

The mean age of patients from the studies selected was 35.6 years (range 31 to 40 years). The mean BMI of patients studied was 27.0kg/m^2. The mean BMI used to separate patients into normal and overweight/ obese was 25.6kg/m^2. The study by Blomqvist had the lowest BMI cut-off with a value of 22kg/m^2 but this was accounted for in the meta-analysis [9] **(III/B)**. The problem with using such a low BMI compared with

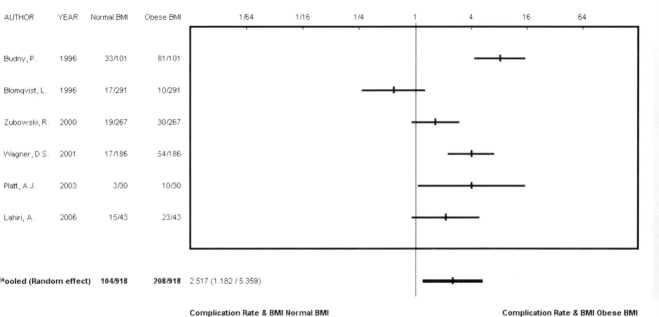

AUTHOR	YEAR	Normal BMI	Obese BMI								
				1/64	1/16	1/4	1	4	16	64	
Budny, P.	1996	33/101	81/101								
Blomqvist, L.	1996	17/291	10/291								
Zubowski, R.	2000	19/267	30/267								
Wagner, D.S.	2001	17/186	54/186								
Platt, A.J.	2003	3/30	10/30								
Lahiri, A.	2006	15/43	23/43								
Pooled (Random effect)		104/918	208/918	2.517 (1.182 / 5.359)							

Complication Rate & BMI Normal BMI   Complication Rate & BMI Obese BMI

Figure 1. Forest plot for meta-analysis: complication rates in reduction mammaplasty - obese versus non-obese.

the other studies was that the overweight group was comparable to the normal weight group of patients in the other studies. So, if a complication did occur in the Blomqvist 'overweight' group, one had to analyse this group in comparison with the 'normal weight' groups in the other studies. The range of BMIs in the studies selected was 18-46kg/m². None of the studies documented how many smokers were in each group or any other comorbidity, for example, diabetes. The mean sample number of patients was 212 with a range of 30 to 780 patients examined. Complication rates were for one patient and not for one breast. The type of pedicle used was clearly stated in four studies [9-12], but only one study documented the use of adrenaline since this was a study variable anyway [8]. Only two studies documented whether the same surgeon was used throughout [11, 12].

The mean weight of breast tissue resected from both breasts was 1236.4g (range 148-8132g). The percentage range of complications in each of the studies is shown in Table 4.

The follow-up time was only noted in two studies by Budny **(III/B)** and Wagner **(IIa/B)** [10, 11]. Unfortunately, not all the studies documented the percentage complication rate for normal weight, overweight and obese patients separately. So it was not possible to state whether a particular complication, for example, fat necrosis, occurred more frequently in patients with a higher BMI.

No studies documented whether blood transfusion was a complication or not and only two studies defined their complications explicitly. A minor complication was defined as one needing outpatient treatment. A major complication was defined as one needing an operation [10, 12]. As a result, the higher overall complication rates documented in some studies may reflect stricter and more meticulous reporting of any wound not perfectly healed at two weeks.

The Forest plot (Figure 1) shows on the x-axis, the increased odds of having a complication with an increase in BMI. Odds greater than 1.0 indicate that

Table 4. Complication rates for reduction mammaplasty. (Studies in italics were excluded).

Author	Delayed healing	Wound breakdown	Infection	Fat necrosis	Nipple loss	Haematoma	Seroma	DVT/ PE
Budny	56	44	8	12	8	0	-	0
Blomqvist	-	-	-	0.01	0.03	-	-	-
Zubowski	-	-	-	-	-	-	-	0.3
Wagner	-	3	-	-	-	2	38.2	-
Platt	-	-	-	-	-	-	-	-
Lahiri	8	0	6	2	2	3	1	-
Dabbah	-	10	-	-	4	-	1	-
Maxwell - Davis	19	-	-	12	6	18	-	-

there is an increased likelihood of a patient having a complication with an increase in BMI. The horizontal line illustrates the confidence interval.

All studies apart from Blomqvist showed that a BMI greater than 25.6 was associated with an increase in complications [9]. The Zubowski study only showed a small increase in the probability of a complication with increasing BMI [12] **(IIa/B)**. This study was of the highest quality with the most robust statistical analysis to justify its findings. There was no evidence to support the idea that the weight of tissue excised may be used to predict the postoperative complications in a patient undergoing reduction mammaplasty. The Wagner study found no significant link between an increased resection weight of breast tissue and an increase in fat necrosis or nipple death [11] **(IIa/B)**. This has been supported by the Zubowski study which found that although there was a slightly higher complication rate in patients who had undergone greater resections, this was not statistically significant [12]. This has been supported by the Blomqvist Study [9]. Budny *et al* found that as the weight of the tissue excised increased, there was an increase in complication rate [10] **(III/B)**. There was no evidence to inform us by what percentage the complication rate increased with each incremental increase in BMI or weight of tissue resected.

Budny *et al* found the BMI was the only factor predictive of postoperative complications using a robust statistical analysis. A BMI of 19-25kg/m^2 was associated with a 30% complication rate. This increased to 70% in patients with a BMI range of 26-30 and was over 80% in patients having a BMI greater than 31. Age, drain use, local anaesthetic infiltration, oral contraceptive pill use, prophylactic heparin, grade of surgeon, smoking status and technique of reduction were all shown to be insignificant [10].

In the Budny *et al* study, measures of outcome included both complications and the time to healing. This study had the most rigorous definition of a complication out of all the papers studied. When sought carefully, the complication rate seemed to be surprisingly high at nearly 60%. However, time to healing is not commonly referred to. The average for the Budny *et al* cohort was four and a half weeks, with a maximum of over four months. Most complications were minor and have been ignored in the other studies but, nevertheless, have considerable practical implications for the patient and those treating them. Major complications were acceptably low in number.

A systematic review with a meta-analysis looking at clinical outcomes of reduction mammaplasty by Chadbourne showed that "women undergoing reduction mammaplasty for breast hypertrophy had a significant improvement in pre-operative signs and symptoms, quality of life or both" [13] **(Ia/A)**. These findings have not been disputed by the studies analysed here. Although a patient may be obese, the evidence strongly suggests a clear physical and psychological benefit. A patient should not be refused a reduction mammaplasty solely on the basis of their BMI. The patient's BMI should be viewed in context with their other comorbidities and psychological status. The balance of factors can allow a more informed discussion and consent process. Health economists may press for cut-off levels for financial rather than clinical reasons.

Abdominoplasty and BMI

In 1890, Demars and Marx in France described the resection of a panniculus (abdominal dermolipectomy) with repair of large umbilical hernias. The technique of abdominoplasty was originally described by Kelly in 1899 who was working at The John Hopkins Hospital in North America. Kelly was the first to suggest the pannus to be "a storehouse of useless adipose tissue" and suggested the removal of the pannus for aesthetic reasons. Regnault, in 1975 **(III/B)**, described what we now know as abdominoplasty and the complications of abdominoplasty were first described by Grazer and Goldwyn in 1977 [14, 15] **(III/B)**. The study was based on a survey of the experiences of 958 surgeons, but did not consider BMI as a contributory factor.

BMI and complications following abdominoplasty

Vastine et al performed a retrospective case note study of 90 patients undergoing abdominoplasty, specifically focusing upon obesity [16]. Vastine et al did not use BMI to categorise their patients but recorded patient weight divided by height. Patients were divided into three different groups: the first group were obese, the second group borderline and the third group non-obese. The results showed that 80% of obese patients had complications compared with 33% in the borderline group and 32.5% in the non-obese group.

Rogliani *et al* performed a retrospective case note study of 80 consecutive abdominoplasties performed by one surgeon over a three-year period [17] **(III/B)**. The study was similar in methodology to the Vastine study, and compared patients in five categories. A normal range of BMI was $18.5\text{-}24.9\text{kg/m}^2$. Overweight patients had a BMI range of $25.0\text{-}29.9\text{kg/m}^2$. Obese class I patients had a BMI range of $30\text{-}34.9\text{kg/m}^2$, obese class II patients had a BMI range of $35\text{-}39.9\text{kg/m}^2$ and those in obese class III had a BMI greater than 40kg/m^2. No liposuction was performed with these abdominoplasties. A major complication was defined as one that resulted in death, required re-hospitalisation or surgical intervention, or resulted in the wound being dressed for more than six months. The obese population (class I, II and III) had a complication rate of 76% compared with 35% in normal weight and overweight groups. Within this 76% complication rate, the percentage complication rates for obesity classes I, II and III were 39%, 52.3% and 8.6%, respectively. Both these papers showed that there was a rise in seromas, haematomas, skin necrosis and wound breakdown in patients with a BMI equal to or greater than 30kg/m^2 [16, 17] **(III/B)**.

Level III/B evidence emerges from the Kim *et al* study regarding seroma formation in 39 patients of varying BMI undergoing abdominoplasty and 79 patients undergoing both abdominoplasty and liposuction [18] **(III/B)**. However, there is no evidence in the literature to suggest that seroma formation increases when liposuction is performed together with an abdominoplasty [19, 20]. Kim's definition of a seroma was a "clinically palpable subcutaneous collection of fluid that could be aspirated at least once". This study showed that patients with a BMI less than 25kg/m^2 had a seroma rate of 18.9%, while patients with a BMI greater than 25kg/m^2 had a seroma rate of 38.3% and those with a BMI range of $30\text{-}34.9\text{kg/m}^2$ or greater had a seroma rate of up to 50%. All other complications (haematoma, partial flap necrosis, wound dehiscence, suture granuloma and wound infection) were similar between the obese and non-obese groups. Kim *et al* concluded that there was a significantly higher risk for developing seromas postoperatively in overweight and obese patients undergoing abdominoplasty regardless of whether liposuction was used or not [18] **(III/B)**.

These slightly disparate findings concur with an earlier report by Chang et al [21] (II/B). This was the only prospective study comparing flap and donor-site complications of free transverse rectus abdominis myocutaneous (TRAM) flap breast reconstruction in non-obese and obese patients. The harvesting of the free TRAM flap incorporating an abdominoplasty technique showed that donor-site complications were significantly more common in obese patients (BMI greater than or equal to 30kg/m^2) than in normal weight patients (BMI less than 25kg/m^2). There was a significantly higher incidence of infection, seroma and hernia formation. However, no statistically significant difference was observed in the rates of abdominal flap necrosis, umbilical necrosis, haematoma or abdominal bulging. Chang supposed that obese patients developed increased abdominal pressure causing tension when closing the rectus fascia, often of poor quality. This may result in the abdominal fascia becoming thin and leading to an abdominal bulge. However, there is strong evidence by Al Basti et al that abdominoplasty does not cause significant changes in intra-abdominal pressure and intrathoracic pressure as measured using an intravesical catheter [22] (III/B).

Panniculus morbidus

In patients with a BMI greater than 40kg/m^2, an abdominal panniculus may be associated with poor hygiene, immobility, chronic back pain and chronic infection secondary to lymphoedema [23-25]. The panniculus may then become the cause of rashes, chronic ulcers, fistulae and poor genital hygiene [26]. In morbidly obese patients, the higher frequency of panniculectomy complication rates (78%) observed by Matory et al included increased blood loss, longer operative time, local tissue trauma from vigorous retraction, difficulty obliterating dead space, fat necrosis and an operation of greater technical difficulty. Matory also stated that anaesthetic complications such as associated cardiovascular disease, aspiration of secretions due to increased gastro-oesophageal reflux, respiratory problems during ventilation, decreased functional residual capacity, aspiration and air trapping lead to ventilation/perfusion mismatch. Consequently the operative mortality rate increases in the morbidly obese [23-25] (III/B). Undermining in thick fat leads to de-vascularisation of

Table 5. Summary of complication rates in abdominoplasty in patients with a BMI >30.

Author of paper	Year	Complication rate (%)
Vastine	1999	80
Rogliani	2006	76
Kim	2006	50
Chang	2000	39

lymphoedematous, ischaemic tissue resulting in infection and necrosis, initially in the fat on the under surface of the flap and later in the skin. Petty stated that the extent of fat necrosis always exceeded the visible extent of skin necrosis which eventually caused wound dehiscence. The incidence of seroma, haematoma, hernias, infection, deep vein thrombosis and blood loss were also reported as higher in the studies by Petty, Matory and Manahan (III/B).

In summary, an increase in complication rate from abdominoplasty has been associated with a BMI greater than 25kg/m^2 [16-18, 21, 23-25]. This complication rate is difficult to quantify with each incremental rise in BMI. In the obese population (BMI greater than 30kg/m^2), the complication rate was between 39.1-80%. An increase in mortality may also occur in morbidly obese patients (BMI greater than 40kg/m^2) (Table 5).

Free tissue transfer and BMI

Very little evidence is available on the effects of obesity on free tissue transfer. What evidence there is comes from the use of the transverse rectus abdominis musculocutaneous (TRAM) flap in breast reconstruction. Obesity was once thought to be an absolute contra-indication to free tissue transfer for breast reconstruction using the TRAM flap. This view was supported by papers from the late 1980s [27] (III/B). However, this view has now softened with the publication of level III/B retrospective studies, such as those from Moran et al, Berrino et al and Chang et al [21, 28, 29] (III/B).

Free TRAM flap complications in obese patients

All papers examining the specific effect of obesity on TRAM flap morbidity were from retrospective case note studies [21, 27-29]. These studies used similar methodologies in that patients were grouped according to their BMI into different categories of: normal weight (BMI <25kg/m^2), overweight (BMI 25-30kg/m^2, obese (BMI >30kg/m^2) and morbidly obese (BMI >40kg/m^2). The study by Kroll et al in the late 1980s demonstrated that patients undergoing free TRAM flap reconstruction with a BMI of less than 25kg/m^2, had complication rates of 15.4%. Complications included flap necrosis, hernia formation, deep vein thrombosis and infected Marlex® meshes. The observed incidence of complications increased to 31.4% in the obese group of patients and 41.7% in the morbidly obese.

The perceived detrimental effect of obesity upon free tissue transfer was challenged by Berrino et al in the early 1990s [29] (III/B). This study suggested that obesity without other comorbidities was not an absolute contraindication to free TRAM flap breast reconstruction, highlighting patient satisfaction with outcomes postoperatively. Results showed that the rate of flap fat necrosis, seroma formation and infection were more than twice that found in those patients with a normal BMI, but for donor-site complications (skin necrosis, umbilical necrosis, seromas and infection), the rates were similar (III/B).

Perhaps the most robust study of the effect of obesity on flap and donor-site complications in free TRAM breast reconstruction, was by Chang et al from the MD Anderson Cancer Centre [21] (II/B). This was a retrospective case note review of 958 patients. The patients were stratified according to their BMI as in previous studies. The complications were sub-divided into those relating to the flap and those relating to the donor site, and overweight and obese patients were compared with those of normal weight. Flap complications included flap loss, seroma formation, mastectomy flap necrosis and haematoma. In both the overweight and obese group of patients, there was a significant increase in flap-related complications compared with those patients of normal weight. In the overweight group this was 27.8% versus 20.4%, and

in the obese group this was 39.1% versus 20.4%. Donor-site complications included umbilical necrosis, infection, seroma, hernia formation and abdominal bulging. Overweight patients had a significantly higher incidence of donor-site complications compared with those of normal weight (23.4% versus 11.1%). Obese patients also had a significantly higher complication rate (19.8% versus 11.1%).

Pedicled TRAM flaps in obese patients

In a retrospective case note study, Moran compared complication rates in obese patients undergoing free and pedicled TRAM flap breast reconstructions with patients of normal weight requiring the same procedures (III/B). In obese patients, the incidence of pedicled flap loss was significantly higher as was the overall complication rate for both free and pedicled flaps. However, Moran et al stated that the BMI alone was not a significant predictor of complication in patients undergoing free TRAM flaps unless the patient was 50 years of age or older based on multivariate analysis of various factors (including age). There was no increase in donor-site morbidity associated with increasing BMI between the two groups but the risk of complications was related to the length of operation. Associated factors such as previous radiotherapy were shown not to be related to any increase in complication rate.

Comorbidities and anaesthetic complications

Wound infection and obesity

Retrospective case studies of median and transverse laparotomy wounds by Roberts et al, Garrow et al and Bates et al (IIa/B) have all shown BMI greater than 30kg/m^2 to be associated with increased wound infection rates [30-32] (II/B). The laparotomy wounds studied differ from abdominoplasty wounds since they did not involve extensive undermining of subcutaneous tissues and were either clean contaminated cases and contaminated or dirty cases invalidating any direct comparison with abdominoplasty wounds [30-32]. Level III/B studies of free TRAM flaps have revealed no

Chapter 4

evidence of increased wound infection in the abdominoplasty wound [28, 29] (III/B), although a more robust study by Chang *et al* showed that there was an increased incidence of infection in the abdominal wound donor site in patients with a BMI greater than 30kg/m^2 [21]. A prospective study of 2964 patients by Thomas *et al* also found that patients undergoing abdominal or gynaecological procedures had a significantly higher infection rate with a BMI greater than 30kg/m^2 compared with overweight or normal weight patients [33] **(IIa/B)**.

What other complications increase with an increase in BMI?

Left ventricular enlargement with systolic and diastolic dysfunction is increased in patients with a BMI greater than 30kg/m^2 [34] **(III/B)**. The risk of atrial fibrillation is increased by 50% and the development of ischaemic heart disease including hypertension, hyperlipidaemia and diabetes mellitus is also increased, but no specific value can be given. ß-blockade may decrease the risk of peri-operative ischaemia, infarction or arrhythmias in patients with coronary artery disease. Cardiac medications should be taken up to the day of surgery [34].

Obstructive sleep apnoea (OSA) has been shown to occur in up to 71% of morbidly obese patients. No correlation exists between BMI and the presence or severity of OSA [35]. The condition is associated with sudden death during sleep resulting from myocardial infarction or arrhythmias. A history of day-time somnolence, disturbance of their partner's sleep due to loud snoring, morning headaches, or frequent nocturnal awakening should be sought. These patients should be referred to a respiratory specialist for sleep polysymmography to confirm the diagnosis, demonstrating cessation of airflow during sleep associated with persistent respiratory efforts. Peri-operative use of continuous positive airway pressure (CPAP) has been shown to reduce hypercarbia, hypoxemia and pulmonary artery vasoconstriction decreasing the incidence of hypoxemic complications. Exertional dyspnoea may indicate pulmonary hypertension and the electrocardiogram (ECG) may show right axis deviation.

Deep vein thrombosis (DVT) and pulmonary embolism (PE) are more frequent in the obese population. Central obesity causing pressure on the inferior vena cava leads to venous stasis in the limbs and pelvis. Obesity is also associated with a hypercoaguable state due to increased levels of fibrinogen, Factor VIII and von Villebrand Factor. A clear association between venous stasis and the development of a PE was shown by Sapala *et al* [36] **(III/B)**. This study recommended that low-molecular-weight heparin administered before surgery may be of benefit and should be continued throughout hospitalisation.

Kranke *et al* conducted a systematic review of the relationship between postoperative nausea and vomiting and an increased BMI [37]. No evidence was found for a positive relationship between an increased BMI as a cause for increased postoperative nausea and vomiting.

An increased BMI (above 30kg/m^2) has been shown to decrease peri-operative lung volumes and increase ventilatory effort in patients undergoing reduction mammaplasty or abdominoplasty [38] **(III/B)**. A randomised controlled trial by Iwuagwu *et al* [39] demonstrated a statistically significant improvement in pulmonary function following reduction mammaplasty that correlated with the specimen weight resected **(IIa/B)**. This finding was also confirmed by a prospective study by Sood *et al* [40] **(IIa/B)**.

Surgery in the obese: financial implications

In a prospective study by Thomas *et al* [33] **(II/B)** of 2964 patients undergoing abdominal or gynaecological procedures with a two-day stay or more, an increased BMI was found to be associated with a significant increase in total costs. This relationship persisted even when patients who had complications were excluded from the study.

Conclusions

The evidence that high BMI causes increased complications in the areas reported comes from mainly level III/B and IIa/B evidence. There is still heterogeneity between the studies. However, recommendations have been based on variables reported in all the studies. Obesity is increasing. Plastic surgeons need evidence to inform overweight and obese patients of the complications that may occur with surgery. This may become more important with economical rationing of health care and rising medico-legal issues surrounding complication rates in overweight and obese patients.

Recommendations

	Evidence level
◆ An increase in BMI is associated with an increased complication rate post-reduction mammaplasty.	IIb/B, III/B
◆ Pulmonary function improves following bilateral reduction mammaplasty.	IV/C
◆ There is an increased risk of seroma formation and infection following abdominoplasty with an increase in BMI.	II/B
◆ Free tissue transfer based on evidence in TRAM flaps in patients with a BMI greater than 30kg/m² shows a clear increase in flap and donor-site mobidity. However, there is a higher flap loss in pedicled TRAMs in these patients.	II/B
◆ The risk of left ventricular enlargement, ischaemic heart disease, obstructive sleep apnoea and poor glycaemic control are greater in the obese patient.	III/B
◆ Surgery in obese patients is more expensive, regardless of whether complications occur.	II/B

Chapter 4

References

1. Rohrich RJ. Obesity in America: an increasing challenge for plastic surgeons. *Plast Reconstr Surg* 2004; 114(7): 1889-91.
2. The Newcastle-Ottawa Scale (NOS) for assessing the quality of non-randomised studies in meta-analyses. http://www.ncbi.nlm.nih.gov/books/bv.fcgi?indexed=google&rid=hstat1a.section.46863 (last accessed 24th October 2007).
3. Strombeck JO. Breast reconstruction. I. Reduction mammaplasty. *Mod Trends Plast Surg* 1964; 16: 237-55.
4. Commissioners of Plastic Surgery Services. www.wise.nhs.uk/sites/clinicalimprovcollab/surgery-plastic/Surgery%20Plastic%20Documents/1/Inclusion.pdf (last accessed 31st October 2007).
5. Lahiri A, Duff CG, Brown TL, Griffiths RW. Anthropometric measurements and their value in predicting complications following reduction mammaplasty and abdominoplasty. *Ann Plast Surg* 2006; 56(3): 248-50.
6. Cruz-Korchin N, Korchin L, Gonzalez-Keelan C, Climent C, Morales I. Macromastia: how much of it is fat? *Plast Reconstr Surg* 2002; 109(1): 64-8.
7. Lejour M. Evaluation of fat in breast tissue removed by vertical mammaplasty. *Plast Reconstr Surg* 1997; 99(2): 386-93.
8. Platt AJ, Mohan D, Baguley P. The effect of body mass index and wound irrigation on outcome after bilateral breast reduction. *Ann Plast Surg* 2003; 51(6): 552-5.
9. Blomqvist L. Reduction mammaplasty: analysis of patients' weight, resection weights, and late complications. *Scand J Plast Reconstr Surg Hand Surg* 1996; 30(3): 207-10.
10. Budny P, Vesly M, Coleman D. The effect of body weight and body mass index on outcome and complication rates in breast reduction surgery. British Association of Plastic Surgeons, Summer Meeting, Leicester, July 1996.
11. Wagner DS, Alfonso DR. The influence of obesity and volume of resection on success in reduction mammaplasty: an outcomes study. *Plast Reconstr Surg* 2005; 115(4): 1034-8.
12. Zubowski R, Zins JE, Foray-Kaplon A, Yetman RJ, Lucas AR, Papay FA, *et al*. Relationship of obesity and specimen weight to complications in reduction mammaplasty. *Plast Reconstr Surg* 2000; 106(5): 998-1003.
13. Chadbourne EB, Zhang S, Gordon MJ, Ro EY, Ross SD, Schnur PL, *et al*. Clinical outcomes in reduction mammaplasty: a systematic review and meta-analysis of published studies. *Mayo Clin Proc* 2001; 76(5): 503-10.
14. Regnault P. Brachioplasty, axilloplasty, and pre-axilloplasty. *Aesthetic Plast Surg* 1983; 7(1): 31-6.

Chapter 4

15. Grazer FM, Goldwyn RM. Abdominoplasty assessed by survey, with emphasis on complications. *Plast Reconstr Surg* 1977; 59(4): 513-7.

16. Vastine VL, Morgan RF, Williams GS, Gampper TJ, Drake DB, Knox LK, *et al*. Wound complications of abdominoplasty in obese patients. *Ann Plast Surg* 1999; 42(1): 34-9.

17. Rogliani M, Silvi E, Labardi L, Maggiulli F, Cervelli V. Obese and nonobese patients: complications of abdominoplasty. *Ann Plast Surg* 2006; 57(3): 336-8.

18. Kim J, Stevenson TR. Abdominoplasty, liposuction of the flanks, and obesity: analyzing risk factors for seroma formation. *Plast Reconstr Surg* 2006; 117(3): 773-9.

19. Dillerud E. Abdominoplasty combined with suction lipoplasty: a study of complications, revisions, and risk factors in 487 cases. *Ann Plast Surg* 1990; 25(5): 333-8.

20. Matarasso A. Liposuction as an adjunct to a full abdominoplasty. *Plast Reconstr Surg* 1995; 95(5): 829-36.

21. Chang DW, Wang B, Robb GL, Reece GP, Miller MJ, Evans GR, *et al*. Effect of obesity on flap and donor-site complications in free transverse rectus abdominis myocutaneous flap breast reconstruction. *Plast Reconstr Surg* 2000; 105(5): 1640-8.

22. Al-Basti HB, El-Khatib HA, Taha A, Sattar HA, Bener A. Intraabdominal pressure after full abdominoplasty in obese multiparous patients. *Plast Reconstr Surg* 2004; 113(7): 2145-50.

23. Matory WE, Jr., O'Sullivan J, Fudem G, Dunn R. Abdominal surgery in patients with severe morbid obesity. *Plast Reconstr Surg* 1994; 94(7): 976-87.

24. Petty P, Manson PN, Black R, Romano JJ, Sitzman J, Vogel J. *Panniculus morbidus*. *Ann Plast Surg* 1992; 28(5): 442-52.

25. Manahan MA, Shermak MA. Massive panniculectomy after massive weight loss. *Plast Reconstr Surg* 2006; 117(7): 2191-7.

26. Meyerowitz BR, Gruber RP, Laub DR. Massive abdominal panniculectomy. *JAMA* 1973; 225(4): 408-9.

27. Kroll SS, Netscher DT. Complications of TRAM flap breast reconstruction in obese patients. *Plast Reconstr Surg* 1989; 84(6): 886-92.

28. Moran SL, Serletti JM. Outcome comparison between free and pedicled TRAM flap breast reconstruction in the obese patient. *Plast Reconstr Surg* 2001; 108(7): 1954-60.

29. Berrino P, Campora E, Leone S, Zappi L, Nicosia F, Santi P. The transverse rectus abdominis musculocutaneous flap for breast reconstruction in obese patients. *Ann Plast Surg* 1991; 27(3): 221-31.

30. Garrow JS, Hastings EJ, Cox AG, North WR, Gibson M, Thomas TM, *et al*. Obesity and postoperative complications of abdominal operation. *Br Med J* 1988; 297(6642): 181.

31. Roberts JV, Bates T. The use of the Body Mass Index in studies of abdominal wound infection. *J Hosp Infect* 1992; 20(3): 217-20.

32. Bates T, Siller G, Crathern BC, Bradley SP, Zlotnik RD, Couch C, *et al*. Timing of prophylactic antibiotics in abdominal surgery: trial of a pre-operative versus an intra-operative first dose. *Br J Surg* 1989; 76(1): 52-6.

33. Thomas EJ, Goldman L, Mangione CM, Marcantonio ER, Cook EF, Ludwig L, *et al*. Body mass index as a correlate of postoperative complications and resource utilization. *Am J Med* 1997; 102(3): 277-83.

34. Wong CY, O'Moore-Sullivan T, Leano R, Hukins C, Jenkins C, Marwick TH. Association of subclinical right ventricular dysfunction with obesity. *J Am Coll Cardiol* 2006; 47(3): 611-6.

35. Frey WC, Pilcher J. Obstructive sleep-related breathing disorders in patients evaluated for bariatric surgery. *Obes Surg* 2003; 13(5): 676-83.

36. Sapala JA, Wood MH, Schuhknecht MP, Sapala MA. Fatal pulmonary embolism after bariatric operations for morbid obesity: a 24-year retrospective analysis. *Obes Surg* 2003; 13(6): 819-25.

37. Kranke P, Apefel CC, Papenfuss T, Rauch S, Lobmann U, Rubsam B, *et al*. An increased body mass index is no risk factor for postoperative nausea and vomiting. A systematic review and results of original data. *Acta Anaesthesiol Scand* 2001; 45(2): 160-6.

38. von Ungern-Sternberg BS, Regli A, Schneider MC, Kunz F, Reber A. Effect of obesity and site of surgery on perioperative lung volumes. *Br J Anaesth* 2004; 92(2): 202-7.

39. Iwuagwu OC, Platt AJ, Stanley PW, Hart NB, Drew PJ. Does reduction mammaplasty improve lung function test in women with macromastia? Results of a randomized controlled trial. *Plast Reconstr Surg* 2006; 118(1): 1-6.

40. Sood R, Mount DL, Coleman JJ, III, Ranieri J, Sauter S, Mathur P, *et al*. Effects of reduction mammaplasty on pulmonary function and symptoms of macromastia. *Plast Reconstr Surg* 2003; 111(2): 688-94.

41. Dabbah A, Lehman JA, Jr., Parker MG, Tantri D, Wagner DS. Reduction mammaplasty: an outcome analysis. *Ann Plast Surg* 1995; 35(4): 337-41.

Chapter 5

Prophylaxis to prevent venous thrombo-embolic disease in plastic surgery patients

James Seaward MRCS

Specialist Registrar, Plastic Surgery

Andrew Watts FRCS (Plast.)

Consultant Plastic and Hand Surgeon

ROYAL DEVON AND EXETER HOSPITAL, EXETER, UK

Introduction

In the UK, pulmonary embolism (PE) following deep vein thrombosis (DVT) in hospitalised patients causes between 25,000 and 32,000 deaths each year [1]. Collectively, PE and DVT are known as venous thrombo-embolism (VTE) and a clear link between the development of DVT and fatal PE has been established [2]. A variety of methods, both physical and pharmacological, have been shown to reduce the incidence of DVT in hospitalised patients. The Department of Health commissioned the National Institute for Health and Clinical Excellence to produce a set of guidelines for the use of these preventative measures in all hospital patients which was published in April 2007 [3].

Plastic surgery encompasses a heterogeneous group of patients and a wide variety of surgical procedures. The outcome of some of these procedures can be adversely affected by the increased haematoma risk of pharmacological thromboprophylaxis.

This chapter aims to review the criteria used for assessing the risk of VTE in plastic surgery patients and to examine the evidence for various regimes of thromboprophylaxis.

Methodology

A PubMed search was employed to gather evidence, using the search terms 'deep vein thrombosis', 'DVT', 'venous thrombo-embolism', 'VTE', 'pulmonary embolus', 'PE', 'prophylaxis', 'plastic surgery', 'cosmetic surgery', 'breast reconstruction', 'reduction mammoplasty', 'abdominoplasty' 'liposuction', 'face lift', 'rhytidectomy', 'head and neck surgery', in a variety of combinations. The evidence presented by the Scottish Intercollegiate Guidelines Network's (SIGN) national clinical guidelines (2002), "Prophylaxis of Venous Thromboembolism", the House of Commons Health Committee second report of session 2004-05, "The Prevention of Venous Thrombo-embolism in Hospitalised Patients" and the American College of Chest Physicians' (ACCP) "Sixth (2000) Guidelines for Antithrombotic Therapy for Prevention and Treatment of Thrombosis", were studied in detail.

patients in either group received any pharmacological thromboprophylaxis, but the incidence of 1.7% in the combined group compared favourably with the incidence of PE reported for gynaecological pelvic surgery alone [26]. A third cohort of 216 patients underwent abdominoplasty in conjunction with one or more, non-abdominal aesthetic procedures such as reduction mammoplasty, augmentation mammoplasty and face lift, with a PE incidence of 0.93% and no fatalities. The authors note that five out of the six patients who suffered a PE were obese and that this may have played a significant role.

In a more recent study, Stevens *et al* analysed the complication rates from 415 sequential abdominoplasty procedures performed by one surgeon over a period of 15 years [27]. In 264 patients, the abdominoplasty was carried out alone and in the remaining 151 it was performed in conjunction with a range of other aesthetic breast surgery procedures. Most patients had a BMI of less than 30 and in all cases patients were treated with compression stockings and early ambulation. There were no cases of DVT or PE, although this outcome was assessed by clinical examination alone.

In 2001, Hughes reported on a national American survey sent to all 1432 active members of ASAPS to assess the complication and mortality rate of liposuction procedures carried out between 1998 and 2000 [28]. Fifty-three percent of the surgeons responded and provided details for 94,159 liposuction procedures. Of these procedures, 66% were liposuction alone, 20% were liposuction with one or more other procedures and 14% involved liposuction with abdominoplasty. The mortality rate of the cohort who underwent liposuction with abdominoplasty was 0.0305% or one per 3,281 procedures. This figure was higher than liposuction alone (0.0021%) or even liposuction together with other procedures, excluding abdominoplasty (0.0137%).

However, the mortality rate for the liposuction combined with abdominoplasty group was lower than that for a group of 26,562 patients studied by Teimourian and Rogers in 1989 who underwent abdominoplasty alone [29]. The mortality rate in this group was 0.0414% or one per 2,415. Sixty percent

of the deaths were due to PE. Unfortunately, the number of fatal PEs is not recorded in Hughes' survey, so it is not possible to compare the figures.

Liposuction (III/B)

VTE mortality associated with liposuction has been reported. Rao *et al* identified five deaths following tumescent liposuction in the City of New York between 1993 and 1998 [30]. Of these, one patient had a fatal PE and calf DVT after tumescent liposuction to the legs.

In 1999, Albin and de Campo reported a series of 181 patients who underwent large-volume liposuction with aspirates of greater than five litres [31]. Of these, 31 patients had tumescent liposuction alone and 150 patients had a combination of tumescent liposuction and ultrasonic liposuction. One patient (0.5%) suffered a DVT and two patients (1.1%) suffered PEs. There were no deaths in the series.

In 2001, the American national survey carried out by Hughes reported on 94,159 liposuction procedures [28]. The overall incidence of DVT was 0.0329% (31 cases) and the overall incidence of non-fatal PE was 0.0266% (25 cases). Unfortunately, there were no details in this survey of the provision of thromboprophylaxis or of other risk factors for VTE. The overall mortality rate for the patients who underwent liposuction alone was 0.0021% (one per 47,415 procedures) and the mortality rate for liposuction carried out with other procedures, excluding abdominoplasty, was 0.0137% (one per 7,314 procedures). Unfortunately, the cause of mortality was not defined and it is not possible to determine how many were due to fatal PE. In the previous survey, covering 1994 to 1998, 95 mortalities were identified in 496,245 liposuction procedures (0.019%) [32]. In this study PE was the single largest cause of mortality accounting for 23% of all deaths or a mortality rate of 0.0046% (one per 21,739 procedures).

Face lift (III/B)

Reinisch *et al* carried out a survey of one third of the randomly selected active members of ASAPS to assess the rate of VTE following face lift procedures over a 12-month period [33]. Two hundred and seventy-three surgeons responded reporting on a total of 9,937 face lift procedures. VTE was only recorded if there was diagnostic proof in the form of either a positive duplex scan, venogram, VQ scan or pulmonary angiogram along with positive clinical findings. DVTs were not recorded separately if the patient also suffered a PE. Sixty-one percent of surgeons used no prophylaxis against VTE, 20% used intermittent compression devices and 20% used compression stockings. Overall, the incidence of DVT was 0.35% and the incidence of non-fatal PE was 0.14%, with one mortality from PE. Only 43.5% of the patients underwent surgery under general anaesthetic, but 83.7% of VTE occurred in this group. Of the patients who developed VTE, 4.1% had received thromboprophylaxis with intermittent compression devices, 36.7% with compression stockings and 59% had no prophylaxis. The use of intermittent compression devices was associated with a reduced rate of PE (p=0.001), whereas the use of compression stockings alone made no significant difference to PE rate.

Concern has been expressed about the use of pharmacological prophylaxis against VTE in face lift patients. The peri-operative use of low-molecular-weight heparin (LMWH) is associated with an increased incidence of postoperative bleeding. Durnig and Jungwirth reported on a group of 126 patients who took part in a retrospective, controlled trial to assess the effect of LMWH on bleeding post-face lift surgery [34]. All patients were treated by the same surgeon under intravenous sedation with compression stockings and were mobilised postoperatively on the day of surgery. Two cohorts were studied. Thirty-seven patients received LMWH two hours before the procedure and then consecutively every 24 hours until hospital discharge. No pharmacological prophylaxis was used in 89 patients. The authors reported that the incidence of postoperative bleeding requiring re-operation was 16.2% in the LMWH group, compared with 1.1% in the control group (p<0.003). There were no cases of DVT or PE in either group. These figures can be compared with a haematoma rate of 4.4% in a large study of 12,325 face-lift patients reported by Matarasso et al in 2000 [35].

Breast reconstruction (IV/C)

There is limited information in the literature regarding VTE following breast reconstruction. Erdmann et al reported a series of 76 consecutive patients who underwent delayed unipedicled TRAM flap reconstruction over a five-year period [36]. One patient suffered a DVT (an incidence of 1.3%) and there were no reported cases of PE. The authors did not indicate whether thromboprophylaxis was used with these patients.

Cosmetic breast surgery (IV/C)

There were no cases of VTE in a series of 151 patients reported by Stevens et al who underwent a variety of cosmetic breast operations in conjunction with an abdominoplasty [27]. Of these patients, 50 patients underwent a breast augmentation, 31 patients underwent a reduction mammoplasty, 28 underwent a mastopexy and 42 patients underwent simultaneous mastopexy and breast augmentation.

Head and neck surgery (III/B)

In a retrospective analysis of 12,805 ENT procedures, 34 patients were identified with postoperative VTE [37]. The incidence of DVT among patients who had undergone elective head and neck surgery was 0.6% and the incidence of PE was 0.4%. The incidence of fatal PEs in the head and neck surgery group was 0.06%. Of the patients who developed a DVT, 35% received no thromboprophylaxis and the remainder received a combination of compression stockings and an intermittent pneumatic compression (IPC) device. This group of patients was compared with a similar control group who had not suffered a VTE. Age and the use of an IPC were the only two factors found to be statistically significant in either increasing or reducing the chances of developing a DVT or PE.

A survey of UK consultant otolaryngologists published in 1997 indicated that only 43% of surgeons who treated head and neck cancer patients routinely used DVT prophylaxis [38].

Chapter 5

Table 2. The evidence for VTE rates in plastic surgery.

Operation type	DVT	PE	Fatal PE	Diagnosis type	Evidence level
Abdominoplasty	0.39%	0.28%	0.05%	Image if suspicious	III/B
Liposuction	0.03%	0.03%	0.002%	Image if suspicious	III/B
Face lift	0.35%	0.14%	0.01%	Image if suspicious	III/B
Breast reconstruction	1.3%	0%	0%	Image if suspicious	IV/C
Cosmetic breast	0%	0%	0%	Image if suspicious	IV/C
Head and neck	0.6%	0.4%	0.06%	Image if suspicious	III/B

Summary

In comparison with orthopaedic and general surgery, the rates of VTE in plastic surgery patients are quite modest (Table 2). Elective hip replacement has an incidence of pulmonary embolus of 2-3% and hip fracture fixation of 4-7% [39]. General surgical procedures, including cancer resections, have a reported incidence of pulmonary embolus of 0.1-0.8%, and this incidence rises to 3.5% in obese patients, even with prophylaxis [40].

DVT prophylaxis

Mechanical methods of DVT prophylaxis

Elastic stockings (Ia/A)

Elastic stockings provide a relatively constant positive pressure to the lower extremity, which acts to reduce venous pooling and increase venous return. Studies on the effectiveness of elastic stockings tend to exclude high-risk patients. Nevertheless, a meta-analysis of 12 controlled studies demonstrated a significant risk reduction (68%) for developing VTE with elastic compression stocking use [41].

There is also evidence to show the benefit of elastic stockings together with other VTE prophylaxis. A randomised trial of 176 patients undergoing major abdominal surgery, comparing the combination of compression stockings with low-dose heparin against low-dose heparin alone, demonstrated that the combination of both methods reduced VTE incidence from 12% to 2%. All patients were screened with the ^{125}I fibrinogen uptake test and VTE was confirmed with either venography or ventilation/perfusion scintigraphy [42].

Intermittent pneumatic compression devices (Ib/A)

Intermittent pneumatic compression (IPC) devices decrease venous stasis, improve the velocity of venous return and induce the fibrinolytic activity of veins [43-45]. There is also evidence that they can stimulate the release of an antiplatelet aggregation factor from vascular endothelial cells [46].

The effectiveness of IPCs to reduce the risk of DVT formation compares well with pharmacological agents. Harris *et al* compared the prophylactic efficacy of aspirin, dextran, heparin and IPCs in patients undergoing THR [47]. The authors reported that the IPC device was associated with the lowest rate of postoperative DVT. The plantar compression device has been shown to be equally effective compared with knee or thigh-length devices at decreasing the risk of

DVT in the postoperative period [48, 49]. Complications of thromboprophylaxis, such as bleeding, are also reduced with IPC, although poor patient compliance may prevent their effective use.

Although the overall rate of DVT is lowest with IPC, this may lead to a false sense of security. A prospective study of 425 patients undergoing elective orthopaedic surgery with a combination of IPC and elastic stockings demonstrated that while the incidence of postoperative distal thrombus was low (0.8%), the rate of the more dangerous proximal thrombus remained considerable (3.8%). All DVTs in this study were asymptomatic and diagnosed by routine ultrasound at six days [50].

Pharmacological methods of DVT prophylaxis

Antiplatelet drugs

Aspirin
Aspirin acts on the cyclo-oxygenase pathway, irreversibly inhibiting the synthesis of thromboxane A2. Because platelets are unable to regenerate cyclo-oxygenase, the effect of aspirin is as long as the lifespan of the platelet, approximately ten days. Doses of aspirin in clinical trials have ranged from 50-1200mg/day with no significant difference in effectiveness [51].

Dipyridamole
Dipyridamole acts to increase intracellular cyclic AMP both by inhibiting adenosine uptake into the cells, which stimulates platelet adenylate cyclase, and by inhibiting phosphodiesterase, preventing the inactivation of intra-platelet cyclic AMP. This inhibits platelet aggregation and adhesion. It is relatively short acting with a half-life of 40 minutes, so most preparations are slow-release formulations [51].

Clopidogrel
Clopidogrel prevents ADP binding at its receptor site, leading to the inhibition of ADP-mediated platelet aggregation. Although the elimination half-life of clopidogrel is eight hours, its effects are irreversible for the life of the platelet, approximately ten days.

Evidence for antiplatelet thromboprophylaxis (Ia/A)
A meta-analysis of 53 randomised controlled trials of antiplatelet prophylaxis comprising a total of 8400 surgical patients, the Antiplatelet Trialists' Collaboration, demonstrated a highly significant (p<0.00001) reduction in DVT rate as detected by ^{125}I-fibrinogen scanning or venography from 35% to 26%. PE rate was reduced from 1.8% to 0.7% and fatal PE rate from 0.9% to 0.2% [52].

A multi-national randomised controlled trial investigating thrombo-prophylaxis with 160mg/day aspirin in 17,444 surgical patients, the Pulmonary Embolism Prevention Trial, demonstrated a significant reduction in clinically detected and radiologically confirmed DVT and PE rate from 2.5% to 1.6% (p<0.0003). The rate of fatal PEs was reduced from 0.5% to 0.2% (p<0.02) [53].

Anticoagulants

Warfarin
Coumarins, of which warfarin is the most popular in the UK, are oral anticoagulants acting as antagonists to Vitamin K. Vitamin K is a co-factor for synthesis of clotting Factors II, VII, IX and X. Warfarin is rapidly absorbed from the GI tract and binds to plasma proteins. Despite its rapid absorption and high bioavailability, up to 72 hours are required to provide a stable level of anticoagulation, due to the long half-life of Factor II. Response to dose is influenced by a wide variety of genetic, environmental and pharmacological factors, requiring repeated measurement of the international normalised ratio (INR) to determine adequate anticoagulant effect.

Unfractionated heparin
Unfractionated heparin (UFH) binds to anti-thrombin III causing a conformational change, the result of which is to markedly enhance inactivation of thrombin (Factor IIa) and Factors IXa, Xa and XIIa. Heparin is a heterogenous mixture of polysaccharides with an average molecular weight of 15,000 Da (3,000-30,000). It is administered either intravenously or subcutaneously and has a short half-life due to rapid liver metabolism. Oral administration is ineffective due to the high first-pass metabolism. The half-life of intravenous heparin is 30 minutes, requiring

Prophylaxis to prevent venous thrombo-
embolic disease in plastic surgery patients

constant infusions for stable anticoagulation. Even when administered subcutaneously, the half-life is 1.5 hours. Due to the short half-life and unpredictable pharmacokinetics of intravenous heparin, regular monitoring of the activated partial thromboplastin time (APTT) is essential to ensure adequate anticoagulant effect.

Low-molecular-weight heparin

Low-molecular-weight heparin (LMWH) is a selection of the lower-molecular-weight (4,000-6,000 Da) polysaccharides from unfractionated heparin. LMWH has a more specific mechanism of action than UFH, inactivating mainly Factor Xa. As thrombin is relatively unaffected by LMWH, the APTT is not significantly prolonged. The lighter molecules are more homogenous and less likely to bind to plasma proteins, resulting in more predictable pharmacokinetics and less variation of effect between individuals. This allows body-weight-based dosing without monitoring. Given subcutaneously, the smaller molecules of LMWH have a higher bioavailability (>90%) than UFH (30%) and a longer half-life (four hours), enabling once daily dosing.

New thromboprophylactic agents are constantly being developed. Direct thrombin inhibitors are a relatively new class of prophylactic agent, with a limited role at present. They may be useful to consider when heparin cannot be given, such as after heparin-induced thrombocytopaenia.

Evidence for anticoagulant thromboprophylaxis (Ia/A)

A meta-analysis of the effectiveness of low-dose heparin in over 8,000 general surgical patients was undertaken by Clagett and Reisch [54]. Control patients were given no thromboprophylaxis and DVT was identified on a positive fibrinogen uptake test. The control group had a DVT rate of 25.2%, a proximal DVT rate of 6.4%, a PE rate of 1.2% and a fatal PE rate of 0.71%. Patients given subcutaneous heparin 5,000 i.u. twice or three times per day had a DVT rate of 8.7%, a proximal DVT rate of 1.4%, a PE rate of 0.52% and a fatal PE rate of 0.21%. These were all statistically significant. Wound haematoma rate increased from 2.3% in the control group to 8.0% (p<0.01).

There is little evidence comparing LMWH against no thromboprophylaxis. However, a meta-analysis of 36 double-blind randomised controlled trials comparing LMWH with UFH in 16,583 surgical patients was undertaken by Koch et al [55]. In all surgical groups, subcutaneous UFH yielded 2.2% distal DVT, 1.5% proximal DVT and 1.2% PE. LMWH prophylaxis resulted in 2.6% distal DVT, 1.1% proximal DVT and 0.8% PE. Wound haematoma rates varied depending on the dose of LMWH: <3400 i.u. LMWH resulted in 4% of patients developing haematoma and 0.9% requiring a return to theatre, whereas >3400 i.u. LMWH resulted in 6.4% of patients developing haematoma and 1.8% requiring a return to theatre.

UFH demonstrated rates between the two doses of LMWH, with 5.3% developing haematoma and 1.2% requiring further surgery. The difference in VTE rates between LMWH and UFH was particularly noticeable in orthopaedic surgery, with UFH prophylaxis resulting in distal DVT, proximal DVT and PE rates of 15.8%, 21.2% and 10.6%, respectively, whereas LMWH prophylaxis resulted in 17.8%, 10.9% and 7.5%. The reduction in the more dangerous proximal DVT rate was statistically significant (p<0.002).

A randomised controlled trial of 145 surgical patients treated with a coumarin, with subcutaneous heparin or with placebo was performed by Taberner et al [56]. All patients were screened for DVT with the ^{125}I-fibrinogen uptake scan. DVT rate in the control group was 23%. Both the coumarin and heparin groups had DVT rates of 6% (p<0.05). There was no significant difference in either the DVT rate or haematoma rate between the two treatment groups.

Guidelines for DVT prophylaxis in plastic surgery

Davison et al devised a scoring system of risk factors for plastic surgery patients based on the 2001 ACCP risk factor assessment guidelines [57]. Factors are considered as predisposing or exposing and each carries a weighting, the sum of which is used to assign a risk category, as illustrated in Table 3. The 7th ACCP conference recommendations for general surgery patients in each risk category is presented in Table 4 [58].

Table 3. VTE risk factor scores and risk categories.

Predisposing factors	Exposing factors
Age 40-60 (1)	Minor surgery (1)
Pregnancy or <1 month post-partum (1)	Major surgery (2)
Obesity >120% ideal weight (1)	Immobilising plaster cast (2)
Oral contraceptive or hormone replacement therapy (1)	Bedrest >72h (2)
Age >60 (2)	Central venous access (2)
Malignancy (2)	Free flap surgery (3)
History of VTE (3)	Previous MI (3)
Genetic hypercoagulable disorders (3)	Congestive cardiac failure (3)
Lupus anticoagulant (3)	Severe sepsis (3)
Antiphospholipid antibodies (3)	Hip, pelvis or leg fracture (5)
Myeloproliferative disorders (3)	Stroke (5)
Heparin-induced thrombocytopaenia (3)	Multiple trauma (5)
Hyperviscosity (3)	Acute spinal cord injury (5)
Homocystinaemia (3)	

Total score	Risk category
1	Low risk
2	Moderate risk
3-4	Higher risk
>4	High risk

Table 4. Current ACCP recommendations for each risk category.

Low-risk category Recommendation Grade B	Early ambulation No pharmacological prophylaxis
Moderate-risk category Recommendation Grade A	Low-molecular-weight heparin (LMWH) 2500 i.u. daily OR 5000 i.u. s/c heparin every 12 hours
Higher-risk category Recommendation Grade A	Low-molecular-weight heparin 3500 i.u. daily OR 5000 i.u. s/c heparin every 8 hours
High-risk category Recommendation Grade B	Low-molecular-weight heparin 3500 i.u. daily COMBINED WITH intermittent pneumatic compression (IPC) OR 5000 i.u. s/c heparin every 8 hours COMBINED WITH intermittent pneumatic compression
General recommendations	Elastic stockings can be used as an adjunct to the above recommendations Patients at high risk of bleeding should use graduated compression stockings (GCS) or IPC until bleeding risk has subsided

Chapter 5

Chapter 5

35. Matarasso A, Elkwood A, Rankin M, Elkowitz M. National plastic surgery survey: face lift techniques and complications. *Plast Reconstr Surg* 2000; 106(5): 1185-95; discussion 1196.

36. Erdmann D, Sundin BM, Moquin KJ, Young H, Georgiade GS. Delay in unipedicled TRAM flap reconstruction of the breast: a review of 76 consecutive cases. *Plast Reconstr Surg* 2002; 110(3): 762-7.

37. Moreano EH, Hutchison JL, McCulloch TM, Graham SM, Funk GF, Hoffman HT. Incidence of deep venous thrombosis and pulmonary embolism in otolaryngology-head and neck surgery. *Otolaryngol Head Neck Surg* 1998; 118(6): 777-84.

38. Ah-See KW, Kerr J, Sim DW. Prophylaxis for venous thromboembolism in head and neck surgery: the practice of otolaryngologists. *J Laryngol Otol* 1997; 111(9): 845-9.

39. McDevitt NB. Deep vein thrombosis prophylaxis. American Society of Plastic and Reconstructive Surgeons. *Plast Reconstr Surg* 1999; 104(6): 1923-8.

40. Most D, Kozlow J, Heller J, Shermak MA. Thromboembolism in plastic surgery. *Plast Reconstr Surg* 2005; 115(2): 20e-30.

41. Wells PS, Lensing AW, Hirsh J. Graduated compression stockings in the prevention of postoperative venous thromboembolism. A meta-analysis. *Arch Int Med* 1994; 10; 154(1): 67-72.

42. Wille-Jorgensen P, Thorup J, Fischer A, Holst-Christensen J, Flamsholt R. Heparin with and without graded compression stockings in the prevention of thromboembolic complications of major abdominal surgery: a randomized trial. *Br J Surg* 1985; 72(7): 579-81.

43. Jacobs DG, Piotrowski JJ, Hoppensteadt DA, Salvator AE, Fareed J. Hemodynamic and fibrinolytic consequences of intermittent pneumatic compression: preliminary results. *J Trauma* 1996; 40(5): 710-6; discussion 716-7.

44. Janssen H, Trevino C, Williams D. Hemodynamic alterations in venous blood flow produced by external pneumatic compression. *J Cardiovasc Surg* 1993; 34(5): 441-7.

45. Kosir MA, Schmittinger L, Barno-Winarski L, *et al.* Prospective double-arm study of fibrinolysis in surgical patients. *J Surg Research* 1998; 74(1): 96-101.

46. Gertler JP, Abbott WM. Prothrombotic and fibrinolytic function of normal and perturbed endothelium. *J Surg Research* 1992; 52(1): 89-95.

47. Harris WH, Athanasoulis CA, Waltman AC, Salzman EW. Prophylaxis of deep vein thrombosis after total hip replacement. Dextran and external pneumatic compression compared with 1.2 or 0.3 gram of aspirin daily. *J Bone Joint Surg Am* 1985; 67(1): 57-62.

48. Few JW, Marcus JR, Placik OJ. Deep vein thrombosis prophylaxis in the moderate- to high-risk patient undergoing lower extremity liposuction. *Plast Reconstr Surg* 1999; 104(1): 309-10.

49. Stannard JP, Harris RM, Bucknell AL, Cossi A, Ward J, Arrington ED. Prophylaxis of deep venous thrombosis after total hip arthroplasty by using intermittent compression of the plantar venous plexus. *Am J Orthop* (Belle Mead, NJ 1996; 25(2): 127-34.

50. Hooker JA, Lachiewicz PF, Kelley SS. Efficacy of prophylaxis against thromboembolism with intermittent pneumatic compression after primary and revision total hip arthroplasty. *J Bone Joint Surg Am* 1999; 81(5): 690-6.

51. Blann AD, Landray MJ, Lip GY. ABC of antithrombotic therapy: an overview of antithrombotic therapy. *Br Med J* (Clinical Research ed) 2002; 325(7367): 762-5.

52. Antiplatelet Trialists' Collaboration. Collaborative overview of randomised trials of antiplatelet therapy - III: Reduction in venous thrombosis and pulmonary embolism by antiplatelet prophylaxis among surgical and medical patients. *Br Med J* (Clinical Research ed) 1994; 308(6923): 235-46.

53. Prevention of pulmonary embolism and deep vein thrombosis with low dose aspirin: Pulmonary Embolism Prevention (PEP) trial. *Lancet* 2000; 355(9212): 1295-302.

54. Clagett GP, Reisch JS. Prevention of venous thromboembolism in general surgical patients. Results of meta-analysis. *Ann Surg* 1988; 208(2): 227-40.

55. Koch A, Ziegler S, Breitschwerdt H, Victor N. Low molecular weight heparin and unfractionated heparin in thrombosis prophylaxis: meta-analysis based on original patient data. *Thrombosis Research* 2001; 102(4): 295-309.

56. Taberner DA, Poller L, Burslem RW, Jones JB. Oral anticoagulants controlled by the British comparative thromboplastin versus low-dose heparin in prophylaxis of deep vein thrombosis. *Br Med J* 1978; 1(6108): 272-4.

57. Davison SP, Venturi ML, Attinger CE, Baker SB, Spear SL. Prevention of venous thromboembolism in the plastic surgery patient. *Plast Reconstr Surg* 2004; 114(3): 43E-51.

58. Proceedings of the seventh ACCP conference on antithrombotic and thrombolytic therapy: evidence-based guidelines. *Chest* 2004; 126(3 Suppl): 172S-696.

Chapter 6

Physiological responses to burn injury and resuscitation protocols for adult major burns

Rob Duncan MB BCh MRCS (Ed)

Burns Research Registrar

Ken Dunn BSc FRCS (Plast.)

Consultant Burns and Plastic Surgeon

WYTHENSHAWE HOSPITAL, MANCHESTER, UK

Introduction

There are approximately 13,000 burn injury admissions per year in the UK, with an overall mortality rate of 2.3%. Approximately 1000 of these admissions are for burns that require fluid resuscitation, half of which are in children [1] **(IV/C)**, in whom mortality is highest.

There are a series of inter-related, complex physiological responses to a major burn injury, which impact upon the function of all organ systems. Major fluid shifts occur between compartments, giving rise to hypovolaemia; large amounts of protein are lost in oedema/exudates and many toxic metabolites, oxidants and inflammatory mediators enter the circulation. The cardiovascular sequellae include hypovolaemia and myocardial depression, at a time when an elevated cardiac output is required. Therefore, intravascular volume must be appropriately supported.

The discovery of the importance of fluid therapy in burn care dates back to 1832, when Baron Dupuytren drew parallels between post mortem findings in fatal burns and cholera (in which O'Shaugnessy had reported successful treatment with intravenous saline). Both conditions shared the findings of congested organs and a high haematocrit [2] **(IV/C)**.

The concept of post-burns hypovolaemic shock appears to have developed towards the end of the 19th century [3] **(IV/C)**, by Neiss (1880), Brown (1896), Tommasoli (1897) and Parascandolo (1901). In 1905, Sneve identified four major determinants of outcome in burns patients, and introduced xenografting [4]. Over the latter half of the 20th century, it was discovered that mortality may be significantly reduced by the rapid delivery of appropriate fluid resuscitation and improvements in wound management.

In the present day, patients with superficial dermal burns or deeper, covering 15% or more of their total body surface area (TBSA) (10% for children), are generally given intravenous resuscitation fluids to replace rapid fluid losses from the circulation. Various regimes are employed and much debate persists as to which is the best, both in terms of infusion rates at different post-burn periods, overall infusion volumes, type of fluid, monitoring techniques and resuscitation goals. There is general acceptance that either too little in an emergency when no venous access can be obtained, the intra-osseous route may be employed.

What size of burn requires fluid resuscitation?

The body has a tremendous capacity to compensate for hypovolaemia. It does so by vasoconstriction, increasing myocardial contractility and heart rate, retaining salt and water, inducing thirst and diverting blood flow to preserve critical organs. Many of the sequellae of large burns impair these compensatory mechanisms. Mediators released following a burn injury induce local vasodilatation and cause myocardial contractile dysfunction [14] **(Ib/A)** Animal and slow isovolaemic diastolic relaxation [15] **(Ib/A)** Animal. The larger and deeper the burn injury, the more profound the fluid loss and the more compromised the endogenous compensatory mechanisms.

Fluid resuscitation should be instituted for any patient considered unlikely to be able to maintain an adequate circulation through oral hydration alone. This depends upon many factors, including injury severity, conscious level, cognition, mobility, age, comorbidities and presence of nausea or vomiting.

By convention, adults with burns covering ≥15% of their skin surface area receive fluid resuscitation, 10% in children. This difference is in part due to the significant differences in body surface area to weight ratios between adults and children. Oedema formation and fluid losses are consequently proportionately greater. Children also have a lesser capacity to compensate for hypovolaemia.

Elderly patients with burns of less than 15% may also require intravenous fluid, as they also exhibit an impaired capacity to compensate for hypovolaemia and are more vulnerable to acute renal failure with any reduction of renal perfusion pressures [16] **(III/B)**.

As understanding of the physiological response to major burn injury increases and more therapeutic opportunities become available (e.g. anti-oxidants, inhibition of inflammatory mediators, immuno-modulation), the size of injury treated by intravenous fluid resuscitation may change.

When should resuscitation fluids be given?

Following burn injury, intravascular fluid volume is lost primarily as oedema. Underhill made the first attempts to temporally quantify volume depletion following burn injury, through measurements of haematocrit, haemoglobin and chloride in blood and burn blister fluid in 1921 [17]. Losses occur very quickly, and if the burn is of a sufficient size, this leads rapidly to hypovolaemic shock, unless fluid losses are expeditiously replaced. Oedema develops more rapidly in partial-thickness burns [11] **(IIb/B)** Animal compared with deeper burns [18] **(Ib/A)** Animal (maximum oedema formation 12h vs. 18h), reflecting greater preservation of vascularity in partial-thickness injuries.

With the increasing passage of time following injury, worsening hypovolaemia results in tissue hypoperfusion. If fluid resuscitation is delayed, tissues suffer a reperfusion-type injury [19] **(Ib/A)** Animal. Reperfusion of hypoxic tissues is believed to generate oxidants by elevating the activity of xanthine oxidase [20] **(Ib/A)** Animal. Oxidants indiscriminately damage cells and macromolecules, including the matrix proteins of the interstitium. This damage leads to cellular dysfunction, capillary leakage, increased interstitial space compliance and macromolecular fragmentation, generating osmotically active particles within the interstitium [21] **(IV/C)**. A healthy adult's interstitium usually occupies a volume of approximately 8L, and accounts for around 10% of the body weight. Following a major burn, this can increase many times due to loss of structural integrity and oedema formation.

Hypoperfusion-related hypoxia can induce apoptosis in certain cells (e.g. myocardium, enterocytes) [22] **(Ib/A)** Animal. This can lead to increased bacterial and endotoxin translocation from the gut (believed to underlie development of multi-organ dysfunction syndrome [MODS]). Evidence from animal studies show that apoptosis may be prevented (or at least attenuated) by prompt administration of fluid resuscitation [23] **(Ib/A)** Animal. Avoidance of significant metabolic lactic acidosis (a sequellae of hypoperfusion) by provision of adequate fluid resuscitation has been demonstrated to reduce both mortality and organ failure rate [24] **(IIb/B)**.

Ninety percent of maximal oedema formation within burned tissue occurs by four hours following a partial-thickness burn [11]. Fluid resuscitation should therefore be started as soon as possible after injury, to avoid hypovolaemia and the secondary injuries resulting from hypoxia, oxidant generation and inducement of apoptosis resulting from delayed resuscitation.

Fluid volume requirements

Numerous factors influence fluid requirements following a major burn including: injury size, depth, distribution, aetiology, patient weight, body habitus, age, comorbidities, pre-morbid hydration, concomitant injuries, type of dressings, body temperature, room temperature, humidity and altitude. Below, we consider the factors influencing fluid requirements in terms of fluid lost in the generation of oedema (in both burned and unburned tissues), insensible losses, as a result of the magnitude of the inflammatory response, variations according to the type of fluid administered and also individual clinician factors.

Oedema formation (Figures 1 and 2)

Oedema formation is primarily governed by the forces outlined by Starling [25], some of which can be defined by the following equation:

$$Q_f \propto (P_c - P_i) - \delta(\pi_c - \pi_i)$$

Where: Q_f = transcapillary fluid flux; P_c = capillary hydrostatic pressure; P_i = interstitial hydrostatic pressure; $(P_c - P_i)$ = hydrostatic pressure gradient; δ = osmotic reflection coefficient; π_c = capillary oncotic pressure; π_i = interstitial oncotic pressure; $(\pi_c - \pi_i)$ = oncotic pressure gradient

The volume and rate of interstitial oedema formation is also influenced by tissue vascularity, interstitial compliance, rate of oedema fluid removal (i.e. density of patent lymphatics and lymph flow rate) and cellular resting membrane potential.

From the above equation, we can predict that mechanical ventilation will increase fluid loss from the capillaries. Upon the change from negative pressure ventilation (physiological) to positive pressure ventilation (mechanical), the intrathoracic pressure is greatly increased, which exerts extrinsic compression upon the great vessels, proportionally having the greatest effect upon the lowest pressure vessels - the great veins. Forward flow is thus impeded and at the capillary level this translates into an increase in P_c, forcing more fluid into the interstitium. Oedema formation due to mechanical ventilation is less problematic on the pulmonary side of the circulation because there is no net rise in pressure gradient ($P_c - P_i$), as the elevated intra-thoracic pressure is applied relatively equally to both the capillary and the interstitium.

Oedema in burned tissues

The post-burn macromolecular leakage from the capillary circulation to the interstitial space is most pronounced in burned tissues. The falling colloid oncotic pressure gradient between capillary and interstitium steadily neutralises the oncotic pull that usually keeps fluid within the circulation, facilitating oedema formation.

The rate of oedema formation is significantly influenced by the depth of the burn. Oedema occurs (and resolves) more rapidly in partial-thickness as opposed to full-thickness injuries. This is thought to be due to the relative differences in vascularity plus the considerably reduced lymphocytic accumulation occurring in deep burns.

The development of heightened capillary permeability to macromolecules is multi-factorial, due both to direct capillary injury within burned tissues and secondary to circulating inflammatory mediators (e.g. histamine, bradykinin). Immediately following injury within the damaged tissues, mast cell degranulation releases large amounts of histamine. Bradykinin is also rapidly formed by the proteolytic cleavage of its plasma pre-cursor, by the action of tissue and plasma kallikrein. Both compounds induce local arteriolar dilatation and increase capillary permeability. In combination with the initial (thermal) injury, these are believed to be the primary contributors to the very rapid phase of oedema formation. Their effects, however, are short-lived, possibly due to tachyphylaxis. Animal studies have shown that maximal albumin extravasation occurs within five minutes of bradykinin injection and within 10 to 20 minutes for histamine, with tachyphylaxis developing at 30 minutes and one hour, respectively [26] **(IIb/B)** Animal.

Chapter 6

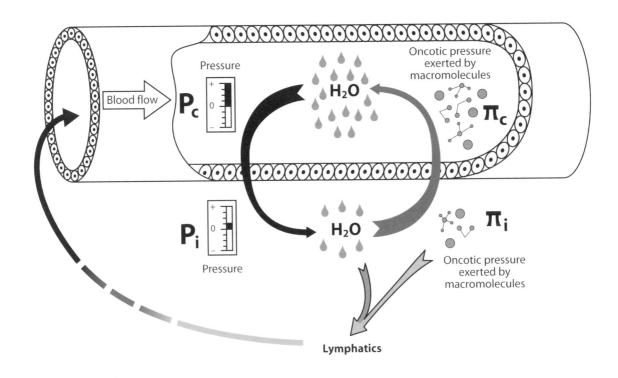

Figure 1. Schematic of normal (post-burn) physiology. The hydrostatic pressure difference (P_c – P_i) causing fluid efflux from the capillary is approximately matched by the oncotic pressure difference (π_c – π_i), maintaining a state of equilibrium of fluid flow to and from the capillary. Water and electrolytes can flow freely across the capillary wall, but macromolecules are mostly prevented from crossing in either direction, but join the circulation via the lymphatics.

Endothelia sustain a further (secondary) injury from oxidants and oxygen-free radicals. This is believed to be responsible for continuing capillary permeability. Chemo-attractants, including interleukin-8, are released by injured tissues, resulting in neutrophil aggregation [27] **(IIb/B)**. Neutrophils are the most potent source of oxidants; however, they may also be produced by induction of xanthine oxidase in any nucleated cell, as a response to cyclical hypoxia-reperfusion.

Delays in restoration of the circulating blood volume result in tissue hypoperfusion and escalate endogenous responses to hypovolaemia (sympathetic outflow, renin-angiotensin-aldosterone system, vasopressin). Hypoperfusion leaves cells hypoxic, inducing anaerobic metabolism. Cellular pH falls, and there is an intracellular accumulation of toxic metabolites and free radicals, damaging cells and impairing cellular function.

Poorly perfused cells swell due to intracellular metabolite accumulation (allowing more sodium and water to enter cells). Furthermore, ATP depletion impairs the Na^+/K^+ ATPase pump, depleting cellular resting membrane potential. Cellular oedema may be limited by prompt fluid resuscitation (thus avoiding hypovolaemia) and by maintaining (or increasing) electrolyte concentrations in administered resuscitation fluids.

Upon restoration of perfusion, a reperfusion-type injury occurs due to toxic metabolites entering the circulation and oedema formation is further increased. This is greater the longer the delay in achieving adequate resuscitation.

The osmotic force exerted by macromolecules is increased by their damage and fragmentation in burned tissue. The more dermis is damaged, the more fragmented macromolecules will exist within the

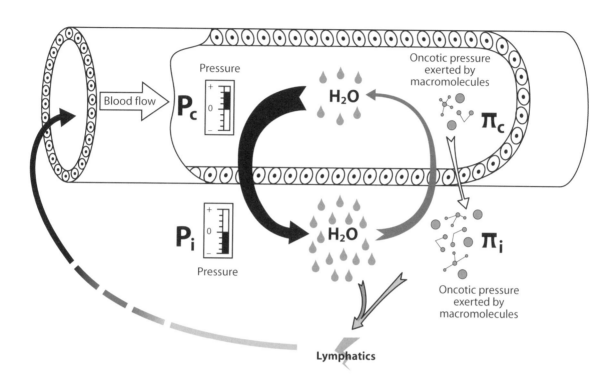

Figure 2. Schematic of acute post-burn physiology. The creation of a significantly negative pressure in the interstitium (P_i) greatly increases the hydrostatic pressure difference and promotes fluid loss from the capillary. The oncotic pressure difference is substantially reduced by macromolecular fragmentation in the interstitium and by heightened capillary permeability to macromolecules. In burned tissue, lymphatics are also often damaged, which restricts clearance of the interstitial macromolecular burden, prolonging oedema. Heightened interstitial compliance also facilitates oedema formation.

interstitial space, amplifying oncotic pressure and generating oedema. This is a particularly prominent feature with hyaluronic acid, which in the dermis is the main generator of tissue oncotic pressure.

Capillary hydrostatic pressure is normally raised shortly after burn injury, primarily due to venoconstriction, but this change is often transient, giving way to venodilation. Meanwhile, interstitial hydrostatic pressure plummets to negative values, due to the sudden increase in osmotically active particles within the interstitial space [21] **(IV/C)**. This negative pressure lasts for 1-2 hours, but takes a long time to be restored to its pre-burn level. The net effect of this huge change in pressure gradient is a significant fluid shift from the intravascular space into the interstitium.

Collagen, hyaluronic acid and other macromolecules serve as dermal scaffolding,

restricting the compliance/expansion of the interstitial space. Damage to this framework allows the space to become dilated more easily, facilitating the ingress of oedema. As the interstitial compartment's volume increases, its compliance increases further, facilitating further oedema formation.

According to Starling's second principle [25], it is not mechanically possible for leaked protein to traverse the capillary wall and return to the circulation. The fourth principle was that proteins within the interstitium must either be utilised by the tissues or cleared by the lymphatic system. Deeper burns, by definition, have more extensively damaged local lymphatics, which impairs the drainage of proteins and oedema fluid. In deeper injuries, macromolecules therefore remain in the interstitium for longer, until lymphatics are repaired or renewed. This prolongs oedema.

Oedema in non-burned tissues

In more extensive burn injuries, oedema formation ceases to be confined to burned tissues, and global oedema develops. This places additional demands upon fluid requirements. Oedema in non-burned tissue typically develops with burns involving greater than 25-30% of the total body surface area. Hence resuscitation fluid requirements are not linearly associated with burn size. Acutely this is due to a transient increase in capillary permeability, which although variable, is of significantly shorter duration than in burned tissues, and estimated to last approximately 8-24 hours post-burn [28] **(III/B)** Animal. Animal model studies suggest that the persistence of oedema in non-burned tissues is predominantly secondary to hypoproteinaemia following the efflux of macromolecules from the circulation and into the interstitium within injured tissues [29] **(III/B)** Animal. This is validated by the finding of significantly lower levels of oedema in patients resuscitated with plasma [30] **(Ib/A)**. Hypoproteinaemia is ubiquitous amongst major burn patients.

Insensible fluid losses

Insensible fluid losses refer to those fluids lost from the body that are difficult to measure in routine practice, including fluids from faeces, perspiration, evaporation and exudation. In health, this accounts for approximately 10ml/kg/day, but in major burns, these losses may equate to many litres. The elevated losses are mainly due to oedema fluid lost through burn wounds. Attempts have been made to estimate the evaporative water loss, and the following equation has been proposed [31]:

$$\text{Evaporative water loss (ml/h)} = (25 + \% \text{ burn TBSA}) \times \text{body surface area (m}^2)$$

It should be remembered that the losses are dependent upon many environmental and patient factors. At higher ambient temperatures, vapour pressures rise, increasing evaporative losses. The magnitude of these losses depends upon ambient humidity and altitude. Patient factors include temperature, hydration, cardiovascular status and wound characteristics. Burn surface area and depth determine oedema formation and consequently losses from exudates or evaporation. The type of dressings applied to burn wounds can reduce evaporative losses by up to 80% [32] **(III/B)**. Evaporation also leaves behind salts and proteins which become increasingly concentrated and exert an osmotic force causing further fluid loss to the surface.

Concomitant inhalation injury elevates fluid requirements, by increasing evaporative losses, elevating both the inflammatory response and oedema formation. Using regression analysis, it is estimated that an inhalational injury increases crystalloid fluid requirements by 30ml/kg/24h [33] **(III/B)**. Others have used their data to re-predict the Parkland formula for patients with inhalational injury, 5.76ml/kg/%, and those without, 3.98ml/kg/% [34] **(III/B)**. However, the severity of inhalational injury is rarely accurately stratified, yet it encompasses a wide spectrum, from those with pure carbon monoxide poisoning or isolated upper airways injury, to severe mucosal damage and particulate contamination of the lower airways. The additional fluid requirements imposed by inhalational injuries are therefore likely to vary considerably and should probably not be pre-empted, but anticipated and responded to appropriately.

Inflammatory response

The systemic inflammatory response has a significant bearing upon fluid requirements, as it is a major determinant of oedema formation and cardiovascular status. It is influenced by injury severity and many other factors. The magnitude of the primary injury is mostly dictated by the quantity and type of tissue burned, and the presence of an inhalation injury or other non-burn injuries. Secondary injuries are exacerbated by delays or inadequacy of fluid resuscitation or the advent of sepsis. There are also patient factors to consider, including comorbidities.

Choice of resuscitation fluid

The fluids used in burns resuscitation can be classified as crystalloids or colloids, either of which can be given as hypo-, iso- or hyper-tonic preparations, which may or may not be physiologically balanced (compared with plasma) with regard to their electrolyte composition. They expand the intravascular compartment to different degrees due to differing osmotic and oncotic properties, and the ease with which they may traverse the capillary wall. Oncotic properties are imparted by the macromolecular content, while the osmotic properties are determined principally by the electrolyte content. Colloids and hypertonic fluids have the greatest volume expansion effect and hypotonic crystalloids the least.

Clinician

There is a delicate balance to be achieved in maintaining adequate tissue perfusion, and avoiding over-treating, and thus escalating oedema and exacerbating cellular hypoxia. The use of predictive equations to estimate resuscitation fluid requirements is almost universal, but they are a guide to requirements only and should be calibrated against

objective outcome measurements. For example, a prospective, randomised study of 50 major burns was undertaken to compare the Parkland formula against cardiac output directed therapy using a thermodilution technique (the latter aiming to normalise the derived intrathoracic blood volume). The Parkland formula resulted in significantly less fluid administration, but interestingly this did not result in worsening of cardiac output parameters, nor measured morbidity and mortality [10] **(Ib/A)**.

Fluid resuscitation formulae (Table 1)

There are a myriad of variables influencing fluid requirements and numerous fluid resuscitation formulae have been devised. The guiding principles of

Table 1. Total fluid provision in the first 24 hours by common fluid resuscitation formulae.

Author	Crystalloid	Colloid
Evans (1952) [7]	NS: 1ml/kg/% plus D5W: 2000ml	Plasma: 1ml/kg/%
Brooke (1953) [8]	RL: 1.5ml/kg/% plus D5W: 2000ml	Plasma: 0.5ml/kg/%
Modified Brooke	RL: 2ml/kg/%	
Baxter/Parkland (1974) [37] **(III/B)**	RL: 4ml/kg/%	
Modified Parkland	RL: 3ml/kg/%	
Muir & Barclay (1974) [38]		Alb: 2.5ml/kg/%
Carvajal (1977) [39] **(III/B)** (Galveston formula)	RL: 2000ml/m^2 (1st 8h) RL: 5000ml/m^2/% (24h)	
Monafo (1984) [40] **(Ib/A)**	HLS (250mEq/l) titrated keep UO (0.5 to 1ml/kg/h)	
Demling (1987) [41] **(IV/C)**	RL titrated to UO (30ml/h)	D40+NS: 2ml/kg/h (1st 8h) FFP: 0.5ml/kg/h (8-24h)
Slater (1991) [30] **(Ib/A)**	RL: 2000ml	FFP 75ml/kg

Key: NS = 0.9% sodium chloride; D5W = 5% glucose; RL = lactated Ringer's solution; Alb = 4.5% human albumin solution; HLS = hypertonic lactated saline; UO = urine output; D40 = Dextran 40; FFP = fresh frozen plasma

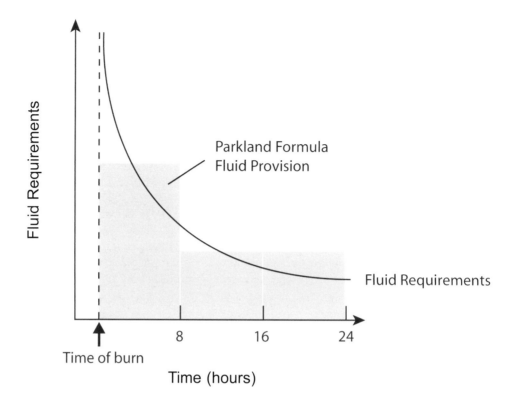

Figure 3. A graph showing theoretical fluid requirements for a generic major burn and the Parkland formula's attempt to provide for this demand. Note that peak fluid requirements occur immediately after the burn, emphasising the need for early fluid resuscitation. The amount of fluid required and its time course depends upon numerous factors, including how promptly fluid resuscitation is started.

fluid resuscitation are to use the least amount of fluid necessary to maintain adequate organ perfusion, and to titrate the infused volumes against individual patient requirements, and to avoid over- or under-resuscitation [35] **(IV/C)**. The formulae, however, remain useful tools in directing early fluid therapy until the patient has been admitted to an appropriate specialist unit and the necessary monitoring established (Figure 3).

A recent multi-centre study [36] **(III/B)** used multi-linear regression analysis to determine the primary variables influencing the required volume of resuscitation fluid. The Parkland formula was used as a guide and the mean infused volume was

5.2ml/kg/%. The major factors determining fluid volumes were:

- Percentage of total body surface area burned.
- Age.
- Weight.
- Intubation status.

Heightened fluid requirements were associated with increased risk of pneumonia, septicaemia, adult respiratory distress syndrome (ARDS), multi-organ failure and death.

Probably the commonest burns fluid resuscitation regime currently in use globally is the Parkland formula (syn. Baxter formula). This was developed by Charles Baxter in the mid-1960s, from retrospective regression analysis studies on adult burn patients at the Parkland Hospital in Dallas, Texas [37] **(III/B)**.

The Parkland formula:

Fluid requirement (1st 24h) =
4 x patient weight (kg) x TBSA (%)

(half given in the 1st 8 h, the
remainder over the last 16 h)

The Parkland formula and its modification (using a multiplication factor of 3 rather than 4) have been adopted by the Advanced Trauma Life Support® (ATLS®) course, the Emergency Management of Severe Burns (EMSB) course, the British Army and most UK burns services. It was derived from data in adult burn resuscitation and was not intended for extrapolation to the resuscitation of children, but it is widely used for this purpose. There have been many critics of its use, some maintaining that it overestimates requirements, others finding it to underestimate them. The reasons for disagreement are numerous, but include the absence of an accepted measurable definition for the adequacy of resuscitation.

Type of resuscitation fluid

Of the available fluids routinely used for burns resuscitation, hypo- and iso-tonic crystalloids require the highest volume infusion and cause the greatest oedema and third space fluid losses. High positive fluid balance correlates with higher mortality, as oedematous tissues function poorly:

* Cerebral oedema causes mental incapacity, delirium and obtunded conscious level (increasing the requirement for sedation and mechanical ventilation) and it can elevate intra-cranial pressure causing long-term damage.
* Pulmonary oedema impairs gas exchange, causing hypoxaemia, prolonging mechanical ventilation and necessitating elevated inspiratory pressures (increasing the incidence of pneumonia, barotrauma, volutrauma and ARDS).
* Myocardial oedema impairs ventricular compliance, escalating myocardial work and compromising cardiac output.

* Cutaneous oedema impairs wound healing and defence from infection and, when circumferential, can act as a tourniquet, impair circulation and lead to compartment syndrome.
* Gastro-intestinal oedema impairs peristalsis and nutrient absorption, and causes expansion of the intra-abdominal contents, which can limit diaphragmatic excursion, impair respiration and may also culminate in abdominal compartment syndrome. Additionally, bacterial translocation from the gut is increased, causing sepsis, escalating the inflammatory response leading to multi-organ failure.

In an attempt to restrict the volume of infused fluid and reduce oedema, there are essentially three treatment strategies, which may be employed either individually or in combination:

* Use less fluid and tolerate a greater degree of hypovolaemia, maintaining minimum cardiovascular parameters with pressors and inotropes.
* Administer fluids containing macromolecules, to increase intravascular oncotic pressure.
* Administer hypertonic fluids to increase intravascular osmotic pressure. In the future this list may be expanded to incorporate pharmacological products which reduce capillary leak, etc.

Crystalloids

Hypotonic and isotonic crystalloids

Historically, burns fluid resuscitation started with crystalloid infusions. Following the work of O'Shaugnessy and Dupuytren, Buhl conducted studies into salt concentrations in the blood and subsequently, in 1855, recommended 0.88% saline solution be given orally, subcutaneously or intravenously to burns patients [42]. This was the first isotonic fluid recommendation for burns treatment.

Work by Davidson (1926) [43] **(IIb/B)** and Moyer (1965) [44] showed that the distribution between intracellular and extracellular compartments is dependent upon the electrolyte content of fluids, as this determines their osmotic potential. The principal contributor to the osmolality of intravenous fluids is sodium chloride. Sodium is the main cation of extracellular fluid, accounting for 90% of the osmotically active solute in plasma and interstitial fluid, thus making it the main determinant of extracellular volume. The lower the electrolyte content of administered fluids, the greater the risk of hyponatraemia and intracellular oedema, most notably in children.

Isotonic crystalloid-based formulae almost exclusively cite Hartmann's solution (or the very similar lactated Ringer's solution). Compared with 0.9% saline, Hartmann's solution is more isotonic (308 vs. 279mOsm/l), less acidic (pH 5.0 vs. 6.5), and carries a lower sodium (154 vs. 131mmol/l) and chloride load (154 vs. 111mmol/l). Instead, it utilises lactate (29mmol/l) as an additional anion and so is associated with a lower risk of hyperchloraemic acidosis. Its composition also more accurately reflects the electrolytes lost from the circulation.

In health, approximately a quarter of the volume of infused isotonic crystalloid remains within the intravascular compartment. In cases of major burns this proportion is lower, due to expansion of the interstitial space.

Of all the fluid resuscitation regimes, those using isotonic crystalloid administer the greatest volume of fluid. The vast majority diffuses to the extravascular space, resulting in heightened interstitial and cellular oedema. Greater interstitial oedema also promotes efflux of endogenous macromolecules from the circulation. The distances between cell and capillary are increased - over which distance oxygen and nutrients must diffuse. The massive increase in interstitial fluid volume also elevates the compliance of this space (as per Laplace's law), facilitating further oedema formation.

Large volume fluid resuscitation has many deleterious effects, including impairment of dynamic functions (joint mobility, intestinal motility, etc.), impaired cellular function and elevation in compartment pressures. Isotonic crystalloid fluid resuscitation is increasingly being recognised as causing various compartment syndromes: intra-abdominal [45] (III/B), [46] (III/B), unburned limbs, and orbital [47] (III/B). Studies on abdominal compartment pressures in major burns have demonstrated a lower incidence of compartment

syndrome with lower volume fluid resuscitation, using either colloids (crystalloid vs. colloid fluid regime, mean intra-abdominal pressures: 26.5 vs. 10.6 mmHg; p<0.0001) [48] (Ib/A) or hypertonic crystalloid solutions [49] (Ib/A). Due to the risk of abdominal hypertension and compartment syndrome, it has been recommended that all adults receiving fluid resuscitation exceeding 500ml/h should receive routine intra-vesicular pressure monitoring [50] (III/B).

In addition to the high volumes of infusions, huge electrolyte loads are provided by crystalloid regimes. Sodium is the principal determinant of extracellular volume and excess must therefore be eliminated from the body before oedema can resolve. Electrolytes are lost through wound exudate, sweat, faeces and urine. However, changes in burn care over recent years have encouraged earlier burn excision and wound closure, thus reducing electrolyte loss via exudates. The main route for electrolyte elimination, therefore, becomes the kidneys. However, the kidneys have a finite concentrating capacity, which serves as a rate limiting step in the resolution of oedema. During the polyuric phase of recovery, the osmotic gradient at the loop of Henle is diluted, further diminishing urinary concentrating capacity.

Physiologically balanced electrolyte solutions are preferable to saline (in both crystalloids and colloids) to avoid the consequences of excess sodium and chloride loading (hyperchloraemic acidosis, renal vasoconstriction and reduced glomerular filtration rate).

Children (unlike adults) have low glycogen reserves and it is often therefore recommended that the infused fluids should contain glucose to prevent critical hypoglycaemia, but not to the exclusion of sodium, as children are particularly vulnerable to hyponatraemia and the consequent problem of cellular oedema.

Colloids

A colloid is a homogeneous non-crystalline substance consisting of large molecules or ultra-microscopic particles of one substance dispersed through a second substance. The particles do not settle and cannot be separated out by ordinary filtering or centrifuging as can those of a suspension such as blood [51] (IV/C).

The use of colloid solutions for resuscitation has a long history. One of the first records of its use in burns dates back to 1881 when von Tappeiner experimented with the use of human plasma [52], but the practice did not start to become more widely adopted until the late 1930s when safe methods were developed to process, store and infuse plasma [53] **(IV/C)** Animal.

Intravascular colloids exert oncotic pressure which draws fluid from the interstitial space, thus expanding and maintaining intravascular volume. In normal plasma, albumin contributes 60-80% of this oncotic pressure. Human studies have demonstrated that within 24 hours the entirety of the body's serum proteins can be lost from the wound exudates of a 20% TBSA burn due to capillary leakage [54] **(IIb/B)**. This diminishes the intravascular oncotic force, whilst at the same time, the interstitial oncotic pressure is increased, due both to intravascular macromolecular efflux and fragmentation of interstitial macromolecules. These major changes in the oncotic gradient promote further volume loss from the circulation. It therefore appears logical to administer colloids as part of the resuscitation fluid regime. This would replace macromolecules lost by capillary leak, and therefore restore the oncotic gradient and reduce oedema in unburned tissues (which is predominantly due to hypoproteinaemia [55] **(Ib/A)** Animal) and minimise the fluid volume required for effective resuscitation. However, there is evidence to suggest that colloid administration further increases protein loss via exudates from burned tissues [56] **(Ib/A)** Animal.

In practice, there are pitfalls to using colloids. As identified by Baxter, almost any colloid administered acutely following a major burn will leak from the circulation [57]. At peak capillary permeability within burned tissue, macromolecules up to approximately 300kDa can traverse the capillary wall (c.f. mean albumin size = 69kDa, mean erythrocyte size 350kDa). This leak persists for a variable time depending upon the degree of tissue damage. A similar picture is seen in unburned tissue with burns of >25% TBSA, although it resolves more quickly - being estimated to last approximately 8-24 hours post-burn [28] **(III/B)** Animal.

Using colloids as opposed to crystalloids, however, indisputably reduces required fluid volumes, mainly due to a reduction in the oedema affecting non-burned tissues. Its use inevitably increases the quantity of leaked colloid within the interstitium, which exacerbates and prolongs oedema (including pulmonary oedema [58] **(Ib/A)**), imparting significant morbidity. All extravasated colloids must eventually be removed from the interstitium. Smaller molecules are drained by the lymphatics, while larger exogenous macromolecules are phagocytosed which causes the additional problem of impaired reticulo-endothelial function [59] **(Ib/A)** Animal and hence immunity.

A few colloids are available that are comprised of molecules with weights in excess of 300kDa. These consequently extravasate to a lesser degree, but their promise has disappointed in clinical use, as they are associated with a higher incidence of coagulopathy and hypersensitivity reactions.

As a result of the inevitable capillary leakage and other inescapable problems with currently available colloids, there has been a shift away from their use in the first 24 hours of burn resuscitation over the last couple of decades both in the UK and globally.

The most recent Cochrane systemic review [60] **(Ia/A)** upon the use of crystalloids versus colloids for the resuscitation of critically ill patients, analysed 46 published studies, although made no distinction between critical illness, trauma and burns. It broadly concluded that there was no evidence to demonstrate that colloids improved survival and the added expense of their use was therefore difficult to justify. However, this meta-analysis incorporated many studies comparing colloids with hypertonic fluids, included disparate patient groups (elective abdominal surgery, sepsis, cardiac bypass surgery, etc.) and out of several thousand total patients, there were only four studies in burns, which included a total of 308 patients, half of which were comparing colloids with hypertonic solutions.

Available colloids (Table 2)

Starches

Hydroxyethyl starches were developed in the 1960s as an alternative to albumin and dextrans. They are derived from amylopectin, a naturally occurring and highly branched glucose polymer, which is the

Chapter 6

Chapter 6

Table 2. Available colloids.

Class	Colloid	Volume expansion (%)	Weight averaged mean Mol.Wt. (kDa)	Number averaged mean Mol.Wt. (kDa)	Colloid oncotic pressure (mmHg)	Anaphylaxis risk (%)	Plasma $T_{1/2}$
Starch	Tetrastarch (Voluven®, Venofundin®)		130	60		0.06	8-12
	Hexastarch (eloHAES®)		200	60			
	Pentastarch (HAES-steril®/Hemohes®/ Infukoll®)	140	280 (10-1000)	60	40		8-12
	Pentastarch (Pentafraction)	140	280 (100-500)	120	40		8-12
	Hetastarch (Hespan®)	100 - 150	450 (10-1000)	70	30	0.085	17d
	Hetastarch (Hextend®)		670	70			
Succinylated gelatin	Gelofusine® Volplex®	60 - 80	30	22.6		0.35	4-8h
Urea cross-linked gelatin	Haemaccel®	60 - 80	30 (5-50)	24.3	27.2	0.35	5h
Dextran	Dextran 40	130 - 200	40	25		0.27	2-12
	Dextran 70	80 - 120	70	39	60	0.27	9-11
Transfusion products	5% Albumin	80 - 150	69		19.5	0.10	18h
	20% Albumin	450	69		78	0.10	18h
	Fresh frozen plasma				20	0.00005	5-19
	Packed cells					0.00005	Varia

principal component of starch (the other being amylose). The substitution of hydroxyethyl ether groups onto the glucose molecules slows their hydrolysis by plasma amylase. Almost all available starches contain a wide range of molecular sizes, ranging from 1 to 1,000kDa with a typical bell-shaped distribution curve. Molecular weights (MW) of polymers can be described by two averaging methods: weight averaged or number averaged.

Available products vary in their plasma half-life according to variation in their mean molecular weight (130 to 670kDa), the range of molecule sizes contained, the amount of hydroxyethyl group substitution and the position of these substitutions upon the carbon ring. Their volume expansion effect generally lasts 4-8 hours. They are eliminated by a combination of phagocytosis and degradation by plasma amylase, followed by excretion in urine and bile.

Advantages

Starches carry the lowest hypersensitivity risk of all commercially available colloids, with an overall anaphylaxis risk of 0.06%, although the risk escalates slightly with increasing mean molecular size.

Potential advantages (unproven by human burns studies) include:

- Possible anti-inflammatory effects (decreased leukocyte-endothelial adhesion and decreased platelet adhesion) [61] **(IV/C)**, with amelioration of the systemic inflammatory cascade [62] **(IV/C)**.
- Reduced capillary leak, by plugging the gap between endothelia (shown in the rat model [63] **(Ib/A)** Animal, [64] **(Ib/A)** Animal).
- Reduction in vasoactive mediator release (e.g. thromboxane A_2 [65] **(Ib/A)** Animal).
- Postulated membrane stabilisation properties.

Disadvantages
- Dose-related haematological (decreased platelet count and fibrinogen), immunological, renal and reticulo-endothelial dysfunction [59] **(Ib/A)** Animal.
- Dose-dependent coagulopathy (decreased Factor VIIIc, decreased platelet adhesion and inhibition of the release of von Willebrand Factor (vWF) from endothelia), especially products with a larger molecular size.
- Accumulation within tissues.
- Severe pruritis with prolonged use (probably due to accumulation of vacuoles within the cytoplasm of keratinocytes and Schwann cells).
- May impair erythrocyte deformability and promote aggregation (Rouleaux formation), impairing microvascular flow.
- Products with high molecular weight could increase blood viscosity.
- Restricted to a maximum dose of 20ml/kg/24h.
- Increases levels of plasma amylase (impairs interpretation of high levels).

To overcome the post-burns capillary leakage, hetastarch or pentastarch (the starches with the highest molecular weights) would appear to be obvious choices, but they carry a significantly greater risk of complications and appear to offer no tangible advantage over colloids of a smaller molecular size [66]

(III/B). Pentafraction (pentastarch which has been diafiltered to leave a narrower spectrum of molecule sizes) has an improved side effect profile, but in canine post-burns studies, the microcirculatory leak does not appear to be attenuated [67] **(Ib/A)** Animal. Ovine studies, however, have shown reduced oedema formation and improvements in cardiac output and systemic vascular resistance when comparing pentafraction to fresh frozen plasma (FFP) or regular pentastarch [68] **(Ib/A)** Animal.

The smaller starches, notably tetrastarch, offer the best side effect profile. They accumulate less in interstitial tissues, glomeruli and plasma (20 times better plasma clearance than hetastarch), cause the least coagulopathy and (in general critical care) offer equivalence in volume expansion when compared with other available starches [69] **(IV/C)**, although this may not apply in post-burns patients with a significant capillary leak. The smaller starches also appear to be safer when given in doses exceeding the recommended maximum [70] **(Ib/A)**.

In the early post-burns phase, there may be additional benefits from fractionated high-molecular-weight starches containing a narrower range of molecular sizes. These should theoretically result in a greater proportion being retained within the intravascular space (possibly even plugging capillary leaks). There is, however, an absence of human data to confirm this and further research is needed.

Gelatins

These proteinaceous plasma expanders were first introduced during World War I. Their manufacture is by hydrolysis of bovine collagen. They have short plasma half-lives (4-8 hours) and are largely renally excreted but also degraded into small peptides and amino acids by proteolytic enzymes (trypsin, plasmin, cathepsin). Due to their small molecular size (30 to 35kDa), they migrate fairly rapidly out of the intravascular space (volume expansion effect lasts 3-4 hours).

Gelofusine® and Volplex® are products of enzymatic succinylation of hydrolysed collagen. This imparts a negative charge to the molecules and causes a conformational change, increasing their molecular size without significantly increasing weight.

Chapter 6

These products have a significant anticoagulant effect, acting at the cellular phase of clot formation (thus undetectable by PT or APTT) [71] **(III/B)**.

Haemaccel® is a polygeline, formed by urea cross-linking of small gelatin peptides (12-15kDa) to form polymers with a molecular weight of c. 30kDa and a plasma half-life c. eight hours. It has a milder anticoagulant effect than the succinylated gelatins, but has a high calcium and potassium content. The method employed for its manufacture changed in 1981, and subsequently there have been fewer adverse effects than initially reported.

Advantages
* Minimal effect upon reticulo-endothelial function.
* No specific dosage limitations.

Disadvantages
* Highest incidence of hypersensitivity (anaphylaxis risk 0.35%) of all the commercially available colloids, numerous reports of severe anaphylaxis and cross-reactivity between succinylated and urea cross-linked gelatins.
* Stimulates histamine release.
* Inhibits plasma fibronectin binding capacity [72] **(Ib/A)** (fibronectin binds a variety of biological ligands including actin, heparin, collagen and gelatin, and opsonises them for elimination from the circulation by hepatic Kupffer cells and macrophages). This elevates end-organ deposition of post-burn micro-aggregates and impairs wound healing.
* May impair clot strength [73] **(IIb/B)**.
* Anticoagulant effect (undetectable by coagulation screen).
* Complement activation [74] **(IIb/B)**.
* Rouleaux formation.
* Increases urinary excretion of proteins (especially ß2-microglobulin and α1-microglobulin) [75] **(IIb/B)**.
* High calcium content of Haemaccel (blood should therefore not be infused through a line previously used for Haemaccel).
* Theoretical risk of transmission of communicable viruses/prions (derived from bovine collagen).
* Small molecular size, therefore more likely to be lost from the circulation through leaking capillaries.

Dextrans

Dextrans are complex, branched polysaccharides formed by bacterial fermentation of sucrose-containing media, followed by acid hydrolysis then fractionation. They have molecular weights ranging from 1 to 2,000kDa, and fluids are named according to their molecular weight (e.g. Dextran 70 has a weight averaged mean molecular weight of 70kDa). They are used for their volume expansion and anti-thrombotic properties. They bind erythrocytes and platelets, reducing their aggregation and they impede the polymerisation of fibrin. Dextrans are also weakly thrombolytic. The smaller molecules are renally excreted, whilst the remainder undergo hepatic metabolism, biliary excretion or phagocytosis by the reticulo-endothelial system.

There are two dextran products in common use: Dextran 40 and Dextran 70, the former used mostly for its microcirculatory and anti-thrombotic effects, the latter being used for volume expansion.

In 1978, Hall and Sørensen conducted a randomised controlled trial, comparing Dextran 70 against Ringer's lactate for burns fluid resuscitation [76] **(Ib/A)**. Although most physiological variables were improved in the dextran group, this did not translate into any significant difference in mortality.

Advantages
* Improve microcirculatory flow (lower viscosity, reduce leukocyte, erythrocyte and platelet adhesion) (Dextran 40 only - not Dextran 70).
* Possible anti-inflammatory effects (decreased leukocyte-endothelial adhesion and decreased platelet adhesion) [61] **(IV/C)**.
* Scavenger of toxic oxygen metabolites.

Disadvantages
* Routinely cause the greatest coagulopathy of all colloids (platelet function and decreased Factor VIIIc, decreased vWF).
* Interferes with the process of cross-matching blood products.
* Hypersensitivity (anaphylaxis risk 0.27%) (significantly reduced by injection of hapten-dextran 1 prior to infusion).
* Stimulates histamine release.
* Complement activation [74] **(IIb/B)**.

- Hyperglycaemia (glucose liberated as Dextran is metabolised).
- Dextran 70 promotes Rouleaux formation.
- Maximum dose of 1.5-2g/kg.

Transfusion products

Packed cells

Blood transfusion is an inappropriate solution to treat post-burns hypovolaemia. Intravascular fluid losses are almost entirely from the plasma component of blood. Packed cell transfusion increases haematocrit levels, further increasing blood viscosity and impairing microcirculatory flow. Although the half life of packed cells is good, its colloid oncotic pressure is poor, so it pulls relatively little fluid from the interstitium. This does not detract from its ability to restore oxygen-carrying capacity by replacing erythrocytes lost to the circulation as a consequence of burn injury.

Fresh frozen plasma and albumin

It contains albumin and globulins, including fibronectin, which are mostly of low molecular weight and consequently leak from the post-burn circulation. FFP carries the risks of a transfusion product. FFP is supplied in single donor units which are small volume preparations, making it expensive and cumbersome to administer. However, it has been found to reduce oedema formation and deliver outcomes comparable to other colloids [30] **(Ib/A)**.

Albumin has a mean molecular weight c. 69kDa; only c. 43% of the body's albumin is intravascular and crosses capillary walls to the lymphatic circulation under normal physiological conditions at a rate of 4-5%/hour. It is one of the most oncotically active colloids in plasma and accounts for 60-80% of the oncotic pressure of normal plasma (25 to 33 mmHg); this makes it an ideal plasma expander. It also benefits from a long plasma half-life (in health), it is a free-radical scavenger and acts as a carrier molecule for many substances. Albumin solutions are obtained from pooled human plasma which has undergone pasteurisation. They may be given without regard to the recipient's blood group, yet they always carry a small hypersensitivity risk (anaphylaxis risk 0.10%) and the potential for transmission of communicable viruses and prions. The extensive processing of these transfusion products make them the most expensive of all available colloid solutions.

The use of albumin and plasma protein fractions in the management of burns patients was once common. In 1998, a meta-analysis conducted by the Cochrane Injuries Group suggested that the use of albumin in critical care was linked with significant mortality (relative risk of death 2.40) [77] **(Ia/A)**. However, the conclusions were fiercely challenged on account of the type and variety of studies included in the meta-analysis. The Saline versus Albumin Fluid Evaluation (SAFE) study [78] **(Ib/A)** was subsequently undertaken, including 6997 patients. This demonstrated no elevated mortality, differences in organ failure rates or length of ICU stay. Its findings have been included in subsequent updates of the Cochrane review, whose conclusions have been modified to declare only an absence of evidence for reducing mortality [79] **(Ia/A)**. These studies were not specific to burns, but they have been followed by a more recent burns-specific multi-centre trial which found combined albumin and crystalloid resuscitation to offer no improvement in organ dysfunction scores when compared with crystalloid resuscitation alone [80] **(IIa/B)**.

Hypertonic fluids

Fluids with an osmolality greater than human plasma (285-293mOsm/kg) are termed 'hypertonic'; they may be crystalloids or colloids. Sodium and chloride ions are usually the principal contributors to the hypertonicity. Alternative compositions have been used to achieve hypertonicity (adding amino acids and glucose) in order to avoid hypernatraemia, but results have been disappointing - failing to parallel reductions in oedema and having an adverse chronotropic effect [81] **(Ib/A)** Animal. Hypertonic saline solutions are available in concentrations of 1.8%, 3%, 5%, 7.5% and 10%; however, to balance the sodium and reduce chloride load (and its associated problems), some solutions include alternative anions (e.g. lactate) in addition to chloride.

The principal benefit of hypertonic fluids is to reduce the overall fluid volume required thus reducing oedema. If more concentrated saline solutions are given, research suggests that lower fluid volumes can be given without escalating the amount of sodium chloride administered [40] **(Ib/A)**. Hypertonic fluids that have been used commonly in burns include hypertonic saline (HS), hypertonic lactated saline (HLS) and hypertonic saline-dextran (HSD) (2400mOsm/kg sodium chloride, 6% dextran 70).

The infused electrolytes diffuse freely across capillaries to achieve equilibrium throughout the extracellular compartment (intravascular and interstitial). The heightened extracellular osmolality osmotically draws water from the intracellular compartment. Hypertonic fluids also have other physiological effects. The effect of saline upon the central vasomotor areas appears to be an elevation in sympathetic outflow and vasoconstriction independent of vasopressin [82] **(IIb/B)** Animal. The net vasomotor effect of hypertonic saline infusion, however, is a combination of vasoconstriction of arteries and larger arterioles, but vasodilatation of smaller arterioles [83] **(Ib/A)** Animal, the latter likely to be due to local stimulation. This potentially improves microcirculatory flow whilst maintaining systemic vascular resistance and hence, blood pressure. In addition, the osmotic properties reduce capillary endothelial oedema, improving luminal diameter and flow [84] **(IIb/B)** Animal.

The most recent Cochrane systematic review [85] **(Ia/A)** assessed the evidence for hypertonic versus isotonic crystalloid resuscitation for hypovolaemia in trauma, burns and post-op patients, with a combined study population of 956. There was inadequate statistical power to justify recommending the use of one over the other.

Advantages

- Cardiovascular: intrinsic myocardial contractile depression has been shown following thermal injury, peaking at 24 hours [86] **(Ib/A)** Animal. Animal studies using HSD [87] **(Ib/A)** Animal, [88] **(Ib/A)** Animal, [89] **(Ib/A)** Animal, and a human study using HS [90] **(Ib/A)** have reported a direct positive inotropic effect, counteracting the intrinsic depression (however, others found the reverse [91] **(Ib/A)** Animal). This is possibly due to improved calcium uptake facilitated by hypertonic fluids [87] **(Ib/A)** Animal. There is also evidence for a reduction in myocardial oxidative damage with HSD [89] **(Ib/A)** Animal (may be attributable to dextran rather than hypertonicity [91] **(Ib/A)** Animal).
- Inflammation: HSD reduces cardiomyocyte production of pro-inflammatory cytokines: TNF-α, IL-1β and IL-6 [88] **(Ib/A)** Animal and HS reduces neutrophil activation [92] **(Ib/A)** Animal, margination [93] **(Ib/A)** Animal and aggregation [94] **(Ib/A)** Animal.

- Immune system: HS ameliorates post-trauma T-cell immunosuppression [95] **(Ib/A)** Animal and may reduce sepsis rates.
- Microvascular: vasodilatation improves flow in small arterioles and capillaries (see above).
- Oedema: may restore euvolaemia and preload with a lower volume and sodium load than if isotonic crystalloids alone are used [96] **(Ib/A)** Animal, resulting in less oedema and fewer oedema-related complications, such as abdominal compartment syndrome [49] **(Ib/A)**.
- Cerebral protection: distant thermal injury disrupts the blood brain barrier by a systemic mode of action; HS resuscitation reduces leukocytic aggregation around cerebral vessels and reduces oedema by reducing microvascular leak [94] **(Ib/A)** Animal.

Disadvantages

- Several studies have shown an elevated mortality rate in patients treated with hypertonic fluids [97] **(Ib/A)**, [98] **(III/B)**; their use is, therefore, confined to short duration, possibly in divided doses [53] **(IV/C)** Animal.
- Systemic small vessel vasodilatation stimulated by hypertonic solutions can cause hypotension, and in the presence of stiff or diseased vessels may cause a steal phenomenon. Within coronary vasculature, this may exacerbate myocardial ischaemia and depression [99] **(Ib/A)** Animal.
- Electron microscopy (animal studies) has shown that although systemic circulation is improved when HS is compared with isotonic saline resuscitation, at a capillary level, microthrombi are formed, impairing microcirculatory flow [100] **(Ib/A)** Animal.
- Animal studies have linked HS resuscitation with worsening of lung injuries [101] **(Ib/A)** Animal and gut barrier dysfunction [102] **(Ib/A)** Animal. They have found increased neutrophil deposition in the lungs, oxidative damage and hyper-permeability compared to isotonic resuscitation.
- High plasma sodium levels usually indicate dehydration; physiologically, the body therefore responds by stimulating renal vasoconstriction and ADH secretion, reducing urine output (prolonging oedema and reducing toxic metabolite excretion).

- Iatrogenic hypernatraemia has been linked with an elevated rate of apoptosis within burn wounds [103] **(Ib/A)** Animal.
- Risk of central pontine demyelination (especially in children) due to rapid changes in serum osmolality [104] **(III/B)**.
- Risk of arrhythmias.
- Large doses of chloride can cause hyperchloraemic acidosis, limiting its use in acidotic patients.
- Hypertonic solutions can cause thrombophlebitis and haemolysis at the infusion site.

Assessing the adequacy of fluid resuscitation

The determination of what constitutes adequate resuscitation is a perpetual challenge to those involved in the care of major burns victims. Many variables are routinely recorded, and there are many investigations which may be performed in an attempt to evaluate a patient's level of resuscitation and fluid requirements. The relative contribution and usefulness of each measured parameter in providing resuscitation treatment goals must be defined. Resuscitation fluid requirements vary significantly between patients with a comparable size of burn and between burns services, and this complicates the interpretation of published literature.

Haemoconcentration

As fluid leaks from the circulation, haemoconcentration occurs. The haematocrit, haemoglobin and erythrocyte count have therefore all been used as surrogate indicators of circulating blood volume. This method is unfortunately compromised by a variety of factors. Following burn injury, many erythrocytes are sequestered within injured tissues, many are haemolysed, and Rouleaux formation essentially removes others from the circulation. Occult haemorrhage may also have occurred which would clearly impact upon the interpretation of the haematocrit and erythrocyte count. These are, therefore, not sensitive or specific tests and caution must be exercised in their interpretation.

Maintenance of CVS within specific ranges - pressure measurements

Arterial blood pressure

Below a specific arterial pressure, organ function deteriorates (notably the kidney and brain). This critical pressure varies between individuals, but in general, the lower acceptable limit for mean arterial pressure is approximately 70 mmHg (adults and children). The elderly, with a greater incidence of atherosclerosis, who have a lesser capacity for autoregulation, or patients with renal artery stenosis, may require higher target pressures to maintain renal function.

Blood pressure depends upon blood volume, cardiac output and SVR. Major burn injuries affect all these variables. Post-burn hypovolaemia reduces preload and consequently stroke volume, myocardial depressants impair contractility, and vasodilatation reduces systemic vascular resistance. The short-term endogenous mechanisms are excellent at maintaining mean arterial pressure: heightened sympathetic outflow and various vasoactive peptides maintain cardiac output by shifting the distribution of circulating blood, increasing heart rate and myocardial contractility and increasing vascular tone, but they have adverse consequences if employed beyond the short term.

Administered fluid provision replaces losses from oedema and exudates, thereby improving preload. Myocardial depression and sometimes poor tone within systemic vasculature mean that fluids alone may be insufficient to generate adequate mean arterial pressures. In this scenario, further fluid administration compounds problems by escalating systemic and pulmonary oedema, both of which result in worsening cellular hypoxia.

Blood pressure in itself is a poor surrogate measure of tissue perfusion and adequacy of fluid resuscitation. It does not correlate with blood flow, which is an essential determinant of oxygen delivery, and hence adequacy of resuscitation. Studies repeatedly find that fluid management strategies guided by pressures (arterial, central venous pressure [CVP] or pulmonary arterial wedge pressure [PAWP]) are less successful than those targeted at blood flow. However, it remains important to maintain mean arterial pressure ≥70 mmHg to maintain organ function.

Arterial pressure variation with respiration

Pressure variation studies include pulsus paradoxus (clinically) or the observed 'swing' in the arterial pressure waveform trace (variation in absolute pressure or pulse pressure with cycles of inspiration-expiration). Their presence generally indicates hypovolaemia, as under such conditions, the intrathoracic pressure change (which effects respiration) partially collapses the great veins, compromising venous return and over the course of the respiratory cycle, this causes fluctuations in preload. This is translated into variations in cardiac output, recordable by pressure monitoring, although the pressure changes do not correlate well with changes in flow rates. When a patient is receiving mechanical ventilation using high positive pressures, these pressures exert a significantly greater impedance to venous return. To remove the 'swing' phenomenon, fluid is given to augment preload, but blood volume may have to be increased to supra-physiological levels to achieve this, which exacerbates transcapillary flux and oedema formation.

Central venous pressure (CVP)

Central venous access is very commonly required in major burns. This provides an opportunity to measure CVP, which is frequently used as an indicator of intravascular filling status, preload and hence a marker of right ventricular end-diastolic volume.

Prospective studies in major burns have demonstrated that CVP correlates poorly with cardiac output or total circulating blood volume. It is instead most strongly influenced by intra-abdominal pressure [105] (IIb/B). Isolated measurements of CVP that are high or normal, are consequently unreliable indicators of volume status, particularly in the context of large burns where intra-abdominal hypertension is common. Low CVP readings may still be useful to indicate hypovolaemia (or systemic vasodilatation).

Fluid challenges are sometimes given, followed by serial monitoring of the CVP. In major burns, this approach is unfortunately limited on account of the significant influence of intra-abdominal pressure. To observe a rise in CVP, the venous pressure must be elevated above intra-abdominal pressure, which may be considerably higher than physiological values for CVP.

Maintenance of CVS within specific ranges - flow measurements

Cardiac output monitoring

Swann-Ganz catheters have historically been the mainstay for cardiac output monitoring. Over the last decade, however, various new and less invasive options have become available. These techniques work either by venous tracer injection and rapid serial measurement of the rate and concentration of tracer reappearance in the arterial circulation, or by thermodilution - venous injection of boluses of cold fluid and mapping of arterial temperature changes over time. Other methods use values derived from vascular pressure-flow studies (e.g. oesophageal Doppler). Measurements are processed by computerised algorithms to make indirect assessments of stroke volume. Some also estimate vascular resistance, blood volume and extravascular lung water volume, and results can be adjusted for the patient's weight to give indexed values, to simplify interpretation.

Cardiac output monitoring is used in various ways to guide the fluid prescription. A common method is to monitor the stroke volume and determine its response to fluid boluses. An increase in stroke volume is a trigger to give more fluid, whilst no change or a reduction in stroke volume implies filling is complete and further fluid would be detrimental. The problem with this method in major burns is that (to a point) stroke volume will continue to rise with increasing central venous pressures (Frank-Starling law), which increases oedema generation. Maintaining maximal stroke volume, therefore, comes at the price of increased oedema, so this may not be a good endpoint for guiding fluid resuscitation. The aim of fluid resuscitation is to deliver just enough to rapidly restore and maintain perfusion in all tissues. This method (and most others) causes this point to be exceeded.

There have been concerns regarding the use of thermodilution techniques in burns due to levels of oedema and temperature variations. Prospective studies have shown there to be an acceptable level of repeatability from such measurements (variations up to 12.9%), and an absence of significant error being introduced by aberrations in body temperature [106] (IIb/B). However, one study has compared thermodilution with a more precise method and concluded that estimates of preload (intrathoracic blood volume [ITBV]) are significantly inaccurate and should not be used in burns to guide fluid resuscitation [107] **(IIb/B)**. This does not detract from this method being useful for cardiac output monitoring, merely some of its derived values.

Cardiac output monitoring is a useful element in guiding fluid resuscitation, as it gives information upon systemic flow (a more useful measure than pressure). It can help differentiate between cardiogenic and hypovolaemic causes for derangements of flow. However, it does not inform about flow at tissue level and hence the adequacy of oxygen delivery (the goal of fluid resuscitation).

Indicators of end-organ perfusion

Cutaneous perfusion

Capillary return time (CRT) gives a rough guide to the status of cutaneous perfusion. It is, however, prone to misinterpretation as it is influenced by skin temperature. Laser Doppler imaging (LDI) is a more high tech means by which cutaneous perfusion can be quantitatively monitored. It has been shown to correlate with other markers of tissue perfusion [108] **(Ib/A)** Animal, but there is no published evidence regarding its use to guide fluid therapy.

Core-peripheral temperature gradient

A reduction in cutaneous perfusion allows skin to cool, resulting in differences between core and peripheral temperatures. Cutaneous perfusion is determined by circulating blood volume and vasoconstrictor tone within vascular beds. Vasoconstriction may result from hypovolaemia, hypothermia or any other stimulus evoking an increase in sympathetic outflow (pain, distress, nausea, etc.). An increase in temperature gradient between core and periphery is used as a marker of impaired cutaneous perfusion. If there is adequate cutaneous perfusion, the gradient is expected to be <2.5°C. This test has poor sensitivity and specificity and is compromised by a significant latency period before hypoperfusion results in measurable temperature differences. This makes it an unreliable indicator of circulating blood volume [109] **(III/B)**, as it is neither sensitive nor specific and is thus a poor tool for guiding fluid resuscitation.

Indicators of end-organ function

Urine output

Urine output monitoring is one of the commonest and simplest interventions available. In health, the kidneys receive almost a quarter of the cardiac output. The glomerular filtration rate (GFR) and ultimately the urine output is directly influenced by the rate of blood flow in the glomerular capillaries. This flow is normally kept remarkably constant across wide perfusion pressure ranges due to sensitive local autoregulation of renal vascular resistance. Even at relatively low perfusion pressures, GFR is well maintained due to preferential constriction of efferent over afferent vessels, thereby increasing hydrostatic pressure. However, with falling arterial pressure, the internal compensatory mechanisms start to fail, reducing GFR.

The glomerular capillary blood flow is in part regulated by contractile mesangial cells. These contract and reduce glomerular blood flow in response to angiotensin II, vasopressin, noradrenaline, platelet activating factor, thromboxane A2, leukotrienes and histamine. Such substances are present in abundance after a major burn injury, so GFR falls. This causes the physiological oliguria which is to be anticipated after any significant surgery or trauma.

Renin is released by juxtaglomerular cells in response to either ß1-adrenoceptor stimulation, renal artery hypotension and reduced sodium concentration in the distal tubules. It enzymatically converts angiotensinogen to angiotensin. Circulating angiotensin is then converted to angiotensin II by the membrane-bound angiotensin converting enzyme, expressed by certain vascular endothelia (particularly pulmonary).

Angiotensin II has many actions: it causes systemic arteriolar constriction (increasing systemic vascular resistance); it stimulates aldosterone release from the adrenal cortex (increasing renal sodium and water retention); it stimulates vasopressin release from the posterior pituitary (increasing renal fluid retention and causing vasoconstriction); it stimulates hypothalamic thirst centres; and potentiates sympathetic activity.

Chapter 6

inflammatory response, capillary leak, neutrophil activation and the myocardial depression associated with major burn injuries.

Conclusions

Major burn injuries are rapidly followed by major local and systemic changes. These are characterised by the release/generation of osmotically active molecules, damage to the structural integrity of burned tissues, inflammatory cascades, disruption of lymphatic drainage, cellular dysfunction and increased vascular permeability causing leakage of macromolecules from the intra-vascular space. Physiological responses to these changes include increased sympathetic tone, release of renin, angiotensin, vasopressin, plus a huge range of other mediators. These changes are manifested by major compartmental fluid shifts, culminating in hypovolaemia, oedema formation and end-organ hypoperfusion.

With modern advances in monitoring and intensive care, wide ranging measurements can be made of physiological responses to injury and assessment of resuscitation status. This wealth of information better informs clinicians and guides intervention to normalise parameters. This has de-emphasised the importance of fluid resuscitation formulae, but introduced new pitfalls. Modern monitoring allows us to identify hypovolaemia earlier [116] **(IIb/B)**, and there is a growing realisation that the established formulae only partially corrected hypovolaemia.

Each clinician will have a different opinion as to the relative importance of various physiological indicators and will use different thresholds to change therapy. There is currently wide variation in practice and little evidence to support which are the best indicators and what are their optimal endpoints. We are, however, becoming increasingly aware that over-generous fluid resuscitation can be easily precipitated by modern monitoring and this can be as deleterious as under-resuscitation.

The modern trend to aggressively escalate therapy to continually correct measured values to normal or supra-physiological endpoints carries risks. The total volume of administered fluids is increased, oedema worsens and ultimately, tissue hypoxia is exacerbated. The capillary leak and increasing compliance of the interstitial space makes it very difficult to 'overfill' the intravascular compartment using isotonic crystalloids - fluid just leaks out. If we aim to normalise preload, this may result in over-resuscitation. It may be best to adopt a more permissive attitude towards certain predictable aberrations of normal physiology.

Experimentation with colloids and hypertonic fluids has shown that adequate resuscitation can be achieved with smaller fluid volumes, but they carry their own drawbacks. Unfortunately, most of this research has (necessarily) been conducted upon animals and there is little convincing data from human studies to recommend one fluid type over another. When all the risks are balanced, there is probably little difference between various solutions and the crystalloid vs. colloid debate has been won by crystalloids on the basis of little more than cost.

Current resuscitation protocols only address the fluid prescription. It is likely, as evidence and understanding grows, that protocols will also include guidance upon various pharmacological interventions (e.g. anti-oxidants, mediator inhibitors) to minimise secondary injuries and reduce organ dysfunction and fluid requirements.

We are unlikely to substantially improve burn care through the development of additional predictive fluid resuscitation formulae. Instead, advances in monitoring techniques and defining their optimal parameters and drug therapies focused upon ameliorating detrimental pathophysiological processes, are likely to make the most significant contribution to future burns care.

Recommendations	Evidence level
◆ Fluid resuscitation should be started as soon as possible following injury because fluid loss is initially very rapid and prompt resuscitation reduces secondary injuries and mortality.	Ib/A
◆ The intravenous route is the route of choice for fluid resuscitation.	III/B
◆ Oral fluid resuscitation is less appropriate for older patients and those with burns >25%.	III/B
◆ The main factors influencing fluid requirements are TBSA, age, weight and intubation status.	III/B
◆ Resuscitation formulae are only a rough guide to fluid requirements.	III/B
◆ Fluid losses are slower but larger in deeper burns.	Ib/A
◆ Burns larger than 25-30% develop oedema in unburned tissues due to capillary leak (lasting 8 to 24h) and hypoproteinaemia, hence requiring greater resuscitation fluid volumes.	III/B
◆ Inhalational injuries increase required fluid volumes by c. 30ml/kg/24h.	III/B
◆ Children and the elderly require fluid resuscitation for smaller burn injuries than adults.	III/B
◆ Colloids appear not to offer any survival advantage over crystalloids, but burns-specific studies comparing isotonic fluids are limited.	Ia/A
◆ Hypertonic crystalloids should be used sparingly as they have been associated with elevated mortality.	Ib/A
◆ Fluid resuscitation guided by conventional routine monitoring may still result in occult tissue acidosis, particularly in the GI tract and burn wound.	IIb/B
◆ Relative usefulness of different modalities of monitoring to guide fluid resuscitation: • end-organ perfusion (esp. GI); • flow studies / cardiac output; • pressure studies (e.g. blood pressure, CVP); • temperature and haemoconcentration studies.	III/B
◆ Urine output is the best routine measure of end-organ function and is therefore very useful for guiding fluid provision, although there are several potential confounding factors.	IV/C
◆ Physiological oliguria is to be expected following a major burn and does not need to be overcome.	III/B
◆ A low CVP may be a useful indicator of hypovolaemia, but in major burns, a normal or high CVP has no value in estimating intravascular filling status.	IIb/B
◆ Serial blood gas analysis is useful for detecting metabolic lactic acidosis as a consequence of hypoperfusion, but is not infallible and the various causes must be considered.	IV/C
◆ Cardiac output monitoring is a useful adjunct by which to assess adequacy of fluid resuscitation.	IIb/B
◆ Administering fluids to normalise cardiac output parameters results in greater fluid administration than by using the Parkland formula, but without improving outcomes.	Ib/A

Chapter 6

Chapter 6

Recommendations	Evidence level
◆ Thermodilution methods of cardiac output estimation (e.g. PICCO) are sufficiently accurate in major burns, but the derived intrathoracic blood volume index is an unreliable estimate of preload.	IIb/B
◆ pHi is a useful indicator of hypoperfusion in the splanchnic circulation and is more sensitive than either pressure monitoring or serial blood gas analysis.	III/B
◆ pHi correlates well with burn wound perfusion.	Ib/A
◆ Use routine intravesicular pressure monitoring for patients receiving ≥500ml/h to enable early detection of abdominal hypertension and compartment syndrome.	III/B

References

1. National Burn Care Review Committee. Standards and Strategy for Burn Care. A review of burn care in the British Isles, Jan 21, 2001.

2. Cosnett JE. The origins of intravenous fluid therapy. *Lancet* 1989; 1 (8641): 768-71.

3. Hauben DJ, Yanai E, Mahler D. On the history of the treatment of burns. *Burns* 1981; 7 (6): 383-8.

4. Sneve H. The treatment of burns and skin grafting. *JAMA* 1905; 45: 1-8

5. Harkins HN. *The Treatment of Burns.* Illinois: Charles C Thomas, 1942.

6. Cope O, Moore FD. The redistribution of body water and the fluid therapy of the burned patient. *Ann Surg* 1947; 126: 1010-45.

7. Evans EI, Purnell OJ, Robinett PW, Batchelor A, Martin M. Fluid and electrolyte requirements in severe burns. *Ann Surg* 1952; 135 (6): 804-17.

8. Reiss E, Stirmann JA, Artz CP, Davis JH, Mspacher WH. Fluid and electrolyte balance in burns. *JAMA* 1953; 152 (14): 1309-13.

9. Friedrich JB, Sullivan SR, Engrav LH, *et al.* Is supra-Baxter resuscitation in burn patients a new phenomenon? *Burns* 2004; 30 (5): 464-6.

10. Holm C, Mayr M, Tegeler J, *et al.* A clinical randomized study on the effects of invasive monitoring on burn shock resuscitation. *Burns* 2004; 30 (8): 798-807.

11. Demling RH, Mazess RB, Witt RM, Wolberg WH. The study of burn wound edema using dichromatic absorptiometry. *J Trauma* 1978; 18 (2): 124-8.

12. Kim DE, Phillips TM, Jeng JC, *et al.* Microvascular assessment of burn depth conversion during varying resuscitation conditions. *J Burn Care Rehabil* 2001; 22 (6): 406-16.

13. Brown TL, Hernon C, Owens B. Incidence of vomiting in burns and implications for mass burn casualty management. *Burns* 2003; 29 (2): 159-62.

14. Horton JW, Maass DL, White DJ, Sanders B, Murphy J. Effects of burn serum on myocardial inflammation and function. *Shock* 2004; 22 (5): 438-45.

15. Adams HR, Baxter CR, Izenberg SD. Decreased contractility and compliance of the left ventricle as complications of thermal trauma. *Am Heart J* 1984; 108 (6): 1477-87.

16. Herd BM, Herd AN, Tanner NS. Burns to the elderly: a reappraisal. *Br J Plast Surg* 1987; 40 (3): 278-82.

17. Underhill FP. The significance of anhydraemia in extensive superficial burns. *JAMA* 1930; 95: 852-7.

18. Leape IL. Kinetics of burn edema formation in primates. *Ann Surg* 1972; 176 (2): 223-6.

19. Xia ZF, He F, Barrow RE, Broemeling LD, Herndon DN. Reperfusion injury in burned rats after delayed fluid resuscitation. *J Burn Care Rehabil* 1991; 12 (5): 430-6.

20. Demling RH, LaLonde C. Early postburn lipid peroxidation: effect of ibuprofen and allopurinol. *Surgery* 1990; 107 (1): 85-93.

21. Demling RH. The burn edema process: current concepts. *J Burn Care Rehabil* 2005; 26 (3): 207-27.

22. Lightfoot E Jr, Horton JW, Maass DL, White DJ, McFarland RD, Lipsky PE. Major burn trauma in rats promotes cardiac and gastrointestinal apoptosis. *Shock* 1999; 11 (1): 29-34.

23. Zhang C, Sheng ZY, Lu Y, *et al.* (Change in apoptosis rate and expression of apoptosis-related gene of lamina propria lymphocyte and intra-epithelial lymphocyte after burn and delayed resuscitation). *Zhongguo Wei Zhong Bing Ji Jiu Yi Xue* 2003; 15 (5): 284-7.

24. Cartotto R, Choi J, Gomez M, Cooper A. A prospective study on the implications of a base deficit during fluid resuscitation. *J Burn Care Rehabil* 2003; 24 (2): 75-84.

25. Starling EH. On the absorption of fluids from the connective tissue spaces. *J Physiol* 1896; 19 (4): 312-26.

26. Colditz IG. Kinetics of tachyphylaxis to mediators of acute inflammation. *Immunology* 1985; 55 (1): 149-56.

27. Garner WL, Rodriguez JL, Miller CG, *et al.* Acute skin injury releases neutrophil chemoattractants. *Surgery* 1994; 116 (1): 42-8.

28. Harms BA, Bodai BI, Kramer GC, Demling RH. Microvascular fluid and protein flux in pulmonary and systemic

circulations after thermal injury. *Microvasc Res* 1982; 23 (1): 77-86.

29. Harms BA, Kramer GC, Bodai BI, Demling RH. Effect of hypoproteinemia on pulmonary and soft tissue edema formation. *Crit Care Med* 1981; 9 (7): 503-8.

30. Du GB, Slater H, Goldfarb IW. Influences of different resuscitation regimens on acute early weight gain in extensively burned patients. *Burns* 1991; 17 (2): 147-50.

31. Majid AA, Kingsnorth AN. *Burns. Fundamentals of Surgical Practice,* 1st Ed. London: Greenwich Medical Media Ltd., 1998: 127-34.

32. Wu P, Nelson EA, Reid WH, Ruckley CV, Gaylor JD. Water vapour transmission rates in burns and chronic leg ulcers: influence of wound dressings and comparison with *in vitro* evaluation. *Biomaterials* 1996; 17 (14): 1373-7.

33. Inoue T, Okabayashi K, Ohtani M, Yamanoue T, Wada S, Lida K. Effect of smoke inhalation injury on fluid requirement in burn resuscitation. *Hiroshima J Med Sci* 2002; 51 (1): 1-5.

34. Navar PD, Saffle JR, Warden GD. Effect of inhalation injury on fluid resuscitation requirements after thermal injury. *Am J Surg* 1985; 150 (6): 716-20.

35. Schwartz SI. Supportive therapy in burn care. Consensus summary on fluid resuscitation. *J Trauma* 1979; 19 (11 Suppl): 876-7.

36. Klein MB, Hayden D, Elson C, *et al.* The association between fluid administration and outcome following major burn: a multi-centre study. *Ann Surg* 2007; 245 (4): 622-8.

37. Baxter CR. Fluid volume and electrolyte changes of the early postburn period. *Clin Plast Surg* 1974; 1 (4): 693-703.

38. Muir IFK, Barclay TL. *Burns and their Treatment,* 1st Ed. London: Lloyd Luke Ltd., 1974.

39. Carvajal HF. A physiologic approach to fluid therapy in severely burned children. *Surg Gynecol Obstet* 1980; 150 (3): 379-84.

40. Monafo WW, Halverson JD, Schechtman K. The role of concentrated sodium solutions in the resuscitation of patients with severe burns. *Surgery* 1984; 95 (2): 129-35

41. Demling RH. Fluid Resuscitation. In: *The Art and Science of Burn Care,* 1st Ed. Boswick JA, Jr, Ed. Rockville: Aspen Publishers Inc., 1987: 189-302.

42. Buhl L. Mitteilungen aus der Pfeufer'schen Klinik: Epidemische Cholera. *Zeitschrift F Rationelle Med* 1855; 6: 1-105.

43. Davidson EC. Sodium chloride metabolism in cutaneous burns and its possible significance for a rational therapy. *Arch Surg* 1926; 13: 262-77.

44. Moyer CA, Margraf HW, Monafo WW, Jr. Burn shock and extravascular sodium deficiency - treatment with Ringer's solution with lactate. *Arch Surg* 1965; 90: 799-811.

45. Jensen AR, Hughes WB, Grewal H. Secondary abdominal compartment syndrome in children with burns and trauma: a potentially lethal complication. *J Burn Care Res* 2006; 27 (2): 242-6.

46. Oda J, Yamashita K, Inoue T, *et al.* Resuscitation fluid volume and abdominal compartment syndrome in patients with major burns. *Burns* 2006; 32 (2): 151-4.

47. Sullivan SR, Ahmadi AJ, Singh CN, *et al.* Elevated orbital pressure: another untoward effect of massive resuscitation after burn injury. *J Trauma* 2006; 60 (1): 72-6.

48. O'Mara MS, Slater H, Goldfarb IW, Caushaj PF. A prospective, randomized evaluation of intra-abdominal pressures with crystalloid and colloid resuscitation in burn patients. *J Trauma* 2005; 58 (5): 1011-8.

49. Oda J, Ueyama M, Yamashita K, *et al.* Hypertonic lactated saline resuscitation reduces the risk of abdominal compartment syndrome in severely burned patients. *J Trauma* 2006; 60 (1): 64-71.

50. Britt RC, Gannon T, Collins JN, Cole FJ, Weireter LJ, Britt LD. Secondary abdominal compartment syndrome: risk factors and outcomes. *Am Surg* 2005; 71 (11): 982-5.

51. Grocott MP, Mythen MG, Gan TJ. Perioperative fluid management and clinical outcomes in adults. *Anesth Analg* 2005; 100 (4): 1093-106.

52. Tappeiner HA. Veränderungen des Blutes und der Muskeln nach ausgedehnten Hautverbrennungen. *Zentralbl F D Med Wissensch* 1881; 31: 385.

53. Elgjo GI. Small volume hypertonic fluid treatment of burns. *J Burns & Surg Wound Care* 2003; 2 (5): 1-26.

54. Lehnhardt M, Jafari HJ, Druecke D, *et al.* A qualitative and quantitative analysis of protein loss in human burn wounds. *Burns* 2005; 31 (2): 159-67.

55. Demling RH, Kramer GC, Gunther R, Nerlich M. Effect of nonprotein colloid on postburn edema formation in soft tissues and lung. *Surgery* 1984; 95 (5): 593-602.

56. Kramer GC, Gunther RA, Nerlich ML, Zweifach SS, Demling RH. Effect of dextran-70 on increased microvascular fluid and protein flux after thermal injury. *Circ Shock* 1982; 9 (5): 529-41.

57. Baxter CR, Marvin J, Curreri PW. Fluid and electrolyte therapy of burn shock. *Heart Lung* 1973; 2 (5): 707-13.

58. Goodwin CW, Dorethy J, Lam V, Pruitt BA, Jr. Randomized trial of efficacy of crystalloid and colloid resuscitation on hemodynamic response and lung water following thermal injury. *Ann Surg* 1983; 197 (5): 520-31.

59. Schildt B, Bouveng R, Sollenberg M. Plasma substitute induced impairment of the reticuloendothelial system function. *Acta Chir Scand* 1975; 141 (1): 7-13.

60. Roberts I, Alderson P, Bunn F, Chinnock P, Ker K, Schierhout G. Colloids versus crystalloids for fluid resuscitation in critically ill patients. *Cochrane Database Syst Rev* 2004; (4): CD000567.

61. Haljamäe H, Dahlqvist M, Walentin F. Artificial colloids in clinical practice: pros and cons. *Baillière's Clin Anaesthesiol* 1997; 11: 49-79.

62. Traylor RJ, Pearl RG. Crystalloid versus colloid: all colloids are not created equal. *Anesth Analg* 1996; 83 (2): 209-12.

63. Zikria BA, Subbarao C, Oz MC, *et al.* Macromolecules reduce abnormal microvascular permeability in rat limb ischemia-reperfusion injury. *Crit Care Med* 1989; 17(12): 1306-9.

64. Zikria BA, King TC, Stanford J, Freeman HP. A biophysical approach to capillary permeability. *Surgery* 1989; 105(5): 625-31.

Chapter 6

65. Traber LD, Brazeal BA, Schmitz M, *et al.* Pentafraction reduces the lung lymph response after endotoxin administration in the ovine model. *Circ Shock* 1992; 36 (2): 93-103.

66. Waters LM, Christensen MA, Sato RM. Hetastarch: an alternative colloid in burn shock management. *J Burn Care Rehabil* 1989; 10 (1): 11-6.

67. Ferrara JJ, Dyess DL, Collins JN, *et al.* Effects of pentafraction administration on microvascular permeability alterations induced by graded thermal injury. *Surgery* 1994; 115 (2): 182-9.

68. Brazeal BA, Honeycutt D, Traber LD, Toole JG, Herndon DN, Traber DL. Pentafraction for superior resuscitation of the ovine thermal burn. *Crit Care Med* 1995; 23 (2): 332-9.

69. Jungheinrich C, Neff TA. Pharmacokinetics of hydroxyethyl starch. *Clin Pharmacokinet* 2005; 44 (7): 681-99.

70. Vogt NH, Bothner U, Lerch G, Lindner KH, Georgieff M. Large-dose administration of 6% hydroxyethyl starch 200/0.5 in total hip arthroplasty: plasma homeostasis, hemostasis, and renal function compared to use of 5% human albumin. *Anesth Analg* 1996; 83 (2): 262-8.

71. Coats TJ, Heron M. Does calcium cause the different effects of Gelofusine and Haemaccel on coagulation? *Emerg Med J* 2006; 23 (3): 193-4.

72. Damas P, Adam A, Buret J, *et al.* In vivo studies on Haemaccel-fibronectin interaction in man. *Eur J Clin Invest* 1987; 17 (2): 166-73.

73. Brazil EV, Coats TJ. Sonoclot coagulation analysis of *in vitro* haemodilution with resuscitation solutions. *J R Soc Med* 2000; 93 (10): 507-10.

74. Videm V, Mollnes TE. Human complement activation by polygeline and dextran 70. *Scand J Immunol* 1994; 39 (3): 314-20.

75. ten Dam MA, Branten AJ, Klasen IS, Wetzels JF. The gelatin-derived plasma substitute Gelofusine causes low-molecular-weight proteinuria by decreasing tubular protein reabsorption. *J Crit Care* 2001; 16 (3): 115-20.

76. Hall KV, Sørensen B. The treatment of burn shock: results of a 5-year randomised, controlled clinical trial of Dextran 70 v. Ringer's lactate solution. *Burns* 1978; 5 (1): 107-12.

77. Cochrane Injuries Group Albumin Reviewers. Human albumin administration in critically ill patients: systematic review of randomised controlled trials. *Br Med J* 1998; 317 (7153): 235-40.

78. Finfer S, Bellomo R, Boyce N, French J, Myburgh J, Norton R. A comparison of albumin and saline for fluid resuscitation in the intensive care unit. *N Engl J Med* 2004; 350 (22): 2247-56.

79. Alderson P, Bunn F, Lefebvre C, *et al.* Human albumin solution for resuscitation and volume expansion in critically ill patients. *Cochrane Database Syst Rev* 2004; (4): CD001208.

80. Cooper AB, Cohn SM, Zhang HS, Hanna K, Stewart TE, Slutsky AS. Five percent albumin for adult burn shock resuscitation: lack of effect on daily multiple organ dysfunction score. *Transfusion* 2006; 46 (1): 80-89.

81. Milner SM, Kinsky MP, Guha SC, Herndon DN, Phillips LG, Kramer GC. A comparison of two different 2400 mOsm solutions for resuscitation of major burns. *J Burn Care Rehabil* 1997; 18 (2): 109-15.

82. Gavras H, Bain GT, Bland L, Vlahakos D, Gavras I. Hypertensive response to saline microinjection in the area of the nucleus tractus solitarii of the rat. *Brain Res* 1985; 343 (1): 113-9.

83. Bouskela E, Grampp W, Mellander S. Effects of hypertonic NaCl solution on microvascular haemodynamics in normo- and hypovolaemia. *Acta Physiol Scand* 1990; 140 (1): 85-94.

84. Mazzoni MC, Borgstrom P, Intaglietta M, Arfors KE. Capillary narrowing in hemorrhagic shock is rectified by hyperosmotic saline-dextran reinfusion. *Circ Shock* 1990; 31 (4): 407-18.

85. Bunn F, Roberts I, Tasker R, Akpa E. Hypertonic versus near isotonic crystalloid for fluid resuscitation in critically ill patients. *Cochrane Database Syst Rev* 2004; (3): CD002045.

86. Adams HR, Baxter CR, Parker JL. Contractile function of heart muscle from burned guinea pigs. *Circ Shock* 1982; 9 (1): 63-73.

87. Horton JW, White DJ, Baxter CR. Hypertonic saline dextran resuscitation of thermal injury. *Ann Surg* 1990; 211 (3): 301-11.

88. Horton JW, Maass DL, White J, Sanders B. Hypertonic saline-dextran suppresses burn-related cytokine secretion by cardiomyocytes. *Am J Physiol Heart Circ Physiol* 2001; 280 (4): H1591-601.

89. Elgjo GI, Mathew BP, Poli de Figueriedo LF, *et al.* Resuscitation with hypertonic saline dextran improves cardiac function *in vivo* and *ex vivo* after burn injury in sheep. *Shock* 1998; 9 (5): 375-83

90. Zhou J, Liu D, Wang Z, Zhu P. Effect of hypertonic saline solution on the left ventricular functions of isolated hearts from burned rats. *Chin J Traumatol* 2002; 5 (3): 151-5.

91. Brown JM, Grosso MA, Moore EE. Hypertonic saline and dextran: impact on cardiac function in the isolated rat heart. *J Trauma* 1990; 30 (6): 646-50.

92. Angle N, Hoyt DB, Coimbra R, *et al.* Hypertonic saline resuscitation diminishes lung injury by suppressing neutrophil activation after hemorrhagic shock. *Shock* 1998; 9 (3): 164-70.

93. Angle N, Hoyt DB, Cabello-Passini R, Herdon-Remelius C, Loomis W, Junger WG. Hypertonic saline resuscitation reduces neutrophil margination by suppressing neutrophil L selectin expression. *J Trauma* 1998; 45 (1): 7-12.

94. Barone M, Jimenez F, Huxley VH, Yang XF. Morphologic analysis of the cerebral microcirculation after thermal injury and the response to fluid resuscitation. *Acta Neurochir Suppl* 1997; 70: 267-8.

95. Junger WG, Coimbra R, Liu FC, *et al.* Hypertonic saline resuscitation: a tool to modulate immune function in trauma patients? *Shock* 1997; 8 (4): 235-41.

96. Pascual JM, Watson JC, Runyon AE, Wade CE, Kramer GC. Resuscitation of intra-operative hypovolemia: a comparison of normal saline and hyperosmotic/hyperoncotic solutions in swine. *Crit Care Med* 1992; 20 (2): 200-10.

97. Bortolani A, Governa M, Barisoni D. Fluid replacement in burned patients. *Acta Chir Plast* 1996; 38 (4): 132-6.

98. Huang PP, Stucky FS, Dimick AR, Treat RC, Bessey PQ, Rue LW. Hypertonic sodium resuscitation is associated with renal failure and death. *Ann Surg* 1995; 221 (5): 543-54.

99. Kien ND, Moore PG, Pascual JM, Reitan JA, Kramer GC. Effects of hypertonic saline on regional function and blood flow in canine hearts during acute coronary occlusion. *Shock* 1997; 7 (4): 274-81.

100. Chen Y, Hu Y, Sun J. (The effects of hypertonic and balanced saline solutions on burn shock resuscitation in burned rats). *Zhonghua Zheng Xing Shao Shang Wai Ke Za Zhi* 1994; 10 (1): 73-5.

101. Chen LW, Hwang B, Chang WJ, Wang JS, Chen JS, Hsu CM. Inducible nitric oxide synthase inhibitor reverses exacerbating effects of hypertonic saline on lung injury in burn. *Shock* 2004; 22 (5): 472-7.

102. Chen LW, Hwang B, Wang JS, Chen JS, Hsu CM. Hypertonic saline-enhanced postburn gut barrier failure is reversed by inducible nitric oxide synthase inhibition. *Crit Care Med* 2004; 32 (12): 2476-84.

103. Harada T, Izaki S, Tsutsumi H, Kobayashi M, Kitamura K. Apoptosis of hair follicle cells in the second-degree burn wound under hypernatremic conditions. *Burns* 1998; 24 (5): 464-9.

104. McKee AC, Winkelman MD, Banker BQ. Central pontine myelinolysis in severely burned patients: relationship to serum hyperosmolality. *Neurology* 1988; 38 (8): 1211-7.

105. Kuntscher MV, Germann G, Hartmann B. Correlations between cardiac output, stroke volume, central venous pressure, intra-abdominal pressure and total circulating blood volume in resuscitation of major burns. *Resuscitation* 2006; 70 (1): 37-43.

106. Holm C, Mayr M, Horbrand F, *et al.* Reproducibility of transpulmonary thermodilution measurements in patients with burn shock and hypothermia. *J Burn Care Rehabil* 2005; 26 (3): 260-5.

107. Kuntscher MV, Czermak C, Blome-Eberwein S, Dacho A, Germann G. Transcardiopulmonary thermal dye versus single thermodilution methods for assessment of intrathoracic blood volume and extravascular lung water in major burn resuscitation. *J Burn Care Rehabil* 2003; 24 (3): 142-7.

108. Light TD, Jeng JC, Jain AK, *et al.* The 2003 Carl A Moyer Award: real-time metabolic monitors, ischemia-reperfusion, titration endpoints, and ultraprecise burn resuscitation. *J Burn Care Rehabil* 2004; 25 (1): 33-44.

109. Renshaw A, Childs C. The significance of peripheral skin temperature measurement during the acute phase of burn injury: an illustrative case report. *Burns* 2000; 26 (8): 750-3.

110. Gomersall CD, Joynt GM, Freebairn RC, Hung V, Buckley TA, Oh TE. Resuscitation of critically ill patients based on the results of gastric tonometry: a prospective, randomized, controlled trial. *Crit Care Med* 2000; 28 (3): 607-14.

111. Venkatesh B, Meacher R, Muller MJ, Morgan TJ, Fraser J. Monitoring tissue oxygenation during resuscitation of major burns. *J Trauma* 2001; 50 (3): 485-94.

112. Thorniley MS, Sinclair JS, Barnett NJ, Shurey CB, Green CJ. The use of near-infrared spectroscopy for assessing flap viability during reconstructive surgery. *Br J Plast Surg* 1998; 51 (3): 218-26.

113. Edsander-Nord A, Rojdmark J, Wickman M. Metabolism in pedicled and free TRAM flaps: a comparison using the microdialysis technique. *Plast Reconstr Surg* 2002; 109 (2): 664-73.

114. Samuelsson A, Steinvall I, Sjoberg F. Microdialysis shows metabolic effects in skin during fluid resuscitation in burn-injured patients. *Crit Care* 2006; 10 (6): R172.

115. Shah A, Connolly CM, Kirschner RA, Herndon DN, Kramer GC. Evaluation of hyperdynamic resuscitation in 60% TBSA burn-injured sheep. *Shock* 2004; 21 (1): 86-92.

116. Papp A, Uusaro A, Parviainen I, Hartikainen J, Ruokonen E. Myocardial function and haemodynamics in extensive burn trauma: evaluation by clinical signs, invasive monitoring, echocardiography and cytokine concentrations. A prospective clinical study. *Acta Anaesthesiol Scand* 2003; 47 (10): 1257-63.

Chapter 6

Chapter 6

Chapter 7

Improving outcome in paediatric burns

Siobhán O'Ceallaigh MD AFRCSI

Specialist Registrar, Plastic Surgery

Mamta Shah PhD FRCS (Plast.)

Consultant Burns and Plastic Surgeon

BOOTH HALL CHILDREN'S HOSPITAL, MANCHESTER, UK

Introduction

Optimising the management of burn injured paediatric patients is of the utmost importance because the potential sequelae are manifest not only in the critical developmental stages of childhood, but also over the course of their entire adult life with implications for the provision of surgical, medical, psychological and rehabilitation services. Much of paediatric burn care has traditionally been based upon experience and anecdotes rather than a high level of evidence. However, in recent times, there has been a move towards evidence-based practices with emerging randomised controlled trials (RCT), particularly in the critical care setting.

The role of this chapter is to review the available practices pertaining to paediatric burn care which impact upon outcome and to ascertain the levels of evidence to justify their continuation.

Methodology

PubMed and EMBASE searches were employed to collect the evidence using the search terms 'paediatric burn' and 'outcome'. This was supplemented by hand searches of references in the collected articles.

In 2003, the American Burn Association identified a number of key areas where improvements in paediatric burn outcomes could be made and compiled a research programme to promote evidenced-based research into these areas [1]. They included critical care and ventilation issues, psychosocial factors of child and family, and cost-effectiveness in burn care delivery.

Airway management

Inhalational injury remains a major cause of morbidity, prolonged ICU and hospital stay, and mortality in paediatric burns patients.

Prolonged airway access for mechanical ventilation of critically ill children can be provided by the translaryngeal route or by tracheostomy. Airway management in children can be difficult as the paediatric trachea is relatively short. This increases the incidence of endotracheal tube malpositioning or

Chapter 7

displacement. The more anteriorly-placed vocal cords in the child also make intubation problematic, with the diameter of the airway being smaller and more likely to obstruct as a result of inhalation injury.

Prolonged translaryngeal intubation can be associated with subglottic and laryngeal stenosis, vocal cord ulceration, accidental extubation and tracheomalacia. A potential solution to this problem is tracheostomy. However, in the past, tracheostomy has been blamed for a higher incidence of tracheostomy site infections and pneumonia in adults [2], and tracheal stenosis requiring reconstruction in younger children [3].

The literature is generally lacking in high level evidence-based data clearly supporting either tracheostomy or translaryngeal intubation as the optimum mode of prolonged airway access in children. Recently, retrospective case studies have been reported supporting the use of early tracheostomy in paediatric inhalation injury. Barret *et al* [4] demonstrated a significantly lower incidence of subglottic stenosis in patients who had translaryngeal intubation converted to tracheostomy before day ten post-injury, compared with those converted after ten days **(III/B)**. Furthermore, tracheomalacia occurred more frequently in patients requiring airway pressures higher than 50cm H_2O (4.9 kPa) for more than ten days. The incidence of pneumonia was similar in intubated and tracheostomy patients. These findings, in support of early tracheostomy, have been corroborated by other studies [5]. However, one recent study has advocated the practice of prolonged translaryngeal intubation [6] citing improvements in the availability of larger low-pressure cuffs, limiting cuff and peak inflating pressures, as the reason for fewer complications with prolonged translaryngeal intubation **(III/B)**.

Ventilation

Advances in burn care, in particular early excision, fluid resuscitation and improved nutritional support, have improved survival and reduced mortality in the paediatric burn population. Unfortunately, respiratory failure continues to represent a major source of morbidity and mortality in children with severe burns. The current standard of care for burned children

requiring artificial ventilation is conventional volume cycled or pressure limited mechanical ventilation. This can exacerbate pulmonary parenchymal injury through oxygen toxicity. Mechanical ventilation may over-distend and/or repeatedly open and close alveoli. It may also play a role in the development of multi-organ failure by amplifying the systemic inflammatory response [7]. The goal of mechanical ventilation is, therefore, to provide adequate gas exchange at the lowest possible inspired oxygen concentration and peak airway pressure.

The development of high frequency percussive ventilation (HFPV) (Figure 1) offers the potential for achieving this goal. HFPV is a hybrid of conventional mechanical ventilation and high-frequency oscillatory ventilation and provides an option to support ventilation at lower airway pressures and mean lung volumes than conventional ventilation in the pressure control mode. This is accomplished by using tidal volumes less than dead space, delivered at supraphysiological frequencies. This ensures a relatively constant lung volume, resulting in a more homogenous gas distribution, a reduction in regional over-inflation and atelectasis, and prevents barotrauma of more compliant lung segments. Cioffi [8] has demonstrated an improvement in survival and a decreased incidence of pneumonia and mortality with prophylactic use of HFPV in adult burn patients with inhalational injury. Other studies [9, 10] compared conventional mechanical ventilation with HFPV in separate randomised controlled trials in children with inhalational injury and demonstrated significantly lower peak inspiratory pressures, and achieved a significantly higher PaO_2/FiO_2 ratio with HFPV. No child demonstrated barotrauma in the HFPV groups **(Ib/A)**.

Burns metabolism

Severe burns are associated with an acute and persistent hyper-metabolic response characterised by pyrexia, a hyperdynamic circulation, changes in vascular permeability, impairment of gut function, and increased circulating levels of catabolic hormones, leading to increased oxygen consumption and protein and fat wasting. This vulnerable hypermetabolic state depresses the immune system and attenuates wound

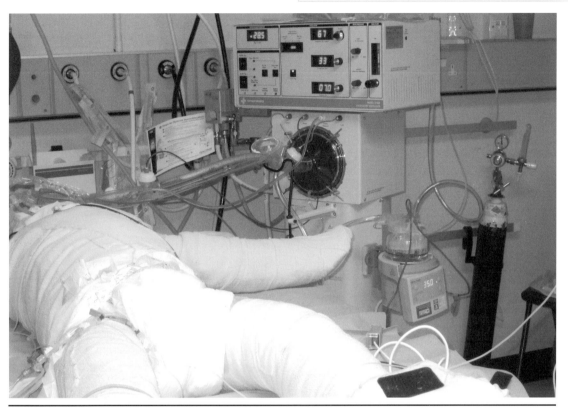

Figure 1. A patient receiving high frequency percussive ventilation (HFPV).

healing. It begins within five hours of injury and can last for up to two years [11], long after the burn wounds have healed. Traditionally, the response was to treat with nutritional support alone, but more recently, recognition of its prolonged detrimental effects has led to the development of measures to try and ameliorate this abnormal physiology. The principal target of these measures is muscle catabolism. Pereira *et al* [12] identified the modulation of the hypermetabolic response as an effective measure of burn care outcome. The approaches used to achieve this are three-fold:

- Firstly, early excision and re-surfacing of the burn wound.
- Secondly, nutritional support to achieve a sufficiently high-caloric enteral intake to ameliorate muscle catabolism.
- Thirdly, limitation of the hypermetabolic response by the administration of pharmacological and hormonal agents.

Early excision and skin grafting

Early burn wound excision is regarded as the main factor in the decline of invasive burn infection and improved survival. With early excision, it is less common for a child to succumb to burn injury of any size even when it is associated with inhalational injury. The burn wound is considered to be a major source of the inflammatory mediators which play an important role in the initiation and maintenance of the post-burn inflammatory response.

A major breakthrough in excisional burn surgery in recent years has been the reduction in the volume of intra-operative blood loss and the amount of blood products administered peri-operatively. Sub-eschar infiltration with adrenaline and the prevention of intra-operative hypothermia have both contributed to this [13]. Early trials by Pietsch *et al* [14] and Tompkins *et al* [15], have shown such excellent mortality statistics in children treated by early excision that it is difficult to contemplate randomisation away from this treatment modality **(Ia/A)**. A more recent paper by Xiao-Wu *et al* [16] demonstrated longer hospital stays and a higher incidence of invasive wound infection and sepsis in patients with delayed wound excision and grafting, although a difference in mortality or number of operations was not seen between early and delayed excision patient groups. Barret *et al* [17], in a case controlled trial of 35 severely burned children, divided the groups into an early excision group and initial conservative management with silver sulphadiazine, and demonstrated a prolongation of the hypermetabolic response in the conservatively treated cohort. A decrease in pro-inflammatory cytokines such as C-reactive protein, TNF-a, IL-6 and IL-10 was seen after early excisional surgery. Also, levels of IGF-1 and growth hormone were significantly lower in the delayed excision group.

Nutrition

Recognition that the hypermetabolic state exists in burn patients for many months after wound closure, and that adverse consequences of inadequately supported catabolism may be encountered, has ensured that nutritional support of burns in children remains at the forefront of the management regimen. It is generally accepted that enteral nutrition is superior to parenteral nutrition, as it maintains gastro-intestinal integrity and function. Enteral nutrition minimises bacterial translocation, suppresses the hypermetabolic response, enhances protein uptake and is associated with a lower incidence of sepsis and length of hospital stay compared with intravenous nutrition. Relative risks of early enteral nutrition include metabolic complications such as hyperglycaemia, electrolyte imbalances, diarrhoea, pulmonary aspiration and intestinal necrosis. Gottschlich *et al* [18] investigated the effectiveness and safety of early enteral feeding in paediatric patients with burns in excess of 25% total body surface area in a randomised controlled prospective study. Seventy-seven patients were randomised to either early enteral feeding (<24 hours post-burn injury) or control (>48 hours). Nutrient intake was measured daily, indirect calorimetry was performed biweekly, and blood and urine samples were obtained for the assay of cortisol, glucagon, insulin, gastrin, epinephrine, norepinephrine, dopamine, triiodothyronine, tetraiodothyronine, albumin, transferrin, prealbumin, retinol-binding protein, glucose, nitrogen balance, and 3-methylhistidine throughout the study period. The delayed feeding group demonstrated a significant caloric deficit during post-burn week one and two. Serum insulin and triiodothyronine were higher in the early fed group during post-burn week one. A decrease in 3-methylhistidine output (suggesting a decrease in protein breakdown) was also evident during that period. No statistically significant difference in the incidence of adverse events occurred between the two groups **(Ib/A)**.

The authors concluded that while provision of enteral nutrients shortly after burn injury reduces caloric deficits and may stimulate insulin secretion and protein retention during the early phase post-burn, their study did not necessarily reaffirm the safety of early enteral feeding, nor could they associate earlier feeding with a direct improvement in endocrine status or a reduction in morbidity, mortality, hypermetabolism, or hospital stay.

Hart *et al* [19], in a study of high carbohydrate diet in severe paediatric burns, demonstrated that carbohydrate is more effective than fat at improving skeletal muscle protein balance due to a reduction in muscle catabolic rate in association with higher insulin concentrations. This supported earlier work by these investigators [20] which showed that insulin could promote muscle anabolism without eliciting a hypoglycemic response.

Glutamine

The non-essential amino acids, glutamine and arginine, appear to play critical roles in paediatric burns [21]. Using stable isotope tracer techniques, studies have demonstrated a relative deficiency in the hypermetabolic burn patient [22] which may have effects on infectious and other complications. To date no randomised controlled trials of significant sample size in paediatric burns have been published, but Sheridan *et al* [23] demonstrated that short-term enteral glutamine (GLN) administration (48 hours) did not result in an immediate whole body protein gain in paediatric burn patients and suggested that several days of supplementation may be required to restore plasma glutamine levels and stimulate protein synthesis. The need for, and safety of, long-term GLN supplementation requires further investigation. Large RCTs may help strengthen recommendations for routine GLN supplementation in paediatric burn patients.

Growth hormone

Recombinant human growth hormone (rHGH) has been shown to have beneficial effects in the treatment of patients with major trauma, sepsis and burns. Improved muscle protein synthesis and preservation of lean body mass, accelerated wound healing, improved height and weight, and elevated bone-mineral content up to one year post-injury are some of the benefits of treatment [24] **(Ib/A)**. Gilpin et al [25] in a randomised controlled trial evaluated two forms of rHGH administered in the acute admission phase and reported that both groups showed a significant reduction in donor-site healing time compared with placebo.

rHGH has been shown to have an increased mortality rate when administered to critically ill adult patients [26], mainly due to the augmentation of the hepatic acute phase. However, in a prospective randomised controlled trial of 28 burned children receiving 0.2mg/kg/day rHGH or placebo, Ramirez et al [27] demonstrated that the increase in mortality seen in adults was not replicated in paediatric burn patients. Concerns about adverse effects on long-term scarring have also been alleviated by Barret et al [28] following a randomised controlled trial showing no difference in scarring intensity between patients receiving 0.2mg/kg/day rHGH and placebo for seven days during hospitalisation. These findings were supported by de Oliveira et al with results from longer-term treatment post-discharge (up to one year post-burn) with rHGH [29].

Androgens

Restoring testosterone levels to normal in young burned adults markedly improves protein synthetic efficiency. Testosterone increases protein synthesis due to its anabolic androgenic effects, but it may result in hepatotoxicity, acne, and, in females, hirsutism and virilisation. Oxandrolone, an oral synthetic analogue of testosterone, has minimal virilising activity and little hepatotoxicity by comparison with testosterone. Oxandrolone improves lean body mass in both adult and paediatric patients by increasing anabolic gene expression and improving net protein balance [30]. When compared with rHGH, fewer complications were noted with oxandrolone.

The research group at Galveston enrolled children with burns greater than 40% total body surface area into a randomised controlled trial to receive oxandrolone as a long-term anabolic agent [31]. Lean body mass (LBM), bone mineral content (BMC) and bone mineral density (BMD) were measured by dual energy X-ray absorptiometry at discharge (95% healed) and at 6, 9, and 12 months after the burn. With oxandrolone, LBM was significantly greater at 6, 9, and 12 months post-burn compared with controls, and BMC significantly greater at 12 months. Liver transaminases were unaffected. This suggests that long-term administration of oxandrolone safely improves LBM, BMC, and BMD in severely burned children **(Ib/A)**.

IGF

Modulation of Types I and II acute phase reactants and attenuation of muscle catabolism has been demonstrated using a combination of insulin-like growth factor-1 (IGF-1) with its binding protein-3 (IGFBP-3) in severely burned children [32, 33]. Animal studies of local liposomal IGF-1 gene transfer have also shown attenuation of mRNA expression of the inflammatory cytokines IL-1beta and TNF-alpha in the burn wound [34].

An increased ratio of (pro-:anti-) inflammatory cytokines may indicate a higher risk for the incidence of multi-organ failure. Jeschke et al [35] administered a continuous infusion of IGF-I/BP-3 (treatment group) or saline (control group) for five days after wound excision and grafting. Serum pre-albumin and cholinesterase increased with IGF-I/BP-3, whereas serum creatinine decreased when compared with controls. IGF-I/BP-3 also significantly improved cardiac index and stroke volume index. These

Chapter 7

improvements in organ homeostasis were associated with decreased ratios of (pro-:anti-) inflammatory cytokines in the IGF-I/BP-3 group when compared with controls, suggesting that such measurement can be used to predict organ function **(IIa/B)**.

Propranolol

Beta-blockade with propanolol has been shown to have anabolic activity, decreasing cardiac work, and increasing expression of anabolic substances in the muscles of burned children. Paediatric burn patients treated with propranolol had significantly reduced resting energy expenditure and predicted resting energy expenditure compared with the control group [36, 37] **(Ib/A)**.

Impact of follow-up by multi-disciplinary team on long-term outcomes

With increased survival of children with massive burns, long-term outcomes are becoming increasingly important. The existent data on children surviving massive burns are compromised by short-term follow-up, small sample size, selection bias, lack of standardised outcome measures, high dropout or non-participation rates, and lack of injury severity adjustments. Few long-term outcome studies of children with massive burns have been published. One study by Sheridan *et al* in 2000 [38] used the Short Form-36 (SF-36) in a retrospective, cross-sectional study in a regional paediatric burn centre of 80 patients younger than 18 years at the time of injury, who survived massive burns involving >70% of the body surface, and who were evaluated an average of 14.7 years after injury. The SF-36 is a generic quality-of-life measurement tool used in a number of chronic diseases and injury disorders. It measures general health, social and emotional roles, and physical roles and functioning. Its main limitation in the study of burns patients is that it does not directly measure quality of life associated with physical appearance. This study found that while 15-20% of children studied demonstrated lower level physical functioning than the general population, the majority had scores comparable with the normal population. Children followed up consistently in the multi-disciplinary burn clinic for two years had higher level physical functioning illustrating the importance of experienced multi-disciplinary aftercare with coordinated physical and occupational therapy, scar management, reconstructive surgery, and family support **(III/B)**.

Psychosocial aspects of paediatric burns

Although it is commonly believed that injury size is the principal determinant of outcome, quality of life, social and emotional factors are also thought to have a major influence. The various psychological reactions to burn injury include depression, anxiety and a broad spectrum of transient and long-term psychological reactions such as body image issues and academic difficulties. Sleep disturbances are also found to be common among burn victims. In addition, El Hamaoui *et al* [39] reported somatic complaints in paediatric burn patients. Finally, burn injury has been found to impact upon social, educational, and occupational functioning as well as medical compliance [40].

Support provided by family and peers appears to play a significant role in youth adjustment after burn injury. It also mediates in helping children cope with stressors. Direct family support and family relationships were found to influence psychological adjustment after burn injury [41].

Pain relief

Burn-related pain includes not only background pain due to the thermal injury, but also the acute pain associated with invasive procedures and exercises, and the chronic itching which develops as the burn wound heals. Significant progress has been made in dealing with the inevitable pain and anxiety associated with burns in children. A number of specific projects have documented both pharmacological and non-pharmacological interventions to improve the quality of pain control for paediatric patients with burn injuries. The availability of validated measures for assessing pain has also increased, allowing for improvements in the evaluation of paediatric pain as well as specific pain control interventions.

Most burn centres have integrated analgesia guidelines into protocols, providing critical pathways for improved care [42]. Multi-disciplinary assessment helps to combine psychological and pharmacological pain-relieving interventions to reduce emotional and mental stress, along with overall family stress. Management of these problems may reduce long-term emotional sequelae [43].

Pharmacological management remains the cornerstone of pain control. The synergistic relationship between opioids and benzodiazepines has become more appreciated in paediatric burns. In a survey of 85 paediatric burn centres, Martin-Herz [44] reported that intravenous morphine was by far the most commonly used analgesic for control of wound care pain in all age groups followed by oral paracetamol and codeine phosphate, then oral morphine.

The use of ketamine [45] and midazolam [46] for children undergoing interventional procedures has been shown to be an effective combination and avoids the gastro-intestinal and respiratory side effects encountered with prolonged opiate use. Humphries *et al* [47] demonstrated the superior effectiveness of oral ketamine over paracetamol and codeine phosphate, for procedural pain in an RCT of 19 paediatric burn patients **(Ib/A)**.

Borland *et al* [48] showed an equivalent analgesic effectiveness of intra-nasal fentanyl (INF) to oral morphine. INF can be titrated during dressing changes and unlike oral morphine, which must be given an hour before dressings, INF may be given just 15 minutes prior to the procedure.

Non-pharmacological adjuvants for pain control include distraction therapy for the very young and music/art therapy and relaxation for older children and adolescents. More recently, hypnosis and virtual reality techniques have been applied; however, their effectiveness has not been convincingly proven.

Functional outcome

Reports of functional outcome following burn injury have primarily focused on isolated components of a child's performance, related to school, activities of daily living, self-esteem, and developmental status. Many studies concentrate on the functional outcome from severe burns (>70% TBSA) with comparatively little attention given to the impact of smaller burns (less than 20% body surface area) on patients' health status after their return to normal life. Small burns can also have significant functional consequences following burns to special areas such as the hands [49].

In a review of the available literature from 1966 to 2003, van Baar *et al* [50] analysed 50 empirical studies, using the International Classification of Functioning, disabilities and health (ICF), as released by the World Health Organisation, as a framework to describe functional consequences of burns. In less than half of the publications, attention was paid to function related solely to movement and to function of the skin, and none of the publications reviewed gave sufficient information to fully estimate the functional consequences of burns. It was recommended that a standard core set for measurement and reporting of functional outcome after burns be developed.

Prevention of hypertrophic scarring (HTS)

There are some data that suggest the application of growth factors to wounds may improve scarring. Basic fibroblast growth factor (bFGF) demonstrates endogenous immunolocalisation in the human dermis in partial-thickness burns from day four to day 11. It is thought that bFGF participates in cutaneous wound healing by activating local macrophages up to the remodelling phase, which occurs several weeks after injury. bFGF in burn wounds may be a presynthesised mediator that is released locally from injury sites and thus may play an important role in early wound healing. Accelerated wound healing may lead to improved scarring. To elucidate the effects of bFGF on second-degree pediatric burn wounds, a recent comparative study was performed by Akita *et al* [51]. Paediatric patients with mixed aetiological burns were divided into two groups: conventional dressings (n=10) and treatment with spray-on bFGF (n=10). A moisture meter, used to objectively measure the stratum corneum and epithelial-mesenchymal functions, was used to assess scars at least one year after wound healing. Children treated with bFGF showed less damaging function of the stratum corneum after healing both in clinical assessment and moisture meter analysis **(III/B)**.

The importance of wound healing time and estimation of burn depth in the prevention of HTS has long been recognised by burns surgeons; however, little mention of this occurs in the literature. Recently, Cubison et al [52] studied 337 children with scalds of intermediate thickness, whose scars were monitored for up to five years. They correlated the relationship between healing time and the development of HTS. For scalds treated with dressings alone there was a direct correlation between length of time to healing and the development of HTS. For those scalds where skin grafting took place there was a much higher incidence of HTS in the 10-14 days group compared with the 15-21 days group. The authors conclude that

there is a low risk of HTS formation in scalds healed before 21 days, and that surgery should be reserved for scalds likely to take more than three weeks to heal.

Conclusions

This chapter has reviewed the available evidence supporting all aspects of the management of children post-burn injury. In no other area of trauma care are the benefits of multi-disciplinary teamwork and comprehensive care, from injury, through recovery and beyond, more evident as in paediatric burn care. Continuing research into improving outcomes is required, with an emphasis on high quality RCTs supplanting more anecdotal and non-evidence-based practices.

Recommendations	Evidence level
◆ Maintenance of airway pressures below 4.9kPa and conversion of the artificial airway to tracheostomy before day ten post-injury may be advisable in patients requiring long-term ventilation to prevent late complications.	III/B
◆ Use of lower pressure cuffs and peak inflationary pressures in prolonged translaryngeal intubation may prevent complications.	III/B
◆ Early enteral nutrition should be instituted to prevent significant caloric deficit in large paediatric burns.	Ib/A
◆ 0.2mg/kg/day rHGH administered as an intramuscular injection has beneficial effects in modulating the catabolic response in major paediatric burns and can be self-administered post-discharge for one year post-injury.	Ib/A
◆ Early excision of full-thickness burns is advocated to ameliorate the hypermetabolic response.	Ia/A
◆ Long-term oxandrolone promotes lean body mass and bone mineral content in children with large burns.	Ib/A
◆ IGF-I/BP-3 administration may have a beneficial effect on organ function by modulating the effect of pro-inflammatory cytokines.	IIa/B
◆ Outcome quality is enhanced by long-term follow-up by a multi-disciplinary specialist burns team.	III/B
◆ Treatment of burns with bFGF may have a preventative effect on the development of problem scarring.	III/B

References

1. American Burn Association. Outcomes measurement in pediatric burn care: an agenda for research: executive summary and final report. *J Burn Care Rehabil* 2003; 24: 269-74.

2. Hunt JL, Purdue GF, Gunning T. Is tracheostomy warranted in the burn patient? Indications and complications. *J Burn Care Rehabil* 1986; 7: 492-5.

3. Prescott CA. Peristomal complications of paediatric tracheostomy. *Int J Pediatr Otorhinolaryngol* 1992; 23: 141-9.

4. Barret JP, Desai MH, Herndon DN. Effects of tracheostomies on infection and airway complications in pediatric burn patients. *Burns* 2000; 26: 190-3.

5. Palmieri TL, Jackson W, Greenhalgh DG. Benefits of early tracheostomy in severely burned children. *Crit Care Med* 2002; 30: 922-4.

6. Kadilak PR, Vanasse S, Sheridan RL. Favorable short- and long-term outcomes of prolonged translaryngeal intubation in critically ill children. *J Burn Care Rehabil* 2004; 25: 262-5.

7. Slutsky AS, Tremblay LN. Multiple system organ failure. Is mechanical ventilation a contributing factor? *Am J Respir Crit Care Med* 1998; 157: 1721-5.

8. Cioffi WG, Jr., Rue LW, III, Graves TA, McManus WF, Mason AD, Jr., Pruitt BA, Jr. Prophylactic use of high-frequency percussive ventilation in patients with inhalation injury. *Ann Surg* 1991; 213: 575-80.

9. Cortiella J, Mlcak R, Herndon D. High frequency percussive ventilation in pediatric patients with inhalation injury. *J Burn Care Rehabil* 1999; 20: 232-5.

10. Carman B, Cahill T, Warden G, McCall J. A prospective, randomized comparison of the volume diffusive respirator vs conventional ventilation for ventilation of burned children. 2001 ABA paper. *J Burn Care Rehabil* 2002; 23: 444-8.

11. Reiss E, Pearson E, Artz CP. The metabolic response to burns. *J Clin Invest* 1956; 35: 62-77.

12. Pereira C, Murphy K, Herndon D. Outcome measures in burn care. Is mortality dead? *Burns* 2004; 30: 761-71.

13. Sheridan RL, Szyfelbein SK. Staged high-dose epinephrine clysis is safe and effective in extensive tangential burn excisions in children. *Burns* 1999; 25: 745-8.

14. Pietsch JB, Netscher DT, Nagaraj HS, Groff DB. Early excision of major burns in children: effect on morbidity and mortality. *J Pediatr Surg* 1985; 20: 754-7.

15. Tompkins RG, Remensnyder JP, Burke JF, Tompkins DM, Hilton JF, Schoenfeld DA, *et al.* Significant reductions in mortality for children with burn injuries through the use of prompt eschar excision. *Ann Surg* 1988; 208: 577-85.

16. Xiao-Wu W, Herndon DN, Spies M, Sanford AP, Wolf SE. Effects of delayed wound excision and grafting in severely burned children. *Arch Surg* 2002; 137: 1049-54.

17. Barret JP, Herndon DN. Modulation of inflammatory and catabolic responses in severely burned children by early burn wound excision in the first 24 hours. *Arch Surg* 2003; 138: 127-32.

18. Gottschlich MM, Jenkins ME, Mayes T, Khoury J, Kagan RJ, Warden GD. The 2002 Clinical Research Award. An evaluation of the safety of early vs delayed enteral support and effects on clinical, nutritional, and endocrine outcomes after severe burns. *J Burn Care Rehabil* 2002; 23: 401-15.

19. Hart DW, Wolf SE, Zhang XJ, Chinkes DL, Buffalo MC, Matin SI, *et al.* Efficacy of a high-carbohydrate diet in catabolic illness. *Crit Care Med* 2001; 29: 1318-24.

20. Ferrando AA, Chinkes DL, Wolf SE, Matin S, Herndon DN, Wolfe RR. A submaximal dose of insulin promotes net skeletal muscle protein synthesis in patients with severe burns. *Ann Surg* 1999; 229: 11-8.

21. Yu YM, Sheridan RL, Burke JF, Chapman TE, Tompkins RG, Young VR. Kinetics of plasma arginine and leucine in pediatric burn patients. *Am J Clin Nutr* 1996; 64: 60-6.

22. Gore DC, Jahoor F. Deficiency in peripheral glutamine production in pediatric patients with burns. *J Burn Care Rehabil* 2000; 21: 171-7.

23. Sheridan RL, Prelack K, Yu YM, Lydon M, Petras L, Young VR, *et al.* Short-term enteral glutamine does not enhance protein accretion in burned children: a stable isotope study. *Surgery* 2004; 135: 671-8.

24. Hart DW, Herndon DN, Klein G, Lee SB, Celis M, Mohan S, *et al.* Attenuation of posttraumatic muscle catabolism and osteopenia by long-term growth hormone therapy. *Ann Surg* 2001; 233: 827-34.

25. Gilpin DA, Barrow RE, Rutan RL, Broemeling L, Herndon DN. Recombinant human growth hormone accelerates wound healing in children with large cutaneous burns. *Ann Surg* 1994; 220: 19-24.

26. Takala J, Ruokonen E, Webster NR, Nielsen MS, Zandstra DF, Vundelinckx G, *et al.* Increased mortality associated with growth hormone treatment in critically ill adults. *N Engl J Med* 1999; 341: 785-92.

27. Ramirez RJ, Wolf SE, Barrow RE, Herndon DN. Growth hormone treatment in pediatric burns: a safe therapeutic approach. *Ann Surg* 1998; 228: 439-48.

28. Barret JP, Dziewulski P, Jeschke MG, Wolf SE, Herndon DN. Effects of recombinant human growth hormone on the development of burn scarring. *Plast Reconstr Surg* 1999; 104: 726-9.

29. de Oliveira GV, Sanford AP, Murphy KD, de Oliveira HM, Wilkins JP, Wu X, *et al.* Growth hormone effects on hypertrophic scar formation: a randomized controlled trial of 62 burned children. *Wound Repair Regen* 2004; 12: 404-11.

30. Barrow RE, Dasu MR, Ferrando AA, Spies M, Thomas SJ, Perez-Polo JR, *et al.* Gene expression patterns in skeletal muscle of thermally injured children treated with oxandrolone. *Ann Surg* 2003; 237: 422-8.

31. Murphy KD, Thomas S, Mlcak RP, Chinkes DL, Klein GL, Herndon DN. Effects of long-term oxandrolone administration in severely burned children. *Surgery* 2004; 136: 219-24.

32. Spies M, Wolf SE, Barrow RE, Jeschke MG, Herndon DN. Modulation of types I and II acute phase reactants with insulin-like growth factor-1/binding protein-3 complex in severely burned children. *Crit Care Med* 2002; 30: 83-8.

33. Herndon DN, Ramzy PI, DebRoy MA, Zheng M, Ferrando AA, Chinkes DL, *et al.* Muscle protein catabolism after severe burn: effects of IGF-1/IGFBP-3 treatment. *Ann Surg* 1999; 229: 713-20.

Chapter 7

Chapter 7

34. Spies M, Nesic O, Barrow RE, Perez-Polo JR, Herndon DN. Liposomal IGF-1 gene transfer modulates pro- and anti-inflammatory cytokine mRNA expression in the burn wound. *Gene Ther* 2001; 8: 1409-15.

35. Jeschke MG, Barrow RE, Suzuki F, Rai J, Benjamin D, Herndon DN. IGF-I/IGFBP-3 equilibrates ratios of pro- to anti-inflammatory cytokines, which are predictors for organ function in severely burned pediatric patients. *Mol Med* 2002; 8: 238-46.

36. Jeschke MG, Norbury WB, Finnerty CC, Branski LK, Herndon DN. Propranolol does not increase inflammation, sepsis or infectious episodes in severely burned children. *J Trauma* 2007, 62(3): 676-81.

37. Herndon DN, Hart DW, Wolf SE, Chinkes DL, Wolfe RR. Reversal of catabolism by beta-blockade after severe burns. *N Engl J Med* 2001; 345: 1223-9.

38. Sheridan RL, Hinson MI, Liang MH, Nackel AF, Schoenfeld DA, Ryan CM, *et al*. Long-term outcome of children surviving massive burns. *JAMA* 2000; 283: 69-73.

39. El Hamaoui Y, Yaalaoui S, Chihabeddine K, Boukind E, Moussaoui D. Post-traumatic stress disorder in burned patients. *Burns* 2002; 28: 647-50.

40. Meyer WJ, III, Blakeney P, Russell W, Thomas C, Robert R, Berniger F, *et al*. Psychological problems reported by young adults who were burned as children. *J Burn Care Rehabil* 2004; 25: 98-106.

41. Tyack ZF, Ziviani J. What influences the functional outcome of children at 6 months post-burn? *Burns* 2003; 29: 433-44.

42. Sheridan RL, Hinson M, Nackel A, Blaquiere M, Daley W, Querzoli B, *et al*. Development of a pediatric burn pain and anxiety management program. *J Burn Care Rehabil* 1997; 18: 455-9.

43. Zeitlin RE. Long-term psychosocial sequelae of paediatric burns. *Burns* 1997; 23: 467-72.

44. Martin-Herz SP, Patterson DR, Honari S, Gibbons J, Gibran N, Heimbach DM. Pediatric pain control practices of North American Burn Centers. *J Burn Care Rehabil* 2003; 24: 26-36.

45. Owens VF, Palmieri TL, Comroe CM, Conroy JM, Scavone JA, Greenhalgh DG. Ketamine: a safe and effective agent for painful procedures in the pediatric burn patient. *J Burn Care Res* 2006; 27: 211-6.

46. Sheridan RL, McEttrick M, Bacha G, Stoddard F, Tompkins RG. Midazolam infusion in pediatric patients with burns who are undergoing mechanical ventilation. *J Burn Care Rehabil* 1994; 15: 515-8.

47. Humphries Y, Melson M, Gore D. Superiority of oral ketamine as an analgesic and sedative for wound care procedures in the pediatric patient with burns. *J Burn Care Rehabil* 1997; 18: 34-6.

48. Borland ML, Bergesio R, Pascoe EM, Turner S, Woodger S. Intranasal fentanyl is an equivalent analgesic to oral morphine in paediatric burns patients for dressing changes: a randomised double blind crossover study. *Burns* 2005; 31: 831-7.

49. Shakespeare V. Effect of small burn injury on physical, social and psychological health at 3-4 months after discharge. *Burns* 1998; 24: 739-44.

50. van Baar ME, Essink-Bot ML, Oen IM, Dokter J, Boxma H, van Beeck EF. Functional outcome after burns: a review. *Burns* 2006; 32: 1-9.

51. Akita S, Akino K, Imaizumi T, Tanaka K, Anraku K, Yano H, *et al*. The quality of pediatric burn scars is improved by early administration of basic fibroblast growth factor. *J Burn Care Res* 2006; 27: 333-8.

52. Cubison TC, Pape SA, Parkhouse N. Evidence for the link between healing time and the development of hypertrophic scars (HTS) in paediatric burns due to scald injury. *Burns* 2006; 32: 992-9.

Chapter 8

Biological skin substitutes

Lachlan Currie MB BS BSc MD FRCS (Plast.)

Fellow in Hand and Microsurgery

THE ROYAL CHILDREN'S HOSPITAL, MELBOURNE, AUSTRALIA

Introduction

Skin replacements have been produced for many years. They have been developed with different combinations of synthetic, dermal and epidermal components. Tissue engineering is generating increasing numbers of matrices that, in combination with different cell types, has the potential to give rise to a wide variety of skin replacement products. These products not only have vastly differing compositions, but they also have different functional roles at the wound bed.

Since 1975 it has been possible to cultivate human keratinocytes *in vitro* using lethally irradiated 3T3 mouse fibroblasts in a specific culture medium [1]. The technique has been refined and it is now possible to culture enough keratinocytes over a five-week period to cover the entire body surface of an adult with sheets of autologous keratinocytes several cells thick. This was a significant advance in the treatment of patients with major burns, with one study showing a reduction in mortality from 48% to 14% by its clinical application [2]. Tissue culture and biomaterial technologies have, over the succeeding 25 years, generated a large number of different approaches to the problem of providing replacement skin for burns. Cuono combined allogeneic cadaveric dermis with cultured keratinocytes [3] to cover burn wounds. Integra® was developed by Burke and Yannas in 1981 as a dermal substitute [4, 5]. The dermal layer of Integra is composed of porous bovine cross-linked collagen and chondroitin-6-sulphate with a defined structure and pore size, which allows the migration of the patient's fibroblasts into it thereby creating a 'neodermis'.

Composite grafts of cultured autologous keratinocytes and fibroblasts attached to an implantable collagen-glycosaminoglycan (C-GAG) substrate have provided promising results in burn patients [6]. More recently, Integra covered with these C-GAG composites has been used on acute minor burn patients with good cosmetic results, and providing early skin coverage for large burns [7]. Other complex structures consisting of cultured fibroblasts and keratinocytes with various dermal analogues have also been extensively investigated both *in vitro* and *in vivo*.

It seems likely that the number of different products and approaches to solving the problems of replacement skin will escalate during the coming years. We consider here what products are currently available to surgeons. This review includes only materials that incorporate a biological component, and excludes non-biological commercially available materials which would be considered as wound dressings.

Methodology

A Medline search was employed using the search words 'skin substitute', 'skin replacement' and 'wound healing'.

What are we substituting?

The skin is the largest organ of the body. It has several homeostatic functions:

- Skin acts as a barrier to the external environment.
- It prevents invasion by pathological micro-organisms.
- It regulates body temperature, controls fluid loss from evaporation, and protects us from ultra-violet radiation.
- Skin produces vitamin D in the epidermal layer.
- It provides us with sensation, and also has mechanical properties which allow it to support other tissues, as well as conveying aesthetic qualities and beauty.

The skin is able to perform all these functions through a relatively simple structure. In order to replace it we must understand this structure at a macroscopic, microscopic and ultra-structural level.

Skin consists of two layers: the dermis, derived from mesoderm, and the epidermis, derived from ectoderm. The epidermis consists mainly of keratinocytes, but also contains melanocytes, Langerhans cells (immune) and Merkel cells (mechanoreceptor). Keratinocytes undergo a transition from relatively immature cells in the basal layer to more differentiated cells in the outer layers. These differentiated cells produce large quantities of the keratin 'family' of proteins and eventually lose their nuclei. The epidermis has been arbitrarily divided into layers: these are the stratum germinativum (the most basal), the stratum granulosum, the stratum lucidum (in which the cells have no nuclei) and the stratum corneum. The stratum corneum consists of dead cells and keratin debris.

Keratinocyte stem cells have an undifferentiated morphology and are slow cycling. However, they have a proliferative reserve which exceeds the life-time of an individual. The stem cells divide producing daughter cells. Some of these replenish the stem cell stocks, whilst others form 'transient amplifying cells' (TA cells) [8]. TA cells are rapidly dividing cells which expand clonally until they undergo terminal differentiation into post-mitotic cells. These in vivo cell types correspond to holoclones, meroclones and paraclones which have been identified in vitro in cell culture studies. Barrandon and Green [9] demonstrated that a clone could be assigned to one of three classes. The holoclone has the greatest reproductive capacity, producing colonies of which less than 5% will abort or terminally differentiate. The paraclone, on the other hand, contains only cells with a short replicative lifespan of less than 15 generations.

The precise position of these stem cells in human skin is unclear, but two models exist with good evidence to back them. Firstly, the 'epidermal proliferative unit' model [10] proposes that a single stem cell lies on the basement membrane at the base of an inverted pyramid of TA cells and post-mitotic cells, which are all derived from that single stem cell. Several studies have supported this theory [11]. An alternative model, the 'deep and shallow rete ridge model' has been proposed [12] in which the stem cells are thought to only exist in the basal layers of the deep rete ridges. The TA cells in the supra-basal layers of the deep ridges, derived from these stem cells are postulated to provide the basal layers of the shallower rete ridges. This theory is supported by research based on pulse-labelled thymidine pick up by the TA cells, which does not occur in the deep rete ridges.

The epidermis is separated from the underlying connective tissue by the basement membrane. The formation of the basement membrane has been shown to depend on keratinocyte-fibroblast interactions [13]. A continuous lamina densa and the formation of hemidesmosomes and anchoring fibrils cannot be identified in co-cultures of fibroblasts and keratinocytes in vitro until after three weeks of culture.

The predominant type of cell in the dermis is the fibroblast. The fibroblast produces elastin, collagen and other extracellular matrix proteins. The elastin and collagen are cross-linked within the semi-fluid ground substance which is composed of macromolecules such as glycosaminoglycan and proteoglycans. The dermis is arbitrarily divided into a superficial papillary and deeper reticular dermis. The reticular layer contains irregular, loosely arranged, coarse elastic fibres interspersed between thick collagen bundles with relatively few fibroblasts and blood vessels compared with the overlying papillary dermis.

Skin also contains blood vessels, melanocytes, sensory receptors, and other adnexal structures such as hair follicles, as well as apocrine and eccrine glands. Skin substitutes rarely attempt to replace these complex anatomical structures and cell types.

Types of skin substitute

An important distinction lies between skin substitutes that provide wound cover, and skin substitutes that achieve wound closure. Wound closure requires a material to restore epidermal barrier function and become incorporated into the healing wound [14], whereas materials used for wound cover rely on in-growth of granulation tissue for adhesion. The ultimate aim of the burn surgeon is to facilitate wound closure, in the fastest possible time, with the optimal cosmetic result. Unfortunately no commercially available product has yet been developed which performs this function better than autologous split skin graft.

Skin substitutes can be divided into four main categories depending on the immunogenicity of the cells they contain (Table 1). All tissue-engineered skin replacements will fit into one of these groups.

Table 1. Types of skin sbstitutes.

Type 1	Acellular
Type 2	Autologous cells only
Type 3	Allogeneic cells only (or xenogenic cells only)
Type 4	Mixed autologous and allogeneic cells

Skin substitutes also differ in their epidermal and dermal composition. Keratinocytes form the commonest epidermal cell population, either as a confluent sheet or as a cell suspension. The alternative is to use a synthetic material such as silicone. Dermal components used in tissue-engineered skin replacements include fibroblasts, extracellular matrix components (such as collagen, fibrin and glycosaminoglycan), or synthetic dermis, such as vicryl mesh. A synthetic biomaterial may act as an epidermis in one skin replacement; however, that same biomaterial may act as a dermis in another skin replacement. Therefore, we need to consider both the content and the proposed function of a skin substitute to consider how it is likely to behave in patients.

Type 1 - acellular skin substitutes

These products do not contain any cells. They rely entirely on repopulation by host cells within the wound bed. When applied to full-thickness wounds they will not provide a viable epidermis without a supplementary procedure (Table 2).

Biobrane® (Dow Hickman/Bertek Pharmaceuticals, Sugar Land, Tx, USA)

Biobrane consists of a nylon mesh which is bonded to a thin layer of silicone. The nylon is covered with porcine collagen. The collagen promotes fibrovascular ingrowth into the material which adheres firmly to the wound bed. The silicone acts as a temporary semi-permeable membrane, protecting the wound and providing an optimal healing environment. Biobrane facilitates wound cover, rather than wound closure. It has been recommended for use in partial-thickness burns (usually due to scalds) within the first 24 hours of injury. It should not be used on potentially contaminated wounds. Some surgeons feel that it reduces the resuscitation requirements, and it may in fact establish temporary wound closure when good adherence is achieved. Several large retrospective studies have confirmed the efficacy of Biobrane use in paediatric scald injuries, with low infection rates, pain-free healing, and good skin recovery with normal

Table 2. The structure, composition and cost of commercially available acellular products.

Trade name	Schematic representation	Layers	Cost per cm²	Website
Biobrane® (Dow Hickman/Bertek Pharmaceuticals, Sugar Land, Texas).		◆ Silicone ◆ Nylon mesh ◆ Collagen	£0.21	http://www.mylan.com
Integra® (Integra Life Science Corporation, Plainsboro, New Jersey)		◆ Silicone ◆ Collagen	£3.05	http://www.integra-ls.com
Alloderm® (LifeCell, Woodlands, Texas.)		◆ Acellular dermis de-epithelialised cadaver	£5.90 (2002 price)	http://www.lifecell.com

pigmentation in over 50% of patients [15] **(III/B)**. However, there is some debate over the cost-effectiveness of Biobrane compared with cheaper alternatives which produce equally good results in this group of patients.

Integra® artificial skin (Integra Life Science Corporation, Plainsboro, New Jersey)

Integra is a synthetic dermal substitute developed for use in burns patients. It was originally described by Yannas [4, 5], and has now become one of the most widely accepted dermal replacements in clinical use. Integra has a bilaminar structure, consisting of a cross-linked bovine collagen and glycosaminoglycan matrix, coated on one side with a silicone membrane that functions as a temporary synthetic epidermal replacement. The collagen layer forms a vascular 'neodermis', a process that takes approximately three weeks in humans. The patient's own endothelial cells and fibroblasts migrate into the matrix through 70-200µm pores. Smaller pores delay migration and prevent bio-integration, whereas larger pores are an

inadequate scaffold for invading host cells. The silicone layer is conventionally removed after three weeks, and an ultra-thin split skin graft applied.

Integra 'take' rates are variable and are dependent on operator experience. A trial involving 106 patients from several centres found the median 'take' was 85%, compared with take rates of 95% in the controls using split skin grafts (SSG) [16]. This trial also highlighted improved cosmetic results, not only of the Integra, but also of the donor sites. The split skin grafts needed to resurface the Integra can be harvested at 0.15mm, rather than the average graft thickness of 0.33mm. Donor sites were shown to heal four days sooner with less hypertrophic scarring.

Long-term results of Integra use are now emerging. A study at the Massachusetts General Hospital and the Boston Unit of the Shriners Burns Institute, which included 121 patients with follow-up as long as ten years, reported successful engraftment rates of over 80% [17]. Hypertrophic scar formation was also reduced with 93% demonstrating absent or minimal hypertrophic scarring. All patients had excellent

Chapter 8

function of involved joints. Interestingly, areas of Integra grafted in children appeared to grow with the child. The general opinion of the patients was that the areas grafted with Integra artificial skin were cosmetically superior to those where split skin autograft was used alone, although in no instances was it felt to be identical to normal skin.

Integra requires a two-stage procedure necessitating a minimum time interval of three weeks between the application of the Integra and the SSG to allow neodemis formation. The use of Integra in combination with cultured epidermal autografts is a very attractive proposition. The three-week time delay would allow for expansion of a skin biopsy into cultured epidermal sheets. However, there are very few reports of the successful combination of cultured epidermal autograft sheets with Integra in clinical use for reasons that are as yet unclear [18].

Integra is relatively expensive when compared with cadaveric allograft skin from skin banks and there is a steep learning curve with initial high failure rates. The advantages are that it provides improved elasticity and cosmesis to an ultra-thin SSG, with reduced donor-site morbidity compared with a standard-thickness SSG. It is available immediately and is without the risks of cross infection related to allograft. Integra has an important role in providing immediate wound closure following early excision for patients with insufficient autograft. However, a new clinical role is emerging for the use of Integra to resurface secondary burn wound deformities, such as neck contractures [19] and upper limb contractures [20].

The safety and effectiveness of the Integra dermal regeneration template was evaluated in a study involving 216 burn patients who were treated at 13 burn care facilities in the US. Integra was applied to surgically excised burn wounds and a thin epidermal autograft was placed after 2-3 weeks. The mean total body surface area burned was 36.5% (range, 1-95%). The incidence of invasive infection at Integra-treated sites was 3.1%. The mean take rate of Integra and epidermal autograft was 76.2% and 87.7%, respectively [21] **(IIb/B)**.

Alloderm® (LifeCell, Woodlands, Tx, USA)

Alloderm is a human cadaveric allograft which has been de-epithelialised and treated to remove the cellular components of the dermis prior to cryopreservation. This renders the skin substitute acellular and non-immunogenic for use as a dermal replacement. Following application to a wound bed, it is re-populated by host cells, revascularised and incorporated into the tissue. Alloderm has been used extensively for abdominal wall fascial reconstruction, but there are only a few reported series demonstrating its use as a dermal replacement. Callcut *et al* recently described its use as a one-stage composite dermal-epidermal replacement using it in conjunction with a thin skin graft [22]. Successful take was observed in 26/27 patients **(III/B)**.

Type 2 - skin substitutes containing autologous cells

These products contain cells (usually fibroblasts or keratinocytes) which are derived from the host by biopsy, developed in culture and returned to the wound bed in vastly increased numbers (Table 3). They enhance wound closure by increasing the number of active cells within the wound bed. However, only a small proportion are stem cells (holoclones), with the majority representing 'transient amplifying cells' (paraclones), which have a short replicating lifespan of less than 15 generations.

Cultured autologous keratinocytes

Cultured keratinocyte sheets are available commercially from a number of companies, e.g. Epicel™ (Genzyme Tissue Repair Corporation, Cambridge, MA), but are relatively straightforward to prepare in suitably equipped university or hospital laboratories. The introduction of cultured epitheial autograft (CEA) was a significant advance in the treatment of patients with major burns, with one study showing a reduction in mortality from 48% to 14% following early CEA application [2] **(IIa/B)**. However, CEA technology is expensive, with a time delay of between three to five weeks to generate sufficient

Table 3. The structure, composition and cost of commercially available autologous products.

Trade name	Schematic representation	Layers	Cost per cm^2	Website
Epicel™ (Genzyme Tissue Repair Corporation, Cambridge, MA.)		• Cultured autologous keratinocytes	Variable	http://www.genzyme biosurgery.com
Cellspray® (Clinical Cell Culture [C3], Perth, Australia)		• Sprayed cultured autologous keratinocytes	Variable	http://www.clinicalcellculture
Myskin™ (Celltran Ltd, Sheffield, UK)		• Silicone • Cultured autologous keratinocytes	Variable	http://www.myskin-info.co
Laserskin™ (Fidia Advanced Biopolymers, Italy)		• Cultured autologous keratinocytes • Hyaluronic acid with laser perforations	Variable	http://www.fidiapharma.it
Hyalograft 3D™ (Fidia Advanced Biopolymers, Italy)		• Hyaluronic acid seeded with autologous fibroblasts	Variable	http://www.fidiapharma.it
Composite autologous epidermal-dermal skin substitutes, e.g. CSS (not commercially availabe)		• Autologous keratinocytes • Collagen seeded with autologous fibroblasts	N/A	

tissue cover for an adult. The longevity of the grafts has also been questioned, with the production of a fragile epithelium which is prone to spontaneous blistering some months after grafting.

Sub-confluent autologous keratinocytes in suspensions

Culturing cells to a non-confluent state *in vitro* for delivery to the wound in suspension can reduce the time needed to cultivate confluent epithelial sheets.

This has the advantage of providing cells that have not undergone the phenotypic changes stimulated by contact inhibition and should therefore have undiminished adhesive and proliferative potential. It also avoids the use of the proteolytic enzyme, Dispase®, required to release epidermal sheets in conventional keratinocyte technology. Dispase may reduce the surface antigen expression of the keratinocytes and reduce their adhesive potential [23].

Many groups are working on the development of keratinocyte delivery systems in the hope that this may reduce costs and improve the take and quality of the resulting epidermis. In order to deliver sub-confluent keratinocytes to a wound bed, they must either be dispersed as a suspension in a suitable medium, or be attached to some form of transferable substrate. Keratinocytes have been attached to hyaluronic membranes (e.g Laserskin™), the polyurethane wound dressing Hydroderm® [24], and a polymer membrane (EpiGen®) [25]. Some of these systems are generally regarded as research materials awaiting further investigation. However, one delivery system which has been used extensively both *in vitro* and *in vivo* studies is fibrin glue.

Fibrin glue as a delivery system for cultured autologous keratinocytes

Hunyadi reported the first use of fibrin glue with cultured keratinocytes in 1988. It was demonstrated that fibrin glue (Beriplast®) could be used to effectively deliver autologous keratinocytes mixed with the fibrinogen component to the wound. A marked increase was found in the rate of leg ulcer healing compared with a control group [26].

Ronfard *et al* developed a technique in 1991 for culturing sheets of autologous keratinocytes on fibrin glue and reported its use in two burn patients. The last subculture prior to grafting was on a petri dish coated with fibrin glue (Biocol®) and seeded with irradiated 3T3 mouse fibroblasts as a standard component of keratinocyte culture [27]. It was found that *in vitro*, there was no destruction of the fibrin matrix for up to 15 days, probably due to the aprotinin in the product. The autologous keratinocytes could then be transferred to the patient on the fibrin sheets

obviating the need for Dispase. Inverted fibrin sheets were used on all but one area, with the keratinocytes closest to the wound. In areas where the graft had been inverted, no deterioration in anchorage or growth of the keratinocytes was observed on histological analysis. This translated into improved graft take. The technique was claimed to accelerate the standard process of handling fragile cultured keratinocyte sheets and permitted the use of subconfluent cells.

The benefit of using fibrin glue to secure sheets of cultured keratinocytes was reiterated in an athymic mouse model [28]. Fibrin glue (Hemaseel®) was sprayed onto the wound bed prior to placement of the epidermal sheets and compared with a control group in which no fibrin glue was used. Seven days after transplantation the percentage of graft take was greater in the tissue sealant group, although no difference was found 14 and 21 days post-grafting. Immunohistological and ultrastructural analysis showed that the evolution of the cultured human epidermis after transplantation was similar in both groups. Ultimately, the application of fibrin sealant probably enhances the mechanical stability of the keratinocyte sheets. Auger *et al* showed a 20% improvement in cultured epithelial graft take in a similar model using Tisseel® fibrin glue [29].

Fibrin glue has also been used to deliver cultured human keratinocytes to a wound in suspension. *In vitro* studies showed that keratinocytes remain viable in suspension in fibrin for at least five days [30]. When compared with standard cultured epidermal sheet grafts in a nude mouse model, re-epithelialisation was similar, but reconstitution of the dermo-epidermal junction zone, as shown by electron microscopy and immunohistochemistry, was significantly enhanced by the fibrin glue suspension technique [31]. It was concluded that the fibrin glue not only delivers highly proliferative keratinocytes but also provides an optimal milieu for their migration, proliferation and differentiation.

The same authors have used cultured autologous keratinocytes suspended in fibrin glue (KFGS) with allogeneic skin overgraft in several burn patients [32-34]. Cultured cells which are 70% confluent prior to trypsinisation were mixed with the fibrin component of the fibrin glue (Tissucol®), and the cell-containing suspension was used to secure the allograft skin to the debrided burn wound. The allogeneic epidermis underwent immunological rejection and cultured autologous keratinocytes replaced them. Pellegrini *et al* showed that keratinocytes cultured on fibrin glue maintained the relative percentage of holoclones, meroclones and paraclones, proving that the fibrin glue technique does not induce clonal conversion and consequent loss of epidermal stem cells [35]. Fibrin glue-cultured keratinocyte autografts bearing stem cells applied 'cells-up' to massive full-thickness burns (initially treated with allo-dermis) displayed a high keratinocyte take rate, which was reproducible, permanent and maintained long-term proliferative potential.

Composite autologous epidermal-dermal skin substitutes

Composites are produced by growing cells on some form of biomaterial. Many variations exist, produced by individual research laboratories. One of the most sophisticated of these has been developed by Boyce *et al*. Patients with major burns are treated with cultured skin substitutes consisting of collagen-glycosaminoglycan substrates populated with autologous fibroblasts and keratinocytes (CSS-cultured skin substitute). The cells are cultured from split skin graft biopsies. In a match pair study involving 40 burn patients with a mean TBSA of 73%, they demonstrated a reduced requirement for donor skin harvesting with the use of CSS [36]. Scar quality was as good as autograft, but pigment remained deficient in wounds covered with CSS **(IIa/B)**.

Type 3 - skin substitutes containing allogeneic cells

These biomaterials contain allogeneic cultured cells, usually fibroblasts or keratinocytes (Table 4), either viable or non-viable, depending upon the techniques involved in production. The allogeneic cells are recognised as foreign by the host and stimulate the production of growth factors at the wound bed, whilst non-cellular components may be

incorporated into the wound with the help of this added stimulus. This effect may be more pronounced in immunosuppressed patients.

Cadaveric allograft

In major burns over 50%, wound closure cannot be rapidly achieved with split skin grafts. Donor sites need to regenerate new epithelium, and new techniques are needed to temporarily close wounds while this happens. This can be achieved with cadaveric allograft. Herndon reported a retrospective study comparing 32 children admitted from 1977 through 1981, treated by serial debridement of their burn wounds, with 32 burned children treated from 1981 to 1984 who were treated by early total excision to fascia with application of autograft and cadaver skin for complete closure. The survivors of the early excision group underwent fewer operative procedures and had a greatly decreased length of hospital stay [37] **(IIb/B)**. The pathological immunosuppression that occurs in the early stages of a severe burn injury protects allografts from rejection during this period. Cadaveric material is supplied by skin banks where it is treated by cryopreservation or glycerolisation. The potential for disease transmission necessitates careful screening of prospective donor material to reduce the risk of transfer of infective agents. However, this risk is never completely eliminated [38]. Cadaveric allograft is a transient means of achieving wound closure, and it is eventually rejected. This has prompted the search for an alternative permanent wound closure material.

Allogeneic keratinocytes

The use of pre-grown allogeneic keratinocytes has been extensively investigated in an attempt to overcome the problem posed by the time delay in growing confluent autologous keratinocytes for wound closure. Allogeneic keratinocyte sheets are not acutely rejected and have been shown to accelerate healing [39]. However, Y chromosome and DNA probes have shown that allogeneic cells survive less than one week when grafted onto tattoo excision wounds or ulcers [40, 41], but over six weeks when applied to a split skin graft donor site [42-44]. The improved wound

Table 4. The structure, composition and cost of commercially available allogeneic cell containing products.

Trade name	Schematic representation	Layers	Cost per cm²	Website
Cadaveric allograft (from not-for-profit skin banks)		• Cryopreserved in order to retain viability • Lyophilised • Glycerolised	£0.60	N/A
Allogeneic keratinocytes (not commercially available)		• Allogeneic keratinocytes	N/A	N/A
TransCyte® (Advanced Tissue Sciences, Inc. La Jolla, California, USA)		• Silicone • Nylon mesh • Collagen seeded with neonatal fibroblasts	£7.87 (2002 price)	http://www.advanced biohealing.com
Apligraf® (Organogenesis Inc, Canton, MA and Novartis Pharmaceuticals Corporation, East Hanover, NJ)		• Allogeneic keratinocytes • Collagen seeded with allogeneic fibroblasts	£14.22	http://www.apligraf.com
Dermagraft® (Advanced Tissue Sciences, Inc. La Jolla, California, USA)		• Polyglycolic acid (Dexon™) or polyglactin-910 (Vicryl™) seeded with neonatal fibroblasts	£7.14 (2002 price)	http://www.advanced biohealing.com
Xenograft e.g. Mediskin® (Brennen Medical Inc. St. Paul, MN, USA).		• Porcine skin		
Orcel® (Ortec International, NY, USA)		• Allogeneic keratinocytes • Collagen seeded with allogeneic fibroblasts		http://www.ortec international.com

healing that is often observed has been attributed to the synthesis of growth factors and cytokines by these cells.

Allogeneic keratinocytes form a temporary and biologically active epidermis until they are progressively replaced [45].

TransCyte™ (Advanced Tissue Sciences, Inc., La Jolla, California, USA)

TransCyte consists of a collagen-coated nylon mesh seeded with neonatal fibroblasts. This mesh is covered with a thin layer of silicone. It was formerly called Dermagraft-TC. As nylon is not biodegradeable, this material can not act as a dermal substitute. Hansbrough [46] performed a clinical trial comparing the use of cryopreserved allograft with TransCyte as a temporary dermal analogue in ten patients. The wounds were closed with meshed split skin autograft. The results showed that autograft adherence and take were at least as good after TransCyte as with allograft. In a larger multi-centre trial with 66 patients, it was noted that as well as showing good adherence, TransCyte was easier to remove resulting in less bleeding than allograft [47]. Histologically, a comparison of TransCyte with allograft in burn wounds showed the only significant difference to be increased granulation tissue with allograft [48], which could translate into better cosmesis after TransCyte. Paediatric burns greater than 7% total body surface area that underwent wound closure with TransCyte, have been shown to subsequently require a lower percentage of split skin autograft, compared with standard therapy consisting of the application of antimicrobial ointments and hydrodebridement [49]. A prospective randomised trial from Australia compared Transcyte, Biobrane and silver sulphadiazine for use in paediatric patients with partial-thickness burns. Mean time to re-epithelialisation was 7.5 days for TransCyte, 9.5 days for Biobrane, and 11.2 days for Silvazine. Patients who received silver sulphadiazine or Biobrane required more autografting than those treated with TransCyte [50] (IIa/B).

Apligraf® (Organogenesis Inc., Canton, MA and Novartis Pharmaceuticals Corporation, East Hanover, NJ)

Apligraf consists of a Type I bovine collagen gel impregnated with living neonatal allogeneic fibroblasts, with an overlying cornified epidermal layer of neonatal allogeneic keratinocytes. It appears to hasten healing particularly in the deeper and more chronic wounds [51], though little experience exists of its use in burns surgery. The potential of Apligraf to improve cosmetic and functional outcomes when applied over meshed split thickness autografts has been evaluated in a multi-centre, randomised controlled clinical trial [52]. There was no difference in the percent take of autograft in the presence or absence of Apligraf. However, in the Apligraf group the cosmetic result in terms of pigmentation, pliability and vascularity of the skin graft was significantly better than in the control group.

Dermagraft® (Advanced Tissue Sciences, Inc., La Jolla, California, USA)

Dermagraft is a cryopreserved living dermal structure, manufactured by cultivating neonatal allogeneic fibroblasts on a biodegradable polymer scaffold (polyglycolic acid or polyglactin-910, marketed as Dexon or Vicryl, respectively) [53]. The fibroblasts become confluent within the polymer mesh, synthesising growth factors and dermal matrix proteins (collagens, tenascin, vitronectin and glycosaminoglycans), thus creating a living dermal structure [54]. This remains viable and metabolically active after implantation into the wound, despite cryopreservation [55]. Although Dermagraft has not been used extensively for burns it has been used as a dermal replacement beneath meshed split skin grafts on full-thickness wounds [53]. The take rate of the SSG was comparable to grafting on the wound bed alone. Wound histology showed extrusion of vicryl fibres from the wound, although this was not clinically apparent. Further studies will be needed to determine any long-term benefits following the application of Dermagraft under meshed split skin grafts.

Xenograft

Xenograft is skin derived from another species. Porcine skin is the most commonly used. It has the advantage of being more readily available than cadaveric allograft. Its applications are similar to those of cadaveric allograft; however, it is more immunogenic. Used in the treatment of partial-thickness wounds, it has been shown to reduce the healing time when compared with paraffin gauze dressings [56]. It provides wound cover, not closure.

Type 4 - Skin substitutes containing autologous and allogeneic cells

Attempts at combining the cultured epidermal autograft (CEA) with the neodermis of artificial skin (Integra) have been largely unsuccessful. This may be due to the complex interactions between the basement membrane proteins and cultured autologous keratinocytes being disrupted by the Dispase used to harvest the cells. Novel techniques to circumvent this problem have been to use allogeneic feeder cells seeded into carrier materials. Lam *et al* [57] used autologous keratinocytes cultivated on a pliable hyaluronate-derived membrane (Laserskin™) which was pre-seeded with allogeneic dermal fibroblasts. In a rat model, 14 of 20 (70%) skin biopsies taken at day 21 from the centre of the grafted wounds revealed regenerated epithelium. This may become a feasible delivery system of cultured keratinocytes on to the neodermis of Integra.

Conclusions

It is still unclear what combinations of constituents of tissue-engineered skin equivalents give the best results in terms of graft take, cosmesis and overall patient survival, both for burns and other areas of cutaneous tissue repair. There are very few randomised controlled trials in the literature. Most trials are retrospective, assessing a cohort of patients before or after a new technique has been introduced. Often comparisons are made between products which clearly have different functions at the wound interface. The cost of some skin substitutes is prohibitive, and for this reason there are still few absolute indications for their use.

Limited resources and the lack of data on clinical effectiveness makes it impossible to set out recommendations for the use of currently available skin substitutes. Clinicians aim to provide patients with the best quality skin cover in the shortest possible time. This will often entail the use of biological skin substitutes, especially when autologous skin is not available. The future will almost certainly involve the use of genetically modified cells or cells derived from pluripotent stem cells, possibly in combination with some of the existing extra-cellular scaffolds available today. Hopefully, market forces will drive down prices and one day we will have a commercially produced 'off the shelf' skin replacement that is readily available, reliable and cosmetically superior to autologous skin grafts.

SLNB has now been incorporated by many melanoma units worldwide, but there remains controversy over its use. The current guidelines from the National Institute for Health and Clinical Excellence recommend that "sentinel node biopsy should only be undertaken in centres where there is clinical experience of the procedure and normally only within the context of ethics-committee-approved clinical trials" [10]. This chapter examines the current levels of evidence surrounding SLNB.

Methodology

A full literature search was carried out using the Medline and EMBASE databases between the periods of May 1990 to September 2006. Search terms included 'sentinel node biopsy', 'sentinel lymphadenectomy', 'melanoma' and relevant subheadings. This identified over 1000 articles. Further articles were identified from the reference lists from the original articles which were deemed to be relevant. The Cochrane Library was also searched but as yet no review has been produced by this collaboration. All articles were evaluated for their relevance, and then assessed on the strength of the study. Where possible for this review, only level one and two evidence has been used.

Literature review

There are a number of issues at this time which remain a subject for debate. Most crucially is whether SLNB is beneficial in terms of both disease-free survival and overall survival. This review aims to address these issues and also some of the criticisms which have been made against SLNB, including the morbidity of the procedure, the potential risk of increased in-transit disease following SLNB and the recognised false negative rate.

Sentinel node theory

The hypothesis underpinning SLNB is that metastatic cells will migrate in an organised fashion through the lymphatics initially to the first 'sentinel'

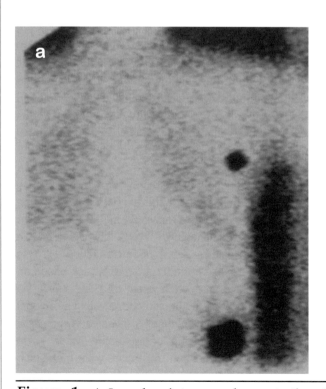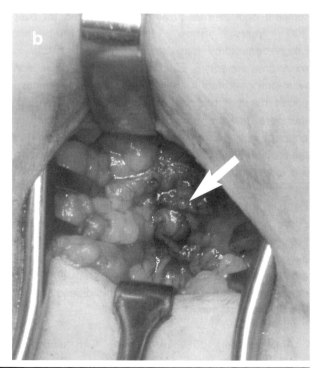

Figure 1. a) **Lymphoscintogram demonstrating the primary injection site on the left flank and subsequent migration of the radioisotope to the sentinel node in the left axilla. b) Intra-operative image of the sentinel node** *in situ* **(white arrow).**

Chapter 9

node prior to spreading to the rest of the basin (Figure 1). Therefore, a negative sentinel node should predict that the whole basin is also disease free. This would then allow those patients with negative nodes to be spared the morbidity of lymphadenectomy.

Within a short time of the sentinel node concept being introduced, the validity of the theory had been confirmed. By removing the sentinel node and then performing an immediate lymphatic clearance it was shown that skip lesions did not occur and that the status of the sentinel node did correlate with the rest of the lymphatic basin [11, 12].

Gershenwald demonstrated a strong correlation between the status of the sentinel node and the long-term prognosis, with only a 55.8% three-year survival for those with a positive node compared with 88.5% for those with a histologically-negative sentinel node [13]. A number of other prospective studies have also shown similar results confirming the validity of the theory [2, 14-16].

It has been shown that whilst sentinel node positivity correlates significantly with Breslow thickness, Clark's level and ulceration, it is individually the most significant predictor of survival [15] **(Ib/A)**.

Overall survival

A key objective of SLNB and early completion lymph node dissection (CLND) was to see if it would improve overall disease survival. This remains a strongly controversial subject. Currently, no conclusive level one evidence exists to show that SLNB followed by CLND is associated with an increased overall survival. There is some lower level evidence that suggests a benefit.

Kretschmer showed a statistically significant survival advantage of 62.5% vs. 50.2% at five years for patients undergoing SLNB [17]. Morton also showed a significant difference in another study examining overall survival comparing matched groups of patients undergoing completion lymphadenectomy after a positive sentinel node with those having a therapeutic lymphadenectomy for clinical nodal disease [2]. Survival differences were 73% versus 51% at five years, 69% versus 37% at ten years, and persisted after long-term follow-up with 69% versus 32% at 15 years.

The only prospective randomised trial data available remains that from the MSLT-1 trial. In that study, overall survival was 87% for the sentinel node arm and 86% for the wide local excision only arm. No statistically significant benefit was seen in the sentinel node arm in terms of overall survival [18] **(Ib/A)**. This is the third interim data analysis with a median follow-up of 59.8 months. Two further analyses remain to be completed and it is felt by the study group that with longer follow-up a small benefit may yet be seen [19].

One important finding from the MSLT-1 study was the difference in survival for those with positive sentinel nodes and CLND compared with those who had only wide local excision and then went on to develop palpable nodal disease. Five-year survival was 72.3% for those having a positive SLNB and 52.4% for those having only wide local excision with development of subsequent nodal disease (p=0.004). Criticism has been made of this comparison as it assumes that all patients with a positive sentinel node would have developed clinical nodal disease [20]. This remains to be proven but the fact that in MSLT-1 the percentage of people with a positive sentinel node was almost exactly equal to the percentage of people who developed nodal disease in the observation group suggests that those with microscopic nodal disease would have progressed to macroscopic clinical disease.

Disease-free survival

There is significant evidence that SLNB improves disease-free survival. The randomised trial data from the MSLT-1 study showed a significant difference in the disease-free survival of 78.3% after SLNB versus 73.1% after wide local excision only [18] **(Ib/A)**. This is partly attributable to the fact that lymph node recurrences were prevented by early lymphadenectomy in the SLNB-positive group. However, the difference between the two groups persisted when loco-regional recurrences were excluded from the analysis [19].

The disease load in the observation group at the time of recurrence was also found to be significantly different from the disease load in those who had an initially positive sentinel node. Histopathological analysis found that after lymphadenectomy the mean number of involved nodes was 1.4 nodes in the sentinel node positive group, with 3.3 nodes involved in the observation group who subsequently developed recurrence. This has a significant effect on prognosis when viewed in association with the current American Joint Committee on Cancer (AJCC) staging classification [21]. In patients with stage III disease with a non-ulcerated primary and one microscopically-involved node, the ten-year survival is 63.0%. If the node is macroscopically involved, the ten-year survival falls to 47.7%, and if there are 2-3 nodes involved it falls further still to 39.2%. This would therefore suggest that those in the sentinel node positive group should potentially have a better prognosis than those detected in the observation group with palpable disease.

Morbidity

The morbidity associated with SLNB has been one of the arguments used against it by its critics [22]. Despite these criticisms, the author quotes relatively low complication rates for seroma (3%) and infection (3%). The Sunbelt Melanoma Trial, which is the largest randomised trial to date, shows a low overall complication rate of 4.6% [15]. The complications could be broken down as haematoma/seroma 2.31%, wound infection 1.08%, and lymphoedema 0.66%. Similar low complication rates were also shown in the MSLT-1 study [23]. This compares to an overall rate of complication for elective lymph node dissection which stands at 36% [5]. SLNB therefore has significantly less morbidity associated with it than lymphadenectomy. It is also generally accepted that a completion lymphadenectomy after SLNB is generally easier to perform and associated with less morbidity than one which is carried out for bulky clinically evident nodal disease. Morbidity should, therefore, not be used as an argument against SLNB **(Ib/A)**.

In-transit disease

In-transit disease drops the five-year survival considerably [21]. Debate exists in the literature as to whether SLNB increases the rate of in-transit disease. Prior to the advent of SLNB the locoregional recurrence rate was reported to range from 0.2% to 6.4% for tumours less than 4mm [24]. However, in a study from Estourgie et al, it was suggested that there was a 23% in-transit rate in sentinel node-positive patients [25]. They postulated that the disruption of lymphatic channels by the SLNB may cause entrapment of melanoma cells in the lymphatics on route to the nodal basin. This study has been criticised due to the small numbers and the high-risk profile of their patients in terms of tumour thickness and ulceration.

A literature overview fuelled the argument by showing an in-transit rate of 20.9% in sentinel node-positive patients. The authors stated that there was a four times greater incidence of in-transit disease in sentinel node patients compared with those who underwent wide local excision alone [26]. This review was pooled from small studies with no controls for confounding factors, for example, Breslow thickness. Three large studies have not confirmed this. Cerovac found only 3.7% developed in-transit disease at a mean follow-up of 42 months after SLNB [27]. The John Wayne Cancer Institute showed an in-transit rate of 3.64% for those undergoing SLNB [28]. Finally, in a large series of 2018 patients from the Sydney Melanoma Unit, the in-transit rate was found to be low (3.6%), with no evidence of an increase since the introduction of SLNB [29]. Interestingly, they also found that the in-transit recurrence rate following elective node dissection was not significantly different from the rate of recurrence following wide local excision alone or wide local excision and SLNB. The MSLT-1 study showed an in-transit rate of 8% in the sentinel node arm compared with 9% in the wide local excision arm, confirming that there is no increased risk of in-transit disease associated with SLNB [23] **(Ib/A)**. The risk of in-transit disease occurrence is related to the original tumour biology [29].

Staging

The role of staging is argued to be one of the most important benefits of SLNB. Whilst many pathological factors are known to predict disease survival, including Breslow thickness, Clark's level and ulceration, SLNB has been shown to be the most powerful predictor of disease survival [13, 21].

Sentinel node status is also known to be a better guide than radiological staging, such as chest X-rays and CT scanning, which rarely reveal evidence of metastatic disease [30, 31].

High resolution ultrasound has also been suggested for the evaluation of the lymphatic basin as an alternative to SLNB. However, it has been shown that it is not sensitive enough to be reliably used, and can only detect deposits greater than 4mm in diameter [32]. Similarly PET-CT has also been suggested for the same purpose. As for ultrasound, it has been found to be not sensitive enough for routine use [33].

SLNB therefore remains the single best staging tool **(Ib/A)**. This importance is highlighted by the major role it has now been given in the current AJCC staging classification for melanoma [21]. This role is crucial to allow correct planning of treatments, access to clinical trials, and to allow patients to be made aware of their likely prognosis such that they can be involved in their own decision making. When proven adjuvant therapy becomes available it will allow patients to be selected for these treatments.

Thin melanomas

Thin melanomas (<1mm Breslow thickness) account for approximately 70% of newly diagnosed cases [34]. Currently, SLNB is generally performed on those melanomas with a Breslow thickness of greater than 1mm or less than 1mm and Clark's level IV or V. It has been generally accepted that below this thickness the number of positive sentinel nodes is too small to allow SLNB to make a difference in this group and be cost-effective. However, recently, a number of studies have suggested that there may be a role for SLNB in thin melanomas. Four studies have shown sentinel node positivity rates of 3% to 10.8% for lesions of 0.75mm to 1.0mm in depth [35-38]. Below this thickness the rates were much less, ranging from 0% to 2.3%.

Thin malignant melanomas with regression have also been investigated. This histological diagnosis reflects an immune response to the tumour causing it to partially or completely disappear. It has been suggested that regression is associated with an increased risk of metastases. Cook found that 50% of metastasising thin lesions had signs of regression [39]. Guitart also found a similar result with 42% of thin metastasising lesions showing regression compared with only 5% for non-metastasising lesions in a matched pairs analysis [40]. However, recently, it has been found in a much larger study that regression does not appear to be a significant predictor of sentinel node involvement [36].

Following these studies, it has been suggested that below 0.75mm it is not worth performing a SLNB but there may be a role for lesions between 0.75mm and 1.0mm Breslow depth. This may be particularly true for thin melanomas with poor prognostic features such as ulceration. As for those lesions which show signs of regression, there is insufficient evidence to use this as a criterion in isolation **(IIa/B)**. Both these areas certainly require further work.

A recent paper has also examined mitotic rate and vertical growth phase in thin melanomas [41]. It was found that a mitotic rate greater than zero and evidence of a vertical growth phase both independently increased the risk of mitoses. This risk was increased further when they occurred in combination, and particularly so in males. Again these are factors which will require further investigation.

Head and neck melanomas

SLNB in head and neck melanomas has a number of factors which make lymphatic mapping more challenging in this area, compared with lympho-scintigraphy of the trunk and extremities. It can be more difficult to detect the sentinel node as the nodes are often close to the site of the tracer injection and, in addition, the tracer travels faster with secondary nodes becoming prominent earlier. Technically, it is a more demanding procedure as the nodes are often smaller than elsewhere and situated around important structures, putting them at risk of injury. Specifically, the peri-parotid nodes and the risk of facial nerve injury have been of concern. These factors have been used to suggest that SLNB should not be carried out in this region. The Sunbelt Melanoma Trial examined this issue as part of the study and found that the incidence of false negatives in the head and neck was only 1.9% at 18 months. Peri-parotid nodes were found in 25% of head and neck melanomas, but there were no cases of facial nerve injury documented. The overall success rate for identification of the sentinel node was 97% [14].

An earlier meta-analysis of head and neck melanomas prior to this trial showed success rates of 95-100% in the head and neck [42]. The average false negative rates ranged between 7.7% and 10.4%.

The results from these studies would suggest that SLNB can be carried out safely in this region with high rates of success (Ib/A). It is, however, essential that those carrying out this procedure are familiar with and used to operating in this region of the body.

False negatives

There has been some criticism of SLNB due to a definite false negative rate. This is defined as the finding of metastases in non-sentinel lymph nodes following a negative sentinel lymph node. A number of factors have been implicated to explain this.

Firstly, the inexperience of the surgeon has been shown to be of importance. Morton initially suggested a minimum of 30 procedures were needed to overcome the learning curve for the procedure [43]. Subsequently, he demonstrated that the learning curve was still significant for up to 50 cases and has since recommended this number as the minimum requirement to minimise false negatives [23].

The second reason for false negatives is a biological failure. This is thought to occur when lymphatics are obstructed by melanoma and secondary drainage channels then later develop to allow cells to spread to nodes other than the sentinel node. This cause of false negatives is thought to be rare [44].

Finally, metastases within the sentinel node may go undetected at histological examination. Gershenwald showed that 'negative' sentinel lymph nodes could often be upstaged by re-examination of the node with serial sections [45].

SLNB has now been in use for a number of years yet no standardised procedure has been agreed for the pathological analysis of the sentinel node. Most pathologists use the technique of Cochran where the node is bivalved through its longest meridian and then ten full-face sections are cut. Half are stained with H&E and half are subjected to immunohistochemical evaluation [46]. If immunohistochemical staining is not used, 5-15% of metastatic nodes may be missed [47].

No agreement has been reached on the number of sections required to fully assess the sentinel node. The Sydney Melanoma Unit routinely samples four sections per paraffin block. Their detection rate for sentinel node metastases has been reported as 15.3% and their false negative rate was 2.66% [48]. On this basis it would be difficult to justify additional sections from a cost-benefit perspective [49].

Conversely, Cook et al in a study for the EORTC using a protocol similar to that of Cochran, produced a metastatic detection rate of 18%. However, by doubling the number of slices taken to 20 they managed to increase their detection rate to 34%. This also doubled the time taken to analyse the nodes and increased the cost by a factor of 1.6 [50]. As part of this study, the role of reverse transcriptase-polymerase chain reaction (RT-PCR) was also assessed. A detection rate of 44% was achieved using this technique compared with the 34% achieved on histological analysis. Further histological analysis of these nodes showed that part of the difference in the results between the two techniques could be attributed to benign naevus cells, melanophages and neural cells within the node making the RT-PCR oversensitive.

The Florida Melanoma Trial also examined the role of RT-PCR and showed that patients who had negative sentinel nodes both histologically and on RT-PCR had a recurrence rate of only 6.6% at three years, but those who were negative histologically and positive on RT-PCR had a recurrence rate of 22% [51]. This would again suggest that histological analysis on its own is not sensitive enough.

It is argued that micrometastases missed on routine histological analysis may have a different biological behaviour when compared to macrometastases. A complex sequence of events needs to occur for tumour cells to develop, and there is no reason to assume that melanoma cells in sentinel nodes will acquire the necessary phenotype to complete the metastatic cascade and progress to clinically significant disease [52]. Cochran agrees that whilst sampling more levels may reveal tiny amounts of melanoma, the clinical significance of these microfoci is unclear. His preliminary data suggest that patients with very small amounts of tumour in the sentinel node are unlikely to have tumour in non-sentinel nodes, to develop recurrence, or to die of melanoma [46].

Despite these debates on histological analysis, low false negative rates were found in two recent randomised trials [15, 18]. MSLT-1 showed that there was no difference in the prognosis of those who presented with false negative sentinel nodes compared with those who were observed and presented with palpable disease. For these reasons the occurrence of false negatives should not be used as a reason not to perform SLNB **(Ib/A)**.

Conclusions

Whilst the evidence continues to accumulate, certain aspects of SLNB remain controversial. The evidence would suggest that it increases disease-free survival but as yet it has not been shown in a randomised trial to have an effect on overall survival. However, at present, it is known that it is the most accurate and reliable test for diagnosing regional node metastases. This allows for accurate staging and the selection of patients for CLND and adjuvant therapy. The authors predict that it will only be a matter of time before entry into clinical trials will require SLNB status. We also believe that it will be the standard of care by 2012.

Recommendations	Evidence level
◆ Sentinel node status is predictive of the status of the rest of the lymphatic basin.	IIa/B
◆ SLNB is the best prognostic indicator for overall survival.	Ib/A
◆ Morbidity is considerably less than elective lymphadenectomy.	Ib/A
◆ SLNB allows improved staging.	Ib/A
◆ SLNB allows identification of patients to be entered in to clinical trials.	Ib/A
◆ There is a probable increase in disease-free survival.	Ib/A
◆ SLNB facilitates early nodal dissection.	Ib/A
◆ Overall survival benefit remains unproven.	Ib/A
◆ There is no evidence of increased in-transit metastatic risk following sentinel node biopsy.	Ib/A
◆ There may be a role for sentinel node biopsy in lesions of 0.75mm to 1.0mm Breslow thickness.	IIa/B
◆ It is safe to carry out sentinel node biopsy in the head and neck region.	Ib/A
◆ More research is required to identify the best histopathological method for identifying metastases.	IIa/B
◆ Currently, SLNB should be carried out in units involved in ongoing research and clinical trials.	IIa/B

References

1. Snow H. Melanotic cancerous disease. *Lancet* 1892; 2: 872.

2. Morton DL, Hoon DS, Cochran AJ, *et al*. Lymphatic mapping and sentinel lymphadenectomy for early-stage melanoma: therapeutic utility and implications of nodal micro anatomy and molecular staging for improving the accuracy of detection of nodal micro-metastases. *Ann Surg* 2003; 238: 538-49.

3. Sim FH, Taylor WF, Irvins JC, Pritchard DJ, Soule EH. A prospective randomized study of the efficacy of routine elective lymphadenectomy in the management of malignant melanoma. *Cancer* 1978; 41: 948-56.

4. Veronesi U, Adamus J, Bandiera DC, *et al*. Delayed regional lymph node dissection in stage 1 melanoma of the skin of the lower extremities. *Cancer* 1982; 49: 2420-30.

5. Balch CM, Soong SJ, Bartolucci DC, *et al*. Efficacy of an elective regional lymph node dissection of 1 to 4mm thick melanomas for patients 60 years of age and younger. *Ann Surg* 1996; 224: 255-66.

6. Cascinelli N, Morabito A, Santinami M, MacKie RM, Belli F. Immediate or delayed dissection of regional nodes in patients with melanoma of the trunk: a randomized trial; WHO melanoma programme. *Lancet* 1998; 351: 793-6.

7. Balch CM, Soong SJ, Ross MI, *et al*. Long-term results of a multi-institutional randomized trial comparing prognostic factors and surgical results for intermediate thickness melanomas (1.0 to 4.0mm). *Ann Surg Oncol* 2000; 7: 87-97.

8. Morton DL, Cagle LA, Wong JH, *et al*. Intraoperative lymphatic mapping and selective lymphadenectomy: technical details of a new procedure for clinical stage I melanoma. Presented at the Annual Meeting of the Society of Surgical Oncology, Washington DC, May 22, 1990.

9. Morton DL, Wen DR, Wong JH, *et al*. Technical details of intraoperative lymphatic mapping for early stage melanoma. *Arch Surg* 1992; 127: 392-9.

10. National Institute for Health and Clinical Excellence. Guidance on cancer services. Improving outcomes for people with skin tumours including melanoma: the manual. February 2006, www.nice.org.uk.

11. Reintgen DS, Cruse CW, Wells K, *et al*. The orderly progression of melanoma nodal metastases. *Ann Surg* 1994; 220: 759-67.

12. Thompson JF, McCarthy WH, Bosch CM, *et al*. Sentinel lymph node status as an indicator of the presence of metastatic melanoma in regional lymph nodes. *Melanoma Res* 1995; 5: 255-60.

13. Gershenwald JE, Thompson W, Mansfield PF, *et al*. Mulit-institutional melanoma lymphatic mapping experience: the prognostic value of sentinel lymph node status in 612 stage I or II melanoma patients. *J Clin Oncol* 1999; 17: 976-83.

14. Chao C, Wong SL, Edwards MJ, *et al*. Sentinel lymph node biopsy for head and neck melanomas. *Ann Surg Oncol* 2003; 10: 21-6.

15. McMasters KM, Noyes RD, Reintgen DS, *et al*. Lessons learned from the Sunbelt Melanoma Trial. *J Surg Oncol* 2004; 86: 212-23.

16. Thompson JF. The Sydney melanoma unit experience of sentinel lymphadenectomy for melanoma. *Ann Surg Oncol* 2001; 8 (Suppl): 445-7S.

17. Kretschmer L, Hilgers R, Mohrle M, *et al*. Patients with lymphatic metastasis of cutaneous malignant melanoma benefit from sentinel lymphadenectomy and early excision of their nodal disease. *Eur J Cancer* 2004; 40: 212-8.

18. Morton DL, Thompson JF, Cochran AJ, *et al*. Sentinel-node biopsy or nodal observation in melanoma. *N Engl J Med* 2006; 355: 1307-17.

19. Morton DL. Prognostic impact of sentinel lymphadenectomy in early-stage melanoma: results of MSLT-I, a phase III international trial. Presented at the 6th World Congress on Melanoma, 10 Sept 2005, Vancouver.

20. Thomas JM. The place of sentinel node biopsy in melanoma after the multicentre selective lymphadenectomy trial. *ANZ J Surg* 2006; 76: 98-9.

21. Balch CM, Buzaid AC, Soong S, *et al*. Final version of the American Joint Committee on Cancer staging system for cutaneous melanoma. *J Clin Oncol* 2001; 19: 3635-48.

22. Thomas JM, Patocskai EJ. The argument against sentinel node biopsy for malignant melanoma. *Br Med J* 2000; 321: 3-4.

23. Morton DL, Cochran AJ, Thompson JF, *et al*. Sentinel node biopsy for early-stage melanoma: accuracy and morbidity in MSLT-I, an international multicenter trial. *Ann Surg* 2005; 242: 302-11.

24. Urist MM, Balch CM, Soong S, Shaw HM, Milton GW, Maddox WA. The influence of surgical margins and prognostic factors predicting the risk of local recurrence in 3445 patients with primary melanoma. *Cancer* 1985; 55: 1398-402.

25. Estourgie SH, Nieweg OE, Valdés Olmos RA, Hoefnagel CA, Kroon BB. Review and evaluation of sentinel node procedures in 250 melanoma patients with a median follow-up of 6 years. *Ann Surg Oncol* 2003; 10: 681-8.

26. Thomas JM, Clark MA. Selective lymphadenectomy in sentinel node-positive patients may increase the risk of local/in-transit recurrence in malignant melanoma. *Eur J Surg Oncol* 2004; 30: 686-91.

27. Cerovac S, Mashhadi SA, Williams AM, Allan RA, Stanley PR, Powell BW. Is there increased risk of local and in-transit recurrence following sentinel lymph node biopsy? *J Plast Reconstr Aesthet Surg* 2006; 59: 487-93.

28. Kang JC, Wanek LA, Essner R, Faries MB, Foshag LJ, Morton DL. Sentinel lymphadenectomy does not increase the incidence of in-transit metastases in primary melanoma. *J Clin Oncol* 2005; 23: 4764-70.

29. Pawlik TM, Ross MI, Thompson JF, Eggermont AM, Gershenwald JE. The risk of in-transit melanoma metastasis depends on tumor biology and not the surgical approach to regional lymph nodes. *J Clin Oncol* 2005; 23: 4588-90.

30. Hafner J, Schmid MH, Kempf W, *et al*. Baseline staging in cutaneous malignant melanoma. *Br J Dermatology* 2004; 150: 677-86.

31. Thompson JF, Shaw HM, Hersey P, Scolyer RA. The history and future of melanoma staging. *J Surg Oncol* 2004; 86: 224-35.

32. Starritt EC, Uren RF, Scolyer RA, Quinn MJ, Thompson JF. Ultrasound examination of sentinel nodes in the initial assessment of patients with primary cutaneous melanoma. *Ann Surg Oncol* 2005; 12: 18-23.

33. Wagner JD, Schauwecker D, Davidson D, *et al*. Inefficacy of F-18 fluorodeoxy-D-glucose-positron emission tomography scans for initial evaluation in early-stage cutaneous melanoma. *Cancer* 2005; 104: 570-9.

34. Wong SL. The role of sentinel node biopsy in the management of thin melanoma. *Am J Surg* 2005; 190: 196-9.

35. Jacobs IA, Chang CK, DasGupta TK, Salti GI. Role of sentinel lymph node biopsy in patients with thin (<1mm) primary melanomas. *Ann Surg Oncol* 2003; 10: 558-61.

36. Wong SL, Brady MS, Busam KJ, Coit DG. Results of sentinel lymph node biopsy in patients with thin melanoma. *Ann Surg Oncol* 2006; 13: 302-9.

37. Hershko DD, Robb BW, Lowy AM, *et al.* Sentinel lymph node biopsy in thin melanoma patients. *J Surg Oncol* 2006; 93: 279-85.

38. Ranieri JM, Wagner JD, Wenck S, Johnson CS, Coleman JJ 3rd. The prognostic importance of sentinel lymph node biopsy in thin melanoma. *Ann Surg Oncol* 2006; 13: 927-32.

39. Cook MG, Spatz A, Brocker EB, Ruter DJ. Identification of histological features associated with metastatic potential in thin (<1.0mm) cutaneous melanoma with metastases. A study on behalf of the EORTC melanoma group. *J Pathol* 2002; 197: 188-93.

40. Guitart J, Lowe L, Piepkom M, *et al.* Histological characteristics of metastasizing thin melanomas: a case control study of 43 cases. *Arch Dermatol* 2002; 138: 603-8.

41. Karakousis GC, Gimotty PA, Botbyl JD, *et al.* Predictors of regional nodal disease in patients with thin melanomas. *Ann Surg Oncol* 2006; 13: 533-41.

42. Davison SP, Clifton MS Kauffman, Minasian L. Sentinel node biopsy for the detection of head and neck melanoma: a review. *Ann Plast Surg* 2001; 47: 206-11.

43. Morton DL, Thompson JF, Essner R, *et al.* Validation of the accuracy of intraoperative lymphatic mapping and sentinel lymphadenectomy for early stage melanoma: a multi-centre trial. *Ann Surg* 1999; 230: 453-63.

44. Vuylsteke RJ, van Leeuwen PA, Statius Muller MG, *et al.* Clinical outcome of stage I/II melanoma patients after selective sentinel lymph node dissection: long-term follow-up results. *J Clin Oncol* 2003; 21: 1057-65.

45. Gershenwald JE, Colome MI, Lee JE, *et al.* Patterns of recurrence following a negative sentinel node biopsy in 243 patients with stage I or II melanoma. *J Clin Onol* 1998; 16: 2253-60.

46. Cochran AJ, Morton DL. Detection of clinically relevant melanoma metastases requires focused, not exhaustive, evaluation of sentinel lymph nodes. *Am J Surg Path* 2006; 30: 419-20.

47. Pawlik TM, Ross MI, Gershenwald JE. Lymphatic mapping in the molecular era. *Ann Surg Oncol* 2004; 11: 362-74.

48. Li LX, Scolyer RA, Ka VS, *et al.* Pathologic review of negative sentinel lymph nodes in melanoma patients with regional recurrence: a clinicopathologic study of 1152 patients undergoing sentinel lymph node biopsy. *Am J Surg Pathol* 2003; 27: 1197-202.

49. Scolyer RA, Thompson JF, McCarthy SW. Sentinel lymph nodes in malignant melanoma: extended histopathologic evaluation improves diagnostic precision. *Cancer* 2004; 101: 2141-2.

50. Cook MG, Green MA, Anderson B, *et al.* The development of optimal pathological assessment of sentinel lymph nodes for melanoma. *J Path* 2003; 200: 314-9.

51. Reintgen DS, Jakub JW, Pendas S, Swor G, Giuliano R, Shivers S. The staging of malignant melanoma and the Florida Melanoma Trial. *Ann Surg Oncol* 2004; 11: 186S-91.

52. Giblin AV, Hayes AH, Thomas JM. The significance of melanoma micrometastases in the sentinel lymph node. *Eur J Surg Oncol* 2005; 31: 1103-4.

Chapter 9

Chapter 9

Chapter 10

Management of inguinal and pelvic nodes in patients with stage III malignant melanoma

Ahmed Ali-Khan MRCS
Specialist Registrar, Plastic Surgery
Christopher Stone FRCS (Plast.)
Consultant, Plastic and Reconstructive Surgery

ROYAL DEVON AND EXETER HOSPITAL, EXETER, UK

Introduction

With the introduction of sentinel lymph node biopsy as a staging tool for lymphatic involvement in patients with malignant melanoma, the debate over superficial inguinal versus extended ilio-inguinal lymphadenectomy for patients with proven nodal metastases has been reignited.

Where there is palpable lymphadenopathy in the groin basin it is accepted that, in the absence of identifiable distant disease, a lymphadenectomy should be undertaken to optimise loco-regional tumour control. However, opinion is divided over the role and efficacy of radical pelvic clearance compared with removal of superficial inguinal nodes only. Evidence of extra-capsular spread of disease may be regarded as a relative indication for adjuvant radiotherapy following lymphadenectomy and this is currently under investigation in the form of a prospective trial (Trans-Tasman Radiation Oncology Group) [1].

The value of completion lymphadenectomy following a positive sentinel node biopsy in the groin is similarly under evaluation within the context of the second Multi-center Selective Lymphadenectomy Trial [2]. It is likely that future nodal staging of microscopic disease will modify our approach to completion lymphadenectomy.

Methodology

Medline and PubMed searches were undertaken to gather evidence using the search terms 'groin', 'ilio-inguinal', 'lymphadenectomy', 'management', 'melanoma', 'metastatic', 'nodal', and 'pelvic'.

Techniques

In the absence of radiologically identifiable distant disease, surgical lymphadenectomy is undoubtedly the treatment modality of choice for melanoma patients with palpable nodal involvement in order to maximise loco-regional tumour control (Figure 1) [3-6]. While many, perhaps most, surgeons limit their dissection to superficial inguinal lymphadenectomy (removing those lymph nodes located within the anatomical boundaries of the femoral triangle only), others clear, or at least sample, the external iliac and obturator nodes (ilio-inguinal or, more accurately, pelvic lymphadenectomy)(Figure 2) [7].

The surgical and oncological principles of superficial inguinal dissection are well established [8-10], although variations in technique have been reported including the choice of incision, thick versus thin flaps, the value of a sartorius switch and the use of drains and fibrin glue.

Open approaches to the iliac and obturator nodes either transgress the inguinal ligament as a continuation of the inguinal incision [8, 11, 12] or preserve it via a separate transverse incision in the iliac fossa [11]. More recently, endoscopic techniques have been described, facilitated either by extra-peritoneal [13] or trans-peritoneal [14] balloon dissection. Endoscopic pelvic node dissection has gained acceptance through the experience of centres caring for patients with urological malignancy [15-18].

Risk factors for pelvic node metastases

It is estimated that of all patients with palpable nodal disease in the groin, between 20% and 40% will have occult melanoma metastases in the pelvic nodes [12, 19] **(III/B)**. The overall tumour burden within the inguinal basin is likely to influence this risk. Mann and Coit [3] reported a 32% risk of pelvic metastases in patients with up to three positive inguinal nodes in the groin, rising to 67% if more than three nodes were involved **(III/B)**. A similar correlation was demonstrated in the Royal Marsden series in which the predictive value for pelvic metastases in the presence of one involved inguinal node compared with more than one involved node was 17% and 51%, respectively [4] **(III/B)**.

However, inguinal metastases are not a prerequisite for pelvic nodal involvement, as evidenced by the elective lymph node dissection (ELND) data, with up to a third of patients harbouring occult pelvic nodal metastases at the time of ELND, despite negative inguinal nodes [7, 20-22] **(III/B)**.

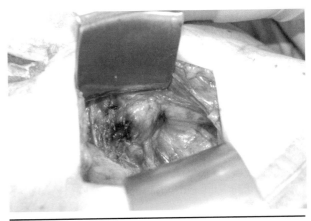

Figure 1. Pelvic lymphadenopathy at open lymphadenectomy.

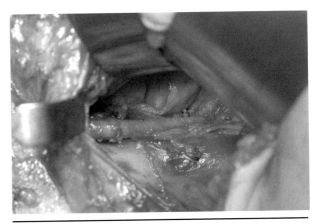

Figure 2. The external iliac vessels cleared of surrounding lymph nodes.

Cloquet's node

Cloquet's node has been defined as the highest inguinal node in the femoral canal [23] and has long been considered to be the 'gatekeeper' between the superficial inguinal and the deeper iliac chain of lymph nodes, essentially acting as sentinel for nodes in the pelvis. This perception allows the assumption that absence of involvement of Cloquet's node correlates with a low risk of pelvic nodal disease.

Shen et al [23] evaluated Cloquet's node in a series of 68 patients undergoing ilio-inguinal lymph-adenectomy for metastatic melanoma. The presence of disease in Cloquet's node had a positive predictive value for pelvic nodal disease of 67%. If Cloquet's node was negative, the pelvic nodes were also found to be negative in 77% of cases. More recently, in a review of 142 patients, Strobbe et al [24] demonstrated similar positive and negative predictive values of 62% and 83%, respectively **(III/B)**.

Hence, the evaluation of Cloquet's node is able to provide useful prognostic information with regard to the risk of pelvic nodal disease, but it is by no means inevitable that the pelvic nodes are free from disease when Cloquet's node is negative. This calls in to question the rather simplistic assertion that lymphatic dissemination of disease from the superficial inguinal node basin can only occur via the femoral canal and Cloquet's node.

Earlier work also found similarly disparate results. Coit and Brennan found sensitivity and specificity values of 90% and 92%, respectively [21], while Illig et al reported values of only 44% and 65%, respectively [25] **(III/B)** demonstrating the uncertainty that still shrouds the usefulness of Cloquet's node.

Radiological staging of pelvic nodes

Computerised tomography (CT) staging for the purpose of identification of cervical, axillary, pelvic and para-aortic lymphadenopathy [8], as well as visceral metastatic disease, is now considered to be a standard of care for melanoma patients.

However, while extensive pelvic involvement may certainly be detected by CT, the risk of understaging remains substantial [8]. In one study [26], CT accurately identified pelvic nodal involvement in only 7% of cases, rather lower than might be expected [9, 11] **(III/B)**. Hence, the positive predictive value of pelvic CT is thought to be low, and false negatives are not uncommon [26, 27] with up to a third of patients harbouring occult metastatic nodal disease despite a normal CT scan [4].

Positron emission tomography (PET) has, in one prospective series, resulted in a change to the proposed management in 15% of patients [28], although of seven patients with increased signal in the iliac lymph nodes, only three had histologically confirmed metastases at lymphadenectomy **(III/B)**, demonstrating false positives can occur and the importance of cytological confirmation of disease before undertaking lymphadenectomy on the basis of CT-PET alone.

Survival following pelvic lymph-adenectomy

Thirty years have elapsed since McCarthy et al advocated inguinal lymphadenectomy alone, without pelvic dissection [29], on the basis that pelvic nodal involvement is essentially indicative of Stage IV [30] disease, and that no surgical cure can be achieved. A number of subsequent studies have corroborated this assertion, with five-year survival rates amongst patients with melanoma metastatic to pelvic nodes consistently less than 20% [21, 22, 29, 31, 32] **(III/B)**. Nevertheless, survival data continue to emerge [3-5, 12, 33] and it would appear that the role of pelvic lymphadenectomy should now be re-appraised [34].

Retrospective reports from Amsterdam [12] and New York [3] suggest that much improved survival can be achieved despite pelvic nodal metastases, with survival at five years comparable with that of patients with inguinal nodal disease only (35% and 40%, respectively) [3]. Karakousis and Driscoll [35] and Jonk et al [36] have reported similar five-year survival rates for patients with pelvic metastases (34% and 33%).

Interestingly, of 71 patients with pelvic disease in Strobbe's series [12], only 24% were alive at five years but 20% were still alive at ten years **(III/B)**. This gives encouragement to the proponents of pelvic lymphadenectomy as it would appear that up to a fifth of patients can be effectively 'cured' by this approach.

Two sizeable retrospective series have published further outcome data within the last seven years. Hughes et al reviewed survival amongst 132 patients requiring therapeutic lymphadenectomy of groin nodes with or without pelvic nodal clearance [4]. Of, the 72 patients subjected to ilio-inguinal lymphadenectomy, 40% were found to have pelvic metastases, consistent with previously published data [12, 19]. Prognostic indicators for survival included the number of inguinal

21. Coit DG, Brennan MF. Extent of lymph node dissection in melanoma of the trunk or lower extremity. *Arch Surg* 1989; 124(2): 162-6.

22. Finck SJ, Giuliano AE, Mann BD, Morton DL. Results of ilioinguinal dissection for stage II melanoma. *Ann Surg* 1982. 196(2): 180-6.

23. Shen P, Conforti AM, Essner R, Cochran AJ, Turner RR, Morton DL. Is the node of Cloquet the sentinel node for the iliac/obturator node group? *Cancer J* 2000; 6(2): 93-7.

24. Strobbe LJ, Jonk A, Hart AA, *et al*. The value of Cloquet's node in predicting melanoma nodal metastases in the pelvic lymph node basin. *Ann Surg Oncol* 2001; 8(3): 209-14.

25. Illig L, Aigner KR, Biess B, *et al*. Diagnostic excision of the Rosenmuller's node. Screening for occult metastases before elective regional lymph node dissection in patients with lower limb melanoma? *Cancer* 1988; 61(6): 1200-6.

26. Kuvshinoff BW, Kurtz C, Coit DG. Computed tomography in evaluation of patients with stage III melanoma. *Ann Surg Oncol* 1997; 4(3): 252-8.

27. Johnson TM, Fader DJ, Chang AE, *et al*. Computed tomography in staging of patients with melanoma metastatic to the regional nodes. *Ann Surg Oncol* 1997; 4(5): 396-402.

28. Tyler DS, Onaitis M, Kherani A, *et al*. Positron emission tomography scanning in malignant melanoma. *Cancer* 2000; 89(5): 1019-25.

29. McCarthy JG, Haagensen CD, Herter FP. The role of groin dissection in the management of melanoma of the lower extremity. *Ann Surg* 1974; 179(2): 156-9.

30. Balch CM, Buzaid AC, Soong SJ, *et al*. Final version of the American Joint Committee on Cancer staging system for cutaneous melanoma. *J Clin Oncol* 2001; 19(16): 3635-48.

31. Fortner JG, Booher RJ, Pack GT. Results of groin dissection for malignant melanoma in 220 patients. *Surgery* 1964; 55: 485-94.

32. Singletary SE, Shallenberger R, Guinee VF. Surgical management of groin nodal metastases from primary melanoma of the lower extremity. *Surg Gynecol Obstet* 1992; 174(3): 195-200.

33. Meyer T, Merkel S, Gohl J, Hohenberger W. Lymph node dissection for clinically evident lymph node metastases of malignant melanoma. *Eur J Surg Oncol* 2002; 28(4): 424-30.

34. Balch CM, Ross MI. Melanoma patients with iliac nodal metastases can be cured. *Ann Surg Oncol* 1999; 6(3): 230-1.

35. Karakousis CP, Driscoll DL. Positive deep nodes in the groin and survival in malignant melanoma. *Am J Surg* 1996; 171(4): 421-2.

36. Jonk A, Kroon BB, Rumke P, van der Esch EP, Hart AA. Results of radical dissection of the groin in patients with stage II melanoma and histologically proved metastases of the iliac or obturator lymph nodes, or both. *Surg Gynecol Obstet* 1988; 167(1): 28-32.

37. Karakousis CP, Emrich LJ, Rao U. Groin dissection in malignant melanoma. *Am J Surg* 1986; 152(5): 491-5.

Chapter 10

Chapter 11

Prognostic indicators in adult soft tissue sarcoma

Paul Wilson FRCS (Plast.)

Specialist Registrar, Plastic and Reconstructive Surgery

Christopher Stone FRCS (Plast.)

Consultant, Plastic and Reconstructive Surgery

ROYAL DEVON AND EXETER HOSPITAL, EXETER, UK

Introduction

Soft tissue sarcomas (STS) are rare tumours accounting for less than 1% of all cancers with an incidence of approximately two per 100,000 population per year. Around 1,200 new cases of STS are diagnosed each year in the UK and 8,000 in the US [1].

Tumour size and grade are well recognised as independent prognostic variables in STS. The depth of the tumour in relation to the deep fascia (intra-compartmental, or deep to fascia, versus supra-fascial) is also prognostic. These variables have been incorporated into the American Joint Committee on Cancer (AJCC) staging classification for STS [2]. Other factors with proven prognostic significance for survival include anatomical site, positive resection margins and locally recurrent disease [3] **(III/B)**.

Extirpative surgery for STS aims to achieve complete tumour resection with negative histological margins, although in recent years tumour resection with planned marginal clearance and the provision of adjuvant therapies has facilitated functional limb salvage in patients who would have previously undergone debilitating amputation [4].

Re-examination of the prognostic variables for STS is therefore important in order to rationalise risks and benefits for different treatment options, as evidenced by local recurrence and survival outcome data, and for stratifying recruitment of patients to clinical trials.

Methodology

A Medline literature search was performed to gather evidence, using the search terms 'prognostic', 'indicators', 'soft tissue', 'sarcoma'.

What factors are predictive of recurrence and survival?

Factors associated with local recurrence

Local recurrence is most commonly predicted by positive resection margins [3, 5-9] and intra-operative tumour violation [7]. Additionally, there are variable associations with patient age (over 50 years) [3, 10] and high grade of tumour [10-11]. Histological subtype may also play a role, with malignant peripheral nerve sheath tumour (MPNST) in particular associated with a high risk for local recurrence [3, 10] while the local recurrence rate for liposarcoma is low [3] **(III/B)**.

In extremity STS, gender [3, 6-8, 10], depth [3, 6] and location on the limb [3, 9, 10] do not appear to influence local recurrence but this is more frequent in the upper extremity compared with the lower extremity [9].

Factors associated with distant recurrence

As for local recurrence, factors prognostic for distant recurrence of disease include high tumour grade, large size (over 5cm diameter) and location beneath the deep fascia [3, 9]. In addition, patients who develop locally recurrent disease are at increased risk of distant metastases. Histological subtypes associated with a low metastatic potential when matched for tumour grade include liposarcoma, whereas the converse is true of leiomyosarcoma [3]. Age [3], gender [3] and tumour location [3, 6-9] do not appear to be independently prognostic for distant spread **(III/B)**.

Predictors of mortality in patients with soft tissue sarcoma

Survival amongst patients with STS correlates closely with distant disease so the same independent prognostic indicators apply to mortality as for distant recurrence [8], including high tumour grade and size over 5cm [3, 6-8, 10, 12]. For patients with established metastatic disease, resectability of metastases, the disease-free interval and local recurrence before or concurrent with distant metastases are associated with poor survival [13].

Lower extremity tumours are associated with worse overall survival compared with upper extremity STS [3, 10], as they are more frequently larger and sub-fascial at presentation. Positive resection margins [3, 12, 14], and high risk histological sub-types (leiomyosarcoma [3, 10] and MPNST [3]) are similarly predictive for disease-specific mortality.

Predictors of survival after local tumour recurrence include size and grade of the primary tumour, development of further local recurrences and male gender [3].

Additional adverse prognostic factors, variably associated with higher mortality, include advancing patient age [5, 10, 12] and proximal location on an extremity [3, 10, 12]. Factors less extensively studied include a high mitotic activity [5], peri-operative blood transfusion [15, 16] and intra-operative tumour violation [7].

Grading in adult soft tissue sarcoma

The histological grade of any STS is the single most important prognostic indicator [17-20]. The two most widely used grading systems for STS are from the US National Cancer Institute (NCI), published in 1984, and the French Federation of Cancer Centres (FNCLCC) published in the same year by Trojani et al [21].

The NCI system is based upon the histological subtype of the tumour, corrected for tumour necrosis, mitotic rate, cellularity and/or pleomorphism.

The French system also proposes a three-tier grading system (low, intermediate and high grade) based upon three independent prognostic factors: necrosis, mitotic activity and degree of tumour differentiation [22].

Both the Trojani and NCI grading systems have demonstrated independent prognostic value [17, 23], although discrepancies in grading occur in approximately one third of cases [23]. An earlier grading classification from the Memorial Sloan Kettering Cancer Centre (MSKCC), was published in 1979 but is less widely used [18].

Clearly a universal grading is not possible for all types of sarcoma. Furthermore, the World Health Organisation has identified over 50 different histological subtypes [19] and many familiar diagnoses, for example, malignant fibrous histiocytoma (MFH), are undergoing re-classification. There is a spectrum of biologic behaviour ranging from the well differentiated liposarcoma (atypical lipomatous tumour), an inherently low grade, non-metastasising lesion, to the high grade round cell sarcomas such as alveolar rhabdomyosarcoma [22].

Staging of adult soft tissue sarcoma

Many staging classifications have been developed for STS, but there is none widely accepted [20], possibly owing to the difficulty in creating a system relevant to all tumours since prognostic factors can vary between histological subtypes [24].

The American Joint Committee on Cancer (AJCC) and the International Union against Cancer (UICC) staging system combine the most important determinants of survival in localised soft tissue sarcomas of the limbs: grade, depth and size of tumour [2]. It is the most widely accepted STS classification system worldwide. Histological grade and tumour size are the most important predictors of distant metastasis and tumour-related mortality in large series [3, 25] **(III/B)**.

Crude five-year survival rates in most series from major STS centres range from 25% to 55% in the retroperitoneum and head and neck sites, versus 60% to 75% or better for stage III extremity STSs [26]. These are further modified by the type and site of the tumour and other factors [27, 28]. The AJCC/UICC staging system is based primarily on the grade of the tumour, with size used to subgroup each stage (Table 1). The classification uses a four-tier system condensed into two tiers for the purposes of stage grouping; there is no allowance for an intermediate grade [29]. A modification of this staging system, based only on grade and four groups of size was proposed by Ramanathan et al [25].

Wunder et al [20] compared four commonly used staging systems for predicting systemic outcomes for patients with localised extremity STS. Those staging systems that made allowance for tumour depth, as proposed by the fourth and fifth editions of the AJCC/UICC staging system and by the MSKCC system, more accurately predicted survival than the Surgical Staging System (SSS) of the Musculoskeletal Tumour Society.

Prognostic factors excluded from the current AJCC STS staging system include site of primary tumour, margin status of the resected tumour, molecular markers, size of soft tissue sarcomas beyond 5cm, and whether the tumour is a *de novo* or recurrent lesion [26].

Histological subtype and prognosis

There has been the assumption that soft tissue sarcomas of the same grade behave similarly with regard to their potential for local recurrence and distant metastasis, despite different tumour types [30]. However, different histological subtypes of STS are associated with different risks for recurrence and death when matched for size, depth, grade and completeness of excision. This lends support to clinical treatment algorithms that include specific assessment of histological subtype in addition to tumor size, grade and depth. These four major prognostic indicators, along with patient age and anatomical site of tumour, have been incorporated into the MSKCC nomogram (Figure 1). This prognostic tool is based upon the experience of 2136 patients and predicts disease-specific death for patients with STS [31]. This has been externally validated by the UCLA and Milan groups [32, 33].

Desmoid tumours, angiosarcomas, dermato-fibrosarcoma protuberans (DFSP), Kaposi sarcoma and sarcoma arising from dura mater, brain parenchymatous organs and hollow viscera are tumour types that are excluded from the AJCC staging system [34] and are frequently excluded from multivariate analyses of sarcoma prognostic indicators.

Well differentiated liposarcoma has a low potential for local recurrence, even when marginally excised, and a very low risk for distant metastasis unless there is de-differentiation. The term 'atypical lipomatous tumour' and well differentiated liposarcoma are synonymous terms associated with similar clinical outcome. Their management should include complete function-preserving excisions with 1cm margins where possible. Adjuvant radiotherapy should be considered for sclerosing sub-types with

Chapter 11

Table 1. **Staging system for soft tissue sarcoma.** *Modified from the American Joint Committee on Cancer, 6th ed* [2].

	Classification
Primary tumour (T)	
TX	Primary tumour cannot be assessed
T0	No evidence of primary tumour
T1	Tumour ≤5cm
	T1a Superficial tumour
	T1b Deep tumour
T2	Tumour >5cm
	T2a Superficial tumour
	T2b Deep tumour
Regional lymph nodes (N)	
NX	Regional lymph nodes cannot be assessed
N0	No regional lymph node metastasis
N1	Regional lymph node metastasis
Distant metastasis (M)	
MX	Distant metastases cannot be assessed
M0	No distant metastasis
M1	Distant metastasis
Histologic grade (G)	
GX	Grade cannot be assessed
G1	Well differentiated
G2	Moderately differentiated
G3	Poorly differentiated
G4	Poorly differentiated or undifferentiated

	Stage grouping			
Stage I	T1a, 1b, 2a, 2b	N0	M0	G1-2
Stage II	T1a, 1b, 2a	N0	M0	G3-4
Stage III	T2b	N0	M0	G3-4
Stage IV	Any T	N0	M0	Any G
	Any T	N0	M1	Any G

microscopically positive surgical margins due to the close proximity of neurovascular structures [35] **(IIa/B)**. Recently, a liposarcoma-specific postoperative nomogram for disease-specific survival has been published by the Memorial Sloan-Kettering Cancer Center [36].

Sarcomas with a high risk for local recurrence but a low risk for distant spread include desmoid tumours and dermatofibrosarcoma protruberans (DFSP). Malignant peripheral nerve sheath tumours (MPNST) [3] and leiomyosarcomas [3,10] are independently associated with an increased risk of local recurrence and worse disease-specific survival. Superficial

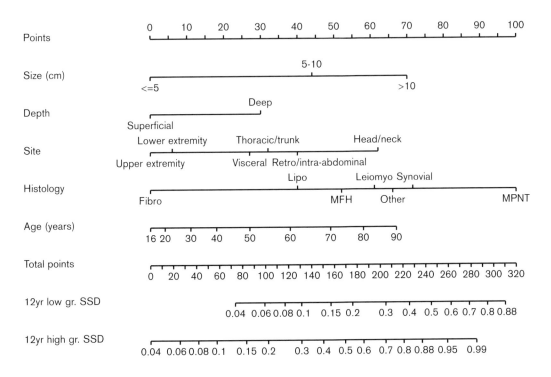

Instructions for physician. Locate the patient's tumour size on the Size axis. Draw a line straight upwards to the Points axis to determine how many points towards sarcoma-specific death the patient receives for his tumour size. Repeat the process for the other axes, each time drawing straight upward to the Points axis. Sum the points achieved for each predictor and locate this sum on the Total Points axis. Draw a line straight down to either the Low grade or High grade axis to find the patient's probability of dying from sarcoma within 12 years assuming he or she does not die of another cause first.

Instruction for patient. "If we had 100 patients exactly like you, we would expect between <predicted percentage from nomogram - 8%> and <predicted percentage + 8%> to die of sarcoma within 12 years if they did not die of another cause first, and death from sarcoma after 12 years is still possible."

Figure 1. Postoperative nomogram for 12-year sarcoma-specific death based on 2163 patients treated at MSKCC. Fibro=fibrosarcoma; Lipo=liposarcoma; Leiomyo=leiomyosarcoma; MFH=malignant fibrous histiocytoma; MPNT=malignant peripheral-nerve tumour; Gr=grade; SSD=sarcoma-specific death. *Reproduced with permission from John Wiley & Sons Ltd. © 2002. Kattan et al* [31].

leiomyosarcomas recur locally, whereas deep sub-fascial leiomyosarcomas are likely to metastasise.

Myxoid liposarcoma has a propensity for extra-pulmonary metastasis [37, 38]. This subgroup of patients should undergo cross-sectional imaging of the chest, abdomen and pelvis as part of their staging evaluation and post-treatment follow-up. Patients who present with localised 'primary' myxoid liposarcoma of the retroperitoneum, thorax, or paraspinal tissues should undergo careful evaluation to exclude an occult primary tumour in an extremity [38].

Nodal metastases in soft tissue sarcoma

Nodal involvement in STS is rare [39], although up to 10% of patients have been shown to develop a regional lymph node recurrence in one series [40]. The incidence of regional nodal metastases in STS of the head and neck is a little higher at 10-12% [41], occurring almost exclusively in high-grade tumours. In these patients, however, elective neck dissection is indicated only if the neck needs to be entered for resection of a high-risk primary lesion [42].

Soft tissue sarcomas associated with a potential for lymphatic metastasis often exhibit a degree of epithelial differentiation. Embryonal rhabdomyosarcoma, angiosarcoma, epithelioid sarcoma, clear cell sarcoma and synovial cell sarcoma are all capable of lymphatic spread and vigilance is warranted [39] **(III/B)**.

Multivariate analysis has demonstrated that the presence of lymph node metastases at presentation is the single most important risk factor for local recurrence [39]. The value of early identification and removal of occult metastatic disease in such patients by sentinel node biopsy has yet to be assessed, although this has been reported in patients with epithelioid sarcoma [40] and clear cell sarcoma [43].

Prognostic relevance of response to neoadjuvant chemotherapy

Tumour shrinkage in response to neoadjuvant chemotherapy facilitates surgical extirpation of the mass with clear margins, thereby reducing the risk of local tumour recurrence [44] and establishing early systemic treatment of occult distant disease.

Tumour chemo-sensitivity, therefore, is indirectly prognostic of outcome but has not correlated consistently with disease-free or overall survival [45-48]. A complete pathological response (more than 95% tumour necrosis) correlates significantly with a lower rate of local recurrence and improved overall survival [49].

Radiological evaluation of STS by positron emission tomography (PET) for both primary and recurrent disease [50] improves staging and treatment planning **(Ia/A)** and may be used to monitor response to chemotherapy in these patients, as for those with other tumour types [51].

Clearly, tumour shrinkage as evidenced by radiological assessment and the degree of tumour necrosis at resection are both relevant when determining chemosensitivity [52].

Marginal disease, local recurrence and re-excision in adult soft tissue sarcoma

The adequacy of surgical resection of the primary tumour has remained a cornerstone to the successful treatment of patients with STS. There does not, however, appear to be a universally accepted definition of what constitutes an adequate margin. Histologically negative but 'close' margins may still be associated with local recurrence, although many patients with microscopically involved margins do not develop locally recurrent disease [27] and margins of only 1mm may be acceptable in some cases [53].

The prognostic implications of re-excision after unplanned surgery have been explored in the literature, with contradictory conclusions in terms of survival [54], [55-57] and the significance of residual disease in the re-resection specimen has not been definitively established [55] (Table 2).

Two large retrospective reviews offer compelling and recent evidence that inadequate resection margins [4] and local tumour recurrence [10], occurring in 70% to 90% of patients undergoing unplanned excisions, impact adversely upon overall survival **(III/B)**. However, local tumour control in patients with re-excised disease appears to be similar to that of patients who received adequate primary resection [29], [57]. Moreover, residual disease at re-excision has not been shown to be prognostic for survival [29], [57] or for further local recurrence [55].

While inadequate resection margins predispose patients to both local [3, 7,16, 27, 29, 44, 58] and distant [4, 8] recurrence and disease-specific death, this may be ameliorated by re-resection, achieving outcomes similar to complete primary resection. Tumour size and grade remain more significant prognostic indicators for distant metastases than positive resection margins and there appears to be little evidence that local tumour recurrence mediates directly in the development of distant disease [29] or that improved local control translates into a survival benefit [7, 59, 60].

Table 2. Rate of re-excision and of residual disease in the re-excised specimen in major published series
Data modified from Fiore et al [64].

Study	No. of patients	Site	Presentation	Re-excision	Residual disease (%)
Giuliano [61] 1985	90	Ext	Primary	90 (100%)	49
Zornig [54] 1995	189	Ext,Tr	NS	67 (35%)	45
Goodlad [62] 1996	236	Ext, Tr, HN	Primary	95 (40%)	58
Davis [55] 1997	239	Ext	Any inc. DFSP	104 (43%)	40
Karakousis [56] 1999	194	Ext	NS	60 (31%)	63
Lewis [57] 2000	1092	Ext	Primary	407 (37%)	39
Chui [63] 2002	116	Any	Primary	69 (59%)	48
Zagars [29] 2003	1225	Any	Any	295 (24%)	46
Fiore [64] 2006	597	Ext	Primary	318 (53%)	24

Ext=Extremity; Tr=Trunk; HN=head and neck; NS=not specified

Where limb-sparing marginal resection of extremity STS is planned in combination with neoadjuvant and adjuvant radiotherapy, local recurrence rates of less than 4% can be achieved [9]. Unplanned positive margins by the sarcoma team or primary surgery upon unrecognised STS results in higher local recurrence rates and decreased overall survival unless residual disease is re-excised [29].

Undoubtedly, positive resection margins predispose to local recurrence, although this may be largely negated by re-resection. Given that local recurrence also occurs in high risk tumours it becomes linked with reduced overall survival, but locally recurrent disease is an unlikely source of distant metastases, reflecting instead the biological aggressiveness of the primary tumour [29, 58].

Molecular markers in soft tissue sarcoma

Recent immunohistochemical studies on STS have shown that over-expression of Ki-67 antigen, p53, proliferating cell nuclear antigen, topo-isomerase IIa, bcl-2, and/or mdm2 are all associated with poor prognosis, and that immunohistochemical detection of fatty acid synthase (FAS) correlates with reduced disease-free and overall survival [65]. The Wilms' tumour gene (WT1) is also variably expressed in STS.

WT1 is a potential molecular marker for predicting prognosis and a promising tumour antigen for targeted tumour-specific immunotherapy [66].

There is some evidence that tumour hypoxia may be associated with poor outcome in patients with STS. Carbonic anhydrase IX activity, as an intrinsic marker of tissue hypoxia, has been detected in high-grade, large and sub-fascial STS, but its value as an independent prognostic indicator has yet to be determined.

Fusion genes as prognostic tools in STS

Chromosomal translocations occur at mitosis to create chimeric or derivative chromosomes. Each chromosomal translocation introduces breaks within two cellular genes and results in the joining of portions of the two genes to create a novel chimeric or fusion gene. The expression of these fusion genes may have prognostic significance in STS [67] and the increased use of the immunohistochemistry and molecular oncology markers is likely to advance the sub-classification of STS [68].

Synovial sarcoma is characterised cytogenetically by the chromosomal translocation t(X;18)(SYT-SSX). In a large multi-centre retrospective study of 243 patients, Ladanyi *et al* [69] showed that tumours with

Chapter 11

SSX1 fusion transcripts were significantly more aggressive than tumours with SSX2, in keeping with previous studies. However, the results of a multi-institutional trial by Guillou et al [70] found no association between the type of fusion gene and clinical outcome, demonstrating instead that the histological grade of the tumour rather than SYT-SSX fusion type was the strongest predictor for survival in a multivariate model.

Other tumour types in which prognostic molecular markers have been studied include Ewing's/peripheral neuroectodermal tumour (EWS-FLI1), alveolar rhabdomyosarcoma (PAX3-FKHR and PAX7-FKHR) and myxoid liposarcoma (TLS-CHOP) [71].

Head and neck soft tissue sarcoma

There have been 19 major reported series of soft tissue sarcomas of the head and neck since 1981, including the recent review by Patel and Shah [42]. Overall five-year survival ranges from 32% to 87% and disease-free survival from 27% to 66%. Effective local tumour control does not, unfortunately, necessarily translate into improved disease-free survival.

As for STS at other sites, tumour grade, size, and surgical margin status are important and independent prognostic factors [72]. Some histological subtypes, including hemangiopericytomas and DFSP, have a significantly better prognosis than others, such as rhabdomyosarcoma and angiosarcoma [68]. The complexity of the local anatomy complicates extirpative surgery and adjuvant radiotherapy is indicated where marginal resection has been undertaken [73]. Unsurprisingly, tumour extension to skin, bone or neurovascular structures has been found to correlate significantly with poor outcome [74].

Conclusions

Tumour size, depth, grade and histological subtype remain the most significant prognostic indicators for patients with STS, although roles are emerging for sentinel lymph node biopsy and molecular marker analysis in predicting outcome. Complete surgical resection should be attempted wherever possible although functional limb salvage surgery in combination with adjuvant therapy is preferable to amputation in most cases. Marginal resection and local recurrence correlate with reduced survival but this may be more of a reflection of biological aggressiveness of the primary tumour rather than being representative of a direct link between persistent local disease and systemic metastases.

Recommendations

	Evidence level
◆ Use of the prognostic nomogram developed by the MSKCC may be useful for patient counselling, follow-up scheduling, and clinical trial eligibility determination.	III/B
◆ The management of well differentiated liposarcomas should include complete function-preserving excisions with 1cm margins where possible.	IIa/B
◆ Sentinel lymph node biopsy should be considered in patients with soft tissue sarcomas with a potential for lymph node metastasis.	III/B
◆ FDG-PET is an effective diagnostic tool for the evaluation of both primary and recurrent soft tissue lesions and is also useful in monitoring the clinical response of chemotherapy.	Ia/A
◆ Patients who either develop a local recurrence or present with locally recurrent disease should be strongly considered for adjuvant systemic therapy.	III/B

References

1. Thomas J. Soft tissue sarcomas. *Curr Pract Surg* 1996; 8: 59-63.

2. Greene FL, Page DL, Fleming FD, *et al*, Eds. American Joint Committee on Cancer: Cancer Staging Manual, 6th ed. New York, NY: Springer, 2002: 221-6.

3. Pisters PW, Leung PH, Woodruff JF, Shi W, Brennan MF. Analysis of prognostic factors in 1041 patients with localized soft tissue sarcomas of the extremities. *J Clin Oncol* 1996; 14: 1679-89.

4. Stojadinovic A, Leung DH, Hoos A, Jaques DP, Lewis JJ, Brennan MF. Analysis of the prognostic significance of microscopic margins in 2,084 localized primary adult soft tissue sarcomas. *Ann Surg* 2002; 235(3): 424-34.

5. Singer S, Corson JM, Gonin R, *et al*. Prognostic factors predictive of survival and local recurrence for extremity soft tissue sarcoma. *Ann Surg* 1994; 219: 165-73.

6. Stotter AT, Ahern RP, Fisher C, *et al*. The influence of local recurrence of extremity soft tissue sarcoma on metastases and survival. *Cancer* 1990; 65: 1119-29.

7. Tanabe KK, Pollock RE, Ellis LM, Murphy A, Sherman N, *et al*. Influence of surgical margins on outcome in patients with preoperatively irradiated extremity soft tissue sarcomas. *Cancer* 1994; 73: 1652-9.

8. Rossi CR, Foletto M, Alessio S, *et al*. Limb-sparing treatment for soft tissue sarcomas: influence of prognostic factors. *J Surg Oncol* 1996; 63: 3-8.

9. Gerrand CH, Bell RS, Wunder JS, *et al*. The influence of anatomic location on outcome in patients with soft tissue sarcoma. *Cancer* 2003; 97: 485-92.

10. Eilber FC, Rosen G, Nelson SD, *et al*. High-grade extremity soft tissue sarcomas: factors predictive of local recurrence and its effect on morbidity and mortality. *Ann Surg* 2003; 237(2): 218-26.

11. Eilber FC, Rosen G, Nelson SD, *et al*. Local recurrences of soft tissue sarcomas in adults: a retrospective analysis of prognostic factors in 102 cases after surgery and radiation therapy. *Eur J Cancer* 1994; 30A: 1636-42.

12. Collin C, Godbold J, Hajdu S, Brennan M. Localized extremity soft tissue sarcoma: an analysis of factors affecting survival. *J Clin Oncol* 1987; 5: 601-12.

13. Grobmyer SR, Brennan MF. Predictive variables detailing the recurrence rate of soft tissue sarcomas. *Curr Opin Oncol* 2003; 15: 319-26.

14. Emrich LJ, Ruka W, Driscoll D, Karakousis CP. The effect of local recurrence on survival time in adult high-grade soft tissue sarcomas. *J Clin Epidemiol* 1989; 42: 105-10.

15. Rosenberg SA, Seipp CA, White DE, Wesley R. Perioperative blood transfusions are associated with increased rates of recurrence and decreased survival in patients with high-grade soft tissue sarcomas of the extremities. *J Clin Oncol* 1985; 3: 698-709.

16. Stefanovski PD Bidoli E, De Paoli A, *et al*. Prognostic factors in soft tissue sarcomas: a study of 395 patients. *Eur J Surg Oncol* 2002; 28: 153-64.

17. Mandard AM, Petiot GF, Marnay J, *et al*. Prognostic factors in soft tissue sarcomas. A multivariate analysis of 109 cases. *Cancer* 1989; 63: 1437-51.

18. Hajdu SI. *Pathology of soft tissue tumors*. Philadelphia: Lea and Febiger, 1979.

19. Fletcher CDM, Unni KK, Mertens F, Eds. *Pathology and genetics of tumors of soft tissue and bone*. Vol 5 of World Health Organisation classification of tumors. Lyon, France: IARC Press, 2002.

20. Wunder JS, Healey JH, Davis AM, Brennan MF. A comparison of staging systems for localized extremity soft tissue sarcoma. *Cancer* 2000; 88(12): 2721-30.

21. Trojani M, Contesso G, Coindre JM, Rouesse J, Bui NB, *et al*. Soft-tissue sarcomas of adults; study of pathological prognostic variables and definition of a histopathological grading system. *Int J Cancer* 1984; 33: 37-42.

22. Deyrup AT, Weiss SW. Grading of soft tissue sarcomas: the challenge of providing precise information in an imprecise world. *Histopathology* 2006; 48(1): 42-50.

23. Guillou L, Coindre JM, Bonichon F, *et al*. Comparative study of the National Cancer Institute and French Federation of Cancer Centers Sarcoma Group grading systems in a population of 410 adult patients with soft tissue sarcoma. *J Clin Oncol* 1997; 15: 350-62.

24. Rydholm A, Gustafson P. Should tumor depth be included in prognostication of soft tissue sarcoma? *BMC Cancer* 2003; 3. http://www.biomedcentral.com/1471-2407/3/17.

25. Ramanathan RC, A'Hern R, Fisher C, Thomas JM. Modified staging system for extremity soft tissue sarcomas. *Ann Surg Oncol* 1999; 6(1): 57-69.

26. Kotilingam D, Lev DC, Lazar AJF, Pollock RE. Soft tissue sarcoma: evolution and change. *CA Cancer J Clin* 2006; 56: 282-91.

27. Stojadinovic A, Leung DHY, Allen P, Lewis JJ, Jaques DP, Brennan MF. Primary adult STS: time-dependent influence of prognostic variables. *J Clin Oncol* 2002; 20(21): 4344-52.

28. Clark MA, Fisher C, Judson I, Thomas M. Soft-tissue sarcomas in adults. *New Engl J Med* 2005; 353: 701-11.

29. Zagars GK, Ballo MT, Pisters PWT, Pollock RE, *et al*. Prognostic factors for patients with localized soft-tissue sarcoma treated with conservation surgery and radiation therapy. *Cancer* 2003; 97(10): 2530-43.

30. Koea JB, Leung D, Lewis JJ, Brennan MF. Histopathologic type: an independent prognostic factor in primary soft tissue sarcoma of the extremity. *Ann Surg Oncol* 2003; 10(4): 432-40.

31. Kattan MW, Leung DHY, Brennan MF. Postoperative nomogram for 12-year sarcoma-specific death. *J Clin Oncol* 2002; 20: 791-6.

32. Eilber FC, Brennan MF, Eilber FR, Dry SM, Singer S, Kattan MW. Validation of the postoperative nomogram for 12-year sarcoma-specific mortality. *Cancer* 2004; 101(10): 2270-5.

33. Mariani L, Miceli R, Kattan MW, *et al*. Validation and adaptation of a nomogram for predicting the survival of patients with extremity soft tissue sarcoma using a three-grade system. *Cancer* 2004; 103(2): 402-8.

Chapter 11

34. AJCC cancer staging manual. American Joint Committee on Cancer, 6th ed. New York: Springer 2002.

35. Kooby DA, Antonescu CR, Brennan MF, Singer S. Atypical lipomatous tumor/well-differentiated liposarcoma of the extremity and trunk wall: importance of histological subtype with treatment recommendations. *Ann Surg Oncol* 2003; 11(1): 78-84.

36. Dalal KM, Kattan MW, Antonescu CR, Brennan MF, Singer S. Subtype specific nomogram for patients with primary liposarcoma of the retroperitoneum, extremity or trunk. *Ann Surg* 2006; 244: 381-91.

37. Estourgie SH, Nielsen GP, Ott MJ. Metastatic patterns of extremity myxoid liposarcoma and their outcome. *J Surg Oncol* 2002; 80: 89-93.

38. Pisters PW. Metastatic patterns of extremity liposarcoma and their outcome: commentary. *J Surg Oncol* 2002; 80: 94-5.

39. Fong Y, Coit D, Woodruff J, et al. Lymph node metastasis from soft tissue sarcoma in adults. Analysis of data from a prospective database of 1772 sarcoma patients. *Ann Surg* 1993; 217: 72-7.

40. Seal A, Tse R, Wehrli B, Hammond A, Temple C. Sentinel node biopsy as an adjunct to limb salvage surgery for epithelioid sarcoma of the hand. *World J Surg Oncol* 2005; 3(1): 41.

41. Farhood A, Hajdu S, Shiu M, et al. Soft tissue sarcomas of the head and neck in adults. *Am J Surg* 1990; 160: 365-9.

42. Patel SG, Shaha AR, Shah JP. Soft tissue sarcomas of the head and neck: an update. *Am J Otolaryngol* 2001; 22: 2-18.

43. Waddah B. Al-Refaie M, Mir W. Clear cell sarcoma in the era of sentinel lymph node mapping. *J Clin Oncol* 2004; 87(3): 126-9.

44. Le Vay J, O'Sullivan B, Catton C, et al. Outcome and prognostic factors in soft tissue sarcoma in the adult. *Int J Rad Oncol Biol Phys* 1993; 27: 1091-9.

45. Schuetze SM, Rubin BP, Vernon C, et al. Use of positron emission tomography in localized extremity soft tissue sarcoma treated with neoadjuvant chemotherapy. *Cancer* 2005; 103(2): 339-48.

46. Meric F, Hess KR, Varma DG, et al. Radiographic response to neoadjuvant chemotherapy is a predictor of local control and survival in soft tissue sarcomas. *Cancer* 2002; 95(5): 1120-6.

47. Pezzi CM, Pollock RE, Evans HL, et al. Preoperative chemotherapy for soft tissue sarcomas of the extremities. *Ann Surg* 1990; 211: 476-81.

48. Pisters PW, Patel SR, Varma DG, et al. Preoperative chemotherapy for stage IIIB extremity soft tissue sarcoma: long-term results from a single institution. *J Clin Oncol* 1997; 15(12): 3481-7.

49. Eilber FC, Rosen G, Eckardt J. Treatment-induced pathologic necrosis: a predictor of local recurrence and survival in patients receiving neoadjuvant therapy for high-grade extremity soft tissue sarcomas. *J Clin Oncol* 2001; 19(13): 3203-9.

50. Ioannidis JPA, Lau J. 18F-FDG PET for the diagnosis and grading of soft-tissue sarcoma: a meta-analysis. *J Nucl Med* 2003; 44(5): 717-24.

51. Schuetze SM, Rubin BP, Vernon C, et al. Use of positron emission tomography in localized extremity soft tissue sarcoma treated with neoadjuvant chemotherapy. *Cancer* 2005; 103(2): 339-48.

52. Wendtner CM, Abdel-Rahman S, Krych M, et al. Response to neoadjuvant chemotherapy combined with regional hyperthermia predicts long-term survival for adult patients with retroperitoneal and visceral high-risk soft tissue sarcomas. *J Clin Oncol* 2002; 20(14): 3156-64.

53. Dickinson IC, Whitwell DJ, Battistuta D, et al. Surgical margin and its influence on survival in soft tissue sarcoma. *ANZ J Surg* 2006; 76: 104-9.

54. Zornig C, Weh HJ, Krull A, Schwarz R, Hilgert RE, Schroder S. Soft tissue sarcomas of the extremities and trunk in the adult: report of 124 cases. *Lagenbecks Arch Chir* 1992; 377: 28-33.

55. Davis AM, Kandel RA, Wunder JS, et al. The impact of residual disease on local recurrence in patients treated by initial unplanned resection for soft tissue sarcoma of the extremity. *J Surg Oncol* 1997; 66(2): 81-7.

56. Karakousis CP, Driscoll DL. Treatment and local control of primary extremity soft tissue sarcoma. *J Surg Oncol* 1999; 71: 155-61.

57. Lewis JJ, Leung D, Espat J, Woodruff JM, Brennan MF. Effect of re-resection in extremity soft tissue sarcoma. *Ann Surg* 2000; 231(5): 655-63.

58. Trovik CS, Bauer HCF, Alvegard TA, et al. Surgical margins, local recurrence and metastasis in soft tissue sarcomas: 559 surgically treated patients from the Scandinavian Sarcoma Group Register. *Eur J Cancer* 2000; 36: 710-6.

59. Li XQ, Parkekh SG, Rosenberg AE, Mankin HJ. Assessing prognosis for high-grade soft-tissue sarcomas. *Ann Surg Oncol* 1996; 3: 550-7.

60. Ueda T, Yoshikawa H, Mori S, et al. Influence of local recurrence on the prognosis of soft-tissue sarcomas. *J Bone Joint Surg* 1997; 79B: 553-7.

61. Giuliano AE, Eilber FR. The rationale for planned re-operation after unplanned total excision of soft tissue sarcomas. *J Clin Oncol* 1985; 3: 1344-8.

62. Goodlad JR, Fletcher CDM, Smith MA. Surgical resection of primary soft-tissue sarcoma. Incidence of residual tumor in 95 patients needing re-excision after local resection. *J Bone Joint Surg Br* 1996; 78: 658-1.

63. Chui CH, Spunt TL, Liu T, et al. Is re-excision in paediatric non-rhabdomyosarcoma soft tissue sarcoma necessary after an initial unplanned resection? *J Pediatr Surg* 2002; 37: 1424-9.

64. Fiore M, Casali PG, Miceli R, et al. Prognostic effect of re-excision in adult soft tissue sarcoma of the extremity. *Ann Surg Oncol* 2006; 13(1): 110-7.

65. Takahiro T, Shinichi K, Toshimitsu S. Expression of fatty acid synthase as a prognostic indicator in soft tissue sarcomas. *Clinical Cancer Research* 2003; 9: 2204-12.

66. Sotobori T, Ueda T, Oji Y, et al. Prognostic significance of Wilms tumor gene (WT1) mRNA expression in soft tissue sarcoma. *Cancer* 2005; 106(10): 2233-40.

67. Eisenberg BL. Sarcomas: editorial overview. *Curr Opin Oncol* 2002; 14(4): 399-400.

Chapter 11

68. Bentz BG, Bhuvanesh S, Woodruff J, Brennan M, Shah JP, Kraus D. Head and neck soft tissue sarcomas: a multivariate analysis of outcomes. *Ann Surg Oncol* 2004; 11(6): 619-28.

69. Ladanyi M, Antonescu CR, Leung DH, Woodruff JM, *et al.* Impact of SYT-SSX fusion type on the clinical behavior of synovial sarcoma: a multi-institutional retrospective study of 243 patients. *Cancer Research* 2002; 62: 135-40.

70. Guillou L, Benhattar J, Bonichon F, *et al.* Histologic grade, but not SYT-SSX fusion type, is an important prognostic factor in patients with synovial sarcoma: a multicenter, retrospective analysis. *J Clin Oncol* 2004; 22(20): 4040-50.

71. Oliveira AM, Fletcher CDM. Molecular prognostication for soft tissue sarcomas: are we ready yet? *J Clin Oncol* 2004; 22(20): 4031-4.

72. Tran LM, Mark R, Meier R, Calcaterra TC, Parker RG. Sarcomas of the head and neck. Prognostic factors and treatment stategies. *Cancer* 1992; 70(1): 169-77.

73. Lewis JJ, Benedetti F. Adjuvant therapy for soft tissue sarcomas. *Surg Oncol Clin North Am* 1997; 6: 847-62.

74. Le Vay J, O'Sullivan B, Catton C, *et al.* An assessment of prognostic factors in soft-tissue sarcoma of the head and neck. *Arch Otolaryngol Head Neck Surg* 1994; 120: 981-6.

Prognostic indicators in adult soft tissue sarcoma

Chapter 12

Evidence-based imaging of soft tissue sarcomas

Alun G Davies MA BM BCh MRCS FRCR

Specialist Registrar, Radiology

David AT Silver FRCR FRCP

Consultant Radiologist

ROYAL DEVON AND EXETER HOSPITAL, EXETER, UK

Introduction

Soft tissue sarcomas are uncommon lesions, representing approximately 1% of all malignant tumours [1, 2]. The annual incidence of soft tissue sarcomas is approximately 1-2/100,000 population. Benign soft tissue tumours, however, far outnumber malignant tumours, with an incidence of around 300/100,000 population [3, 4].

The radiological evaluation of a suspected soft tissue mass has changed dramatically with the advent of computer-assisted imaging. The currently available imaging modalities offer numerous non-invasive methods to diagnose and stage suspected soft tissue sarcomas. This chapter sets out to review the available imaging options and to ascertain the levels of evidence (where appropriate) to substantiate their usage.

Methodology

A Medline and PubMed search was employed to gather evidence using various search terms including 'soft tissue sarcomas/tumours', in combination with 'MRI', 'Ultrasound', 'CT', and 'PET'. Searches were also performed of the Cochrane database, Evidence-based imaging database and NICE guidelines; there were no positive searches from these three.

Purpose of imaging

The main objectives of imaging are:

- To confirm presence of a soft tissue mass.
- Local staging.
- Grading and characterisation.
- Detect regional nodal metastasis.
- Guide biopsy.
- Detect distant metastases, e.g. lung.
- Evaluation of response to neoadjuvant therapy.
- Detection of tumour recurrence.

This information is crucial in guiding patient treatment options.

Initial evaluation

Imaging of soft tissue sarcomas requires a multi-modality approach, with no single imaging modality being ideal for every tumour.

Prior to imaging it is important to obtain an accurate clinical history as this can influence and guide the radiological interpretation. The combination of imaging findings and patient history may allow a specific diagnosis to be made, e.g. muscle haematoma following trauma. Important information that is required includes:

- Is the lesion painful? (Inflammatory process).
- Is there history of trauma?
- Has the lesion remained stable over a long period, or is it growing?
- Has the lesion varied in size over time or activity? (Ganglion or vascular anomaly).
- Is there history of a previous lesion or malignancy?
- Has there been previous surgery or radiotherapy?
- Is the lesion solitary or multiple?

What are the available imaging modalities in the evaluation of soft tissue sarcomas?

Although radiographs are frequently unrewarding, they can provide invaluable information when positive. Radiographs may reveal skeletal deformity that can masquerade as a soft tissue mass or soft tissue mineralisation that may be suggestive, and at times characteristic, of a specific diagnosis. For example, they may reveal the phleboliths within a venous vascular malformation (Figure 1), the osteocartilaginous masses of synovial osteochondromatosis, or the peripherally more mature ossification of myositis ossificans. Radiographs can also provide an excellent method for assessment of osseous involvement by a soft tissue tumour, such as remodelling, periosteal reaction, or overt destruction.

Ultrasound (US) and magnetic resonance imaging (MRI) are the most useful techniques for investigating soft tissue masses. Ultrasound is best suited to superficial lesions and MRI to deep, large or diffuse lesions.

Despite the early optimism for the superiority of MRI in assessing soft tissue tumours, MRI remains relatively limited in its ability to precisely characterise

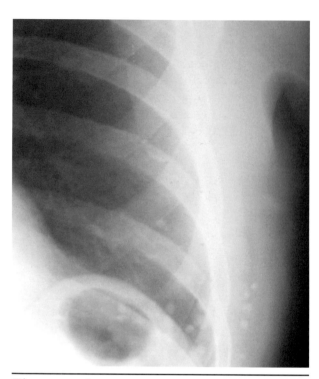

Figure 1. Extensive venous vascular malformation of the lateral chest wall. Note the presence of multiple phleboliths.

these tumours, with a correct histological diagnosis reached upon the basis of imaging studies in only approximately one quarter to one third of cases [5-7].

Role of ultrasound

Sonography is useful in the assessment of musculoskeletal soft tissue masses. It can be a reliable, expedient and readily accessible alternative to other, more costly, imaging techniques such as MR imaging. High frequency probes (9-13MHz) are indicated for the evaluation of superficial structures or subcutaneous masses, and deeper lesions require a lower frequency transducer (3.5-7MHz).

Ultrasound as an initial investigation can confirm or refute the clinical suspicion of a soft tissue mass. In many instances ultrasound can provide a confident diagnosis by taking into account the clinical features along with the ultrasound appearance, and thereby obviate the need for further imaging (Figures 2-4).

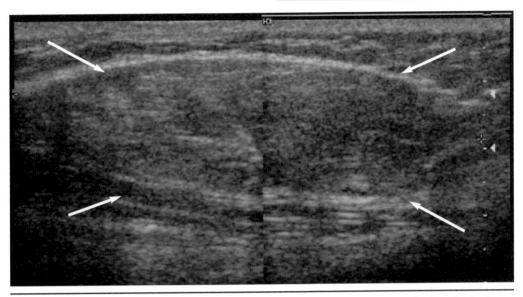

Figure 2. Subcutaneous lipoma. The lesion (arrows) has a typical elliptical shape with multiple linear reflective striations and is slightly hyperechoic compared with adjacent fat.

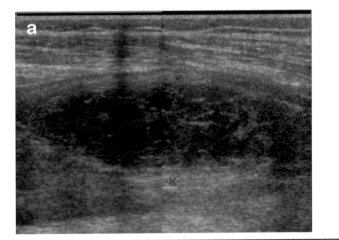
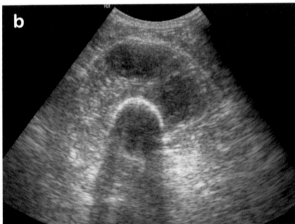

Figure 3. A 38-year-old man with a large haematoma. a) Longitudinal extended field of view ultrasound. b) Transverse ultrasound of the anterior thigh, demonstrating a large complex hypoechoic lesion in the quadriceps muscle compartment consistent with a haematoma.

Chapter 12

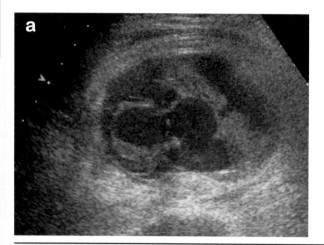
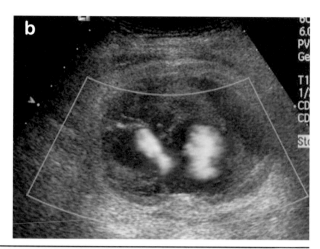

Figure 4. Pseudo-aneurysm. a) Large mainly hypoechoic mass in the groin. b) Power Doppler demonstrates large areas of flow within the lesion.

Ultrasound can readily differentiate solid from cystic lesions. Purely cystic lesions are benign, whereas a minority of solid lesions turn out to be malignant.

Other ultrasound features such as lesion morphology, calcification, compressibility, the presence and type of vascularity and the pattern of internal echoes can all help to narrow the differential diagnosis.

Can ultrasound differentiate benign from malignant solid lesions?

Imaging characteristics of solid masses and complex cystic lesions are generally non-specific and ultrasound has not proven useful in differentiating between benign and malignant solid lesions [8-10] (Figure 5).

Colour, power Doppler and spectral wave analysis may, however, be useful in differentiating benign from malignant tumours. A study by Bodner et al [11] evaluated 79 musculoskeletal tumours: four major (stenosis, occlusions, trifurcations, and vascular patterns) and three minor (shunt, self-loop, and minimum-maximum RI ratio) vessel characteristics were defined. The authors showed that a combination of two major characteristics resulted in the highest sensitivity (94%) and

specificity (93%) in differentiating benign and malignant tumours. However, tumours less than 1.5cm in diameter do not induce ultrasound-detectable malignant neovascularity [12]. Furthermore, completely necrotic tumours also show a lack of vascularisation and thus are not accessible for colour and power

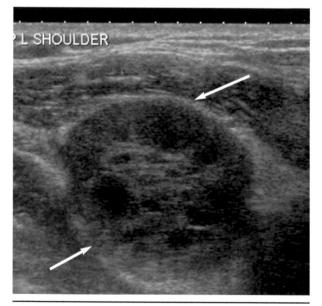

Figure 5. Ultrasound of the anterior chest wall shows a heterogenous low echogenicity lesion (arrows) that has relatively well defined margins. The ultrasound findings are non-specific. The lesion was a leiomyosarcoma.

Doppler ultrasound. The role of ultrasound at present for reliably differentiating benign from malignant lesions is debatable. Colour Doppler ultrasound can be helpful in selecting preferential sites for biopsy by differentiating areas that will most likely represent viable tumour (vascularised) from necrotic areas (avascular).

MRI technique

An outline for imaging of soft tissue sarcomas is provided in the Royal College of Radiologists' booklet 'Recommendations for Cross-sectional Imaging in Cancer Management' [13]. There are a wide array of pulse sequences available utilising spin echo (SE), inversion recovery (IR) and gradient-echo (GE) techniques, with or without fat suppression/saturation. In general, T1-weighted and fast/turbo spin-echo T2-weighted sequences are used for the evaluation of tumours. Tumours should be imaged in at least two planes, firstly, in the coronal or sagittal plane (dependent on the location of tumour), to include the lesion, adjacent joint and regional lymphatic site and, secondly, in the axial plane to cover the lesion. Cod liver oil capsules taped to the skin over the site of the suspected lesion are useful to ensure the correct area has been imaged which is particularly important if no lesion can be identified by palpation.

Fat saturation/suppression sequences

These techniques are useful for characterising soft tissue tumours of fatty origin; they facilitate improved conspicuity of pathology compared with conventional T1- and T2-weighted sequences alone, and are particularly useful in the demonstration of inflammation, infection and post-traumatic changes, e.g. muscle tear.

There are two different ways in which fat signal can be suppressed:

♦ Short tau inversion recovery (STIR).
♦ Frequency-specific (spectral) presaturation sequences.

STIR sequences display additive T1 and T2 contrast with fat suppression. The additive T1 and T2 contrast is a particular advantage with long T1 tissues, e.g. fluid appearing bright, which is opposite to conventional T1-weighted sequences where long T1-weighted tissues are of low signal (Figure 6).

STIR imaging does, however, have a number of disadvantages. The specificity for characterisation of a lesion is reduced when compared to T1- and T2-weighted images. Fat suppression is based upon tissue relaxation times, and lesions with a similar relaxation time will also show suppression of signal. This includes haemorrhage and tissue enhancement following gadolinium contrast injection. There may also be variable fat suppression in different locations within the magnetic field.

Spectral pre-saturation imaging is frequency-specific (dependent on the fact that fat and water protons precess at slightly different frequencies) and can be applied to conventional T1 and T2 sequences. As the reduction in fat signal is based upon a frequency difference and not relaxation time value, the spectral pre-saturation technique is more specific for the diagnosis of haemorrhage, and can be used following gadolinium injection. It is particularly useful when used as a T1 sequence with gadolinium to demonstrate enhancement of lesions in fatty tissues, as without its use the high signal enhancing lesion may become less conspicuous as it is surrounded by high signal fat. As it has to be added to a conventional T1- or T2-weighted sequence, this lengthens the imaging time, especially with a T1-weighted sequence.

The use of contrast

Intravenous gadolinium is helpful if a mass is not pure blood, water or fat. Fat-suppressed T1-weighted images are used for optimum enhancement. In general, MR imaging contrast agents enhance the signal intensity of many tumours on T1-weighted spin echo MR images, in some cases enhancing the demarcation between tumour and muscle, and tumour and oedema, as well as providing information on tumour vascularity [14, 15]. In reality the differentiation between tumour and muscle is quite well delineated

Chapter 12

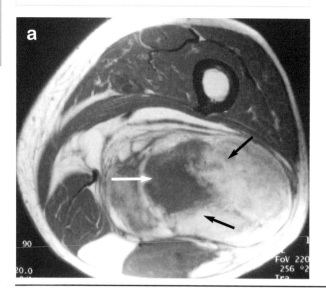

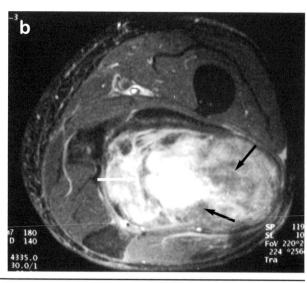

Figure 6. a) Axial T1-weighted spin echo MR image. **b)** Axial STIR MR image. A large tumour is shown within the posterior thigh compartment. On T1-weighted imaging there are areas of high signal corresponding to fatty elements within the tumour; these only partly suppress on STIR imaging (black arrows). The low signal areas on T1-weighted imaging appear as high signal on STIR (white arrows). Histology confirmed a liposarcoma.

without contrast-enhanced imaging on T2-weighted MR images, and the accurate distinction between tumour and oedema is probably of little practical value. Oedema, which is infrequent without superimposed trauma or haemorrhage, is considered to be part of the reactive zone around the neoplasm and as a result, is removed en bloc with the tumour [16]. Gadolinium is useful for the evaluation of haematomas; contrast-enhanced imaging may reveal a small tumour within the haemorrhage on conventional MR imaging [17, 18]. One potential pitfall is the development of fibrovascular tissue within the organising haematoma which may also enhance [19].

Gadolinium-enhanced imaging has also been used to differentiate solid from cystic (or necrotic) areas within solid tumours, with the necrotic or cystic areas showing no enhancement [14]. This distinction is especially important to guide biopsy and may be difficult or impossible to make on conventional T2-weighted MR images, when both tumour and fluid show high signal intensity, well defined margins and homogenous signal intensity. A myxoma and myxoid sarcoma can mimic a cyst (being low and high signal on T1- and T2-weighted sequences, respectively) on unenhanced images, but show soft tissue

enhancement. A cyst does not enhance except for its wall. In general if patients have had an ultrasound examination as a preliminary investigation, then solid and cystic lesions can be readily differentiated.

Local staging

Important considerations in the staging of the local extent of a tumour include:

- Tumour size.
- Location.
- Tumour margin.
- Location relative to the deep fascia.
- Compartmental spread.
- Invasion of adjacent bone and neurovascular structures.

MR imaging has emerged as the preferred imaging modality for the localised staging of soft tissue sarcomas. It provides superior soft tissue contrast, and avoids the use of iodinated contrast agents and ionizing radiation.

Although initial investigations maintained that CT was superior to MR imaging in detecting destruction of cortical bone, later studies suggest that these two studies are comparable [20]. MRI is superior to CT for staging the intramedullary extent of tumour [21].

The location of a tumour relative to major vascular structures can be assessed accurately by MRI. Demas *et al* found MRI to be highly accurate in defining tumour margins relative to the neurovascular bundle [22]. However, adherence of tumour to the neurovascular bundle could not be predicted pre-operatively unless there was encasement.

The superiority of MRI over CT imaging in the local staging of soft tissue sarcomas has, however, been challenged. In a multi-institutional study of a 133 patients with primary soft tissue malignancies, the Radiology Diagnostic Oncology Group found no statistically significant difference between CT and MR imaging in determining tumour involvement of muscle, bone, joint or neurovascular structures [23].

Although this was a very well conducted study, it should be noted that the study was performed between 1991 and early 1995; since then newer CT and MRI equipment and software has become available, which demands comparison. Patients who underwent CT benefited from intravenous contrast for improved characterisation and visualisation of soft tissue tumours, whereas those who underwent MRI did not. This discrepancy in methodology could bias the results towards CT.

The main advantage MRI has over CT is the delineation of the specific muscular compartments, and, in particular, the ability to depict the invasion of individual muscle groups.

CT is occasionally useful to detect subtle calcification or involvement of the underlying bone. CT may also have to be used when there is a contraindication to MRI, e.g. pacemaker fitted or when the patient is unable to tolerate the procedure.

Can MRI differentiate benign from malignant tumours?

Soft tissue tumour staging parameters

Radiological soft tissue tumour staging parameters are:

+ Size.
+ Shape.
+ Margins.
+ Peritumoral oedema.
+ Homogeneity of signal intensity pattern.
+ Contrast enhancement characteristics:
  o static and dynamic studies.
+ Haemorrhage.
+ Distribution:
  o intracompartmental;
  o extracompartmental;
  o neurovascular bundle encasement/ displacement;
  o bone involvement;
+ Growth rate.

Except for a subset of tumours with definitive signal intensity characteristics or morphology that allows for a specific radiological diagnosis, variables such as T1 and T2 homogeneity of signal intensity by themselves are not reliable indications of a benign versus a malignant process (Figure 7).

A combination of different parameters provides for higher sensitivity and specificity. Moulton *et al* [24] analysed the imaging features of 225 soft tissue tumours (179 benign, 46 malignant) to evaluate the efficacy of MR imaging in predicting the pathological diagnosis of soft tissue masses and in distinguishing benign from malignant. Univariate analysis of multiple individual imaging features along with stepwise logistic regression analysis of combinations of imaging features was performed. By quantitative analysis, no single imaging feature or combination of features could reliably be used to distinguish benign from malignant lesions. In addition, they prospectively performed a subjective (group consensus) analysis on

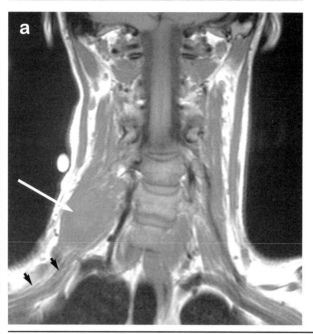

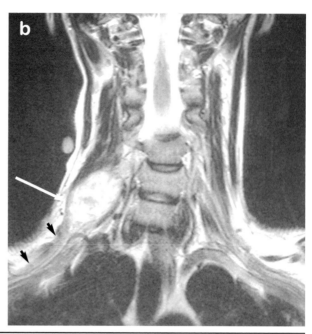

Figure 7. Schwannoma right brachial plexus in a 31-year-old woman. a) T1-weighted spin-echo MRI . b) Coronal turbo spin-echo T2-weighted MRI. An oval tumour (white arrow) extending along the nerves of the brachial plexus (black arrow heads). The lesion returns homogenous low signal on T1-weighted imaging and heterogeneous on T2-weighted imaging but predominantly high signal. Seeing a nerve entering and exiting a mass is pathognomonic of a nerve sheath tumour but it is not demonstrable. Benign peripheral nerve sheath tumours can appear similar on imaging modalities to malignant peripheral nerve sheath tumours (MPNST).

each case. Each tumour was placed into one of three categories:

- Benign, diagnostic of a specific entity.
- Non-specific, most likely benign.
- Non-specific, most likely malignant.

A correct and specific diagnosis of benignity could be made in 44% of the 225 tumours. For the entire cohort the sensitivity was 78% and the specificity was 89% for the diagnosis of malignancy. When the diagnostic benign tumours were excluded, the specificity dropped to 76%. They concluded that the accuracy of MRI declines when characteristic benign tumours are excluded from analysis. A significant percentage of malignant lesions may appear deceptively 'benign' with currently used criteria [24].

DeSchepper *et al* performed a multivariate statistical analysis of ten imaging parameters, individually and in combination. They found that malignancy was predicted with the highest sensitivity when a lesion had a high signal intensity on T2-weighted MR images, was larger than 33mm in diameter, and had a heterogeneous signal intensity on T1-weighted MR images. Signs that conferred the greatest specificity for malignancy included tumour necrosis, bone or neurovascular involvement, and mean diameter of greater than 66mm [25].

In conclusion, many benign soft tissue masses can be correctly and confidently diagnosed with MRI. However, for lesions whose imaging appearances are non-specific, MR imaging is not reliable for distinguishing benign from malignant tumours.

Tumour characterisation

Despite the superiority of MR imaging in delineating soft tissue tumours, it remains limited in its ability to precisely characterise them, with most lesions

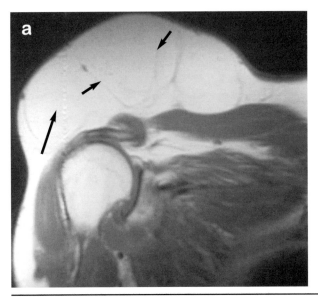
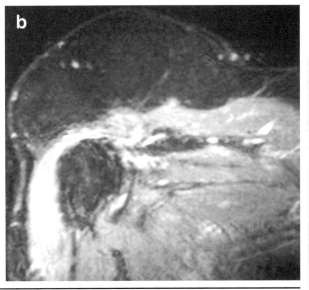

Figure 8. Large left shoulder lipoma. a) Coronal T1-weighted spin-echo MR image of the left shoulder. The lesion (long arrow) is bright and parallels the signal intensity of the subcutaneous fat; fine septations are seen within the lipoma (short arrows). b) STIR coronal image demonstrates complete suppression of the fatty tissue.

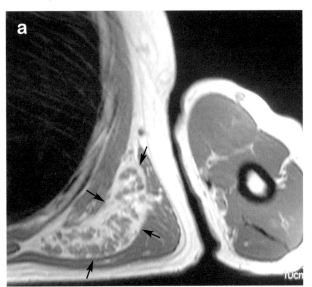
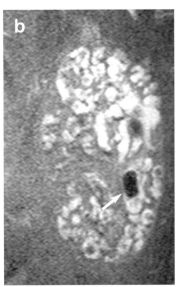

Figure 9. A 66-year-old man with a left lateral chest wall venous vascular malformation. a) Axial T1-weighted spin-echo MRI demonstrates a large mass (arrows) deep to the latissimus dorsi muscle containing areas of intermediate signal surrounded by high signal areas representing the fatty component of the lesion. b) STIR oblique coronal MRI demonstrates serpentine high signal vascular channels. A low signal lesion (arrow) can be seen within the vascular channels; this represents a phlebolith.

showing a non-specific appearance with prolonged T1 and T2 relaxation times (Figure 7). Consequently, a correct histological diagnosis is reached solely on the basis of MR imaging in only 25-44% [24, 26]. There are instances, however, in which a specific diagnosis can be made or strongly suspected on MR imaging features (Figures 8 and 9).

Chapter 12

Image-guided biopsy

Image-guided biopsy is usually performed with CT or US guidance. Several principles are important for biopsy of suspected sarcomatous lesions, particularly co-ordination of the biopsy approach with the surgeon who will perform the definitive resection. An incorrect biopsy violates compartmental anatomy and risks tumour seeding. The biopsy should be performed following completion of adequate imaging studies.

CT is well proven for image-guided biopsy. A large study by Dupuy *et al* [27] found an accuracy rate of 93% for musculoskeletal neoplasms, whilst the fine-needle aspiration rate was only 80%. More recently, studies have shown that ultrasound has a very high accuracy rate [28]. The majority of the studies have used a 14-gauge needle to obtain between 3-5 cores.

The main advantages of ultrasound over CT are:

- ◆ Continuous real-time visualisation of the needle (useful in avoiding neurovascular structures or necrotic areas and highly effective in guiding biopsies to viable areas of the tumour).
- ◆ No risk of ionising radiation.
- ◆ The procedure is performed more quickly than CT, especially when it is necessary to sample several areas of a neoplasm.
- ◆ Sonography is relatively inexpensive and readily available.

Provided the tumour is visible on ultrasound, ultrasound-guided core biopsies should be the preferred method for obtaining tissue diagnoses [28] **(IIb/B)**. CT has a role to play in the biopsy of lesions that are inaccessible to ultrasound biopsy, e.g. deep thigh lesions.

Retroperitoneal sarcomas

CT is the most useful tool in the initial evaluation of retroperitoneal tumours. CT not only allows the assessment of the tumour's location and its relationship to adjacent organs, but also the identification of metastatic lesions in the liver or

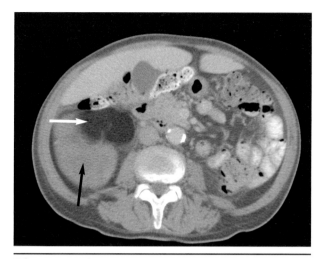

Figure 10. Contrast-enhanced CT of the abdomen demonstrates a large partly solid (black arrow), partly fatty (white arrow) tumour lying within the retroperitoneum on the right. Histology confirmed a liposarcoma.

peritoneal cavity (Figure 10). A high quality MRI can be difficult to obtain, whereas CT is less sensitive to motion artefacts. Currently, large studies comparing MRI of retroperitoneal sarcomas with CT are lacking.

Once a retroperitoneal tumour has been identified, a number of clinical entities must be considered, including adrenal tumours, renal tumours, pancreatic tumours, gastro-intestinal stromal tumours (GIST), advanced gastro-intestinal carcinomas, germ cell tumours and intra-abdominal lymphoma. If imaging is suggestive of a resectable retroperitoneal sarcoma, then biopsy should not be performed, given the potential for transperitoneal spread and track implantation [29]. Where proof of the histological subtype by biopsy is necessary for patients receiving pre-operative chemo- or radiotherapy, CT-guided core biopsy is recommended. When tumours appear to arise from the stomach, pancreas, or duodenum, upper GI endoscopy is indicated. Likewise, colonoscopy with biopsy can be useful in diagnosing tumours arising from the colon. The goal of this strategy is to avoid inappropriate major resection of another tumour, such as an intra-abdominal lymphoma or germ cell tumour.

Systemic staging

Given the risk for haematogenous spread from a high-grade sarcoma to the lungs, chest imaging is key to accurate staging. A chest CT scan should be considered in patients with intermediate- to high-grade lesions that are 5cm or larger because the presence of metastatic disease may change the management of the primary lesion and the overall approach to the patient's disease management [30, 31] (IIb/B). Studies from the MD Anderson Cancer Center have shown that there is no advantage in using CT over CXR for the screening of pulmonary metastases in T1 and low grade T2 soft tissue sarcomas [30, 31]. Abdominopelvic CT, in addition to chest CT, should be undertaken for certain tumour types such as rhabdomyosarcoma, epithelioid sarcoma, and angiosarcoma of the lower limb or pelvis for nodal staging [13, 32] (IV/C). Abdominopelvic CT is also useful in myxoid liposarcoma with its propensity for soft tissue metastases [32] (IV/C).

Response to neoadjuvant therapy

Assessment of response after neoadjuvant chemotherapy is a major factor for determining the overall therapeutic strategy. The aim of monitoring is to predict the percentage of tumour necrosis and differentiate responders from non-responders. Several small studies have reported a decreased FDG-uptake in tumours responsive to chemotherapy [33, 34]. It is suggested that early discrimination between responders and non-responders with PET would be useful to allow adjustment of chemotherapeutic regimes in non-responders.

There are numerous studies assessing the value of dynamic contrast-enhanced MR in monitoring response to pre-operative chemotherapy in osteosarcomas and Ewing's sarcoma, demonstrating high accuracy in distinguishing responders from non-responders. Early rapidly progressive enhancement has been shown to correlate histologically with residual viable tumour. Late and gradual enhancement, or absence of enhancement, is associated with necrosis, or granulation tissue. There is, however, only limited evidence for the use of dynamic MR in soft tissue sarcomas. A small study by

van Rijswijk [35] showed that dynamic contrast-enhanced MR correctly predicted tumour response in eight out of ten patients who had undergone isolated limb perfusion chemotherapy for high-grade sarcomas. Further prospective studies in a larger patient population are required.

Surveillance

It is important to detect locally recurrent disease early to maximise the potential for complete re-resection. Recurrence rates of 5-10% might be expected even after optimal treatment of soft tissue sarcomas. Some two thirds of recurrences occur within the first two years; follow-up should be most intense during this period. Baseline imaging of the primary site is recommended at 3-6 months post-surgery, particularly if the tumour was close to or involving resection margins [13, 32] (IV/C), followed by periodic imaging based upon the estimated risk of local recurrence. In situations where the area is easily monitored by physical examination, imaging may not be required. After ten years, the likelihood of developing a recurrence is small and follow-up should be individualised.

Follow-up surveillance for pulmonary metastases should be with plain chest radiographs [13, 30-32, 36] (IV/C). There is no evidence to direct the frequency or duration of chest imaging, but it should be tailored to the tumour stage, reflecting the relative risk for developing pulmonary metastases. Intervals between CXR can also be increased with time especially after the first two years as the risk of recurrence decreases.

On MRI, a possible local tumour recurrence is shown as a high signal intensity mass on T2-weighted images. A low signal lesion on T2-weighted images following radiation therapy or surgery for malignant soft tissue sarcoma most likely indicates that the patient does not have active tumour. Problems arise in separating high signal tumour from radiation change or early postoperative appearances due to inflammation, haemorrhage or infection.

The evaluation of aggressive soft tissue tumours on follow-up should begin with a T2-weighted sequence. If there is no high signal intensity or a diffuse high signal intensity but no mass, the examination can be considered negative and stopped. If there is a high signal mass, T1-weighted images should be obtained. Seromas do not show change, but the signal intensity of recurrences increases after contrast material injection [37] **(IIb/B)**.

Dynamic gadolinium enhancement (obtaining images within six seconds of the injection) has been found to be helpful in distinguishing recurrent tumour (early enhancement from neoangiogenesis) from radiation-induced inflammation and necrosis (later enhancement via the normal vascular supply) [37].

Sonography has been shown to be as effective as MRI for the assessment of recurrent soft tissue sarcoma [38, 39]. Sonography is not widely used for this purpose because it is operator-dependent, and longitudinal follow-up studies are not easily compared with prior examinations.

Several authors have reported possible detection of recurrent disease with FDG-PET [40-43]. Garcia and co-workers reported a sensitivity of 98% and specificity of 90% for detection of recurrent disease in 48 patients with bone and soft tissue sarcomas [44].

Role of PET imaging

Positron emission tomography (PET) is based upon the use of radioisotopes that undergo positron emission decay; the paired gamma photons released as a consequence of decay are received by a ring detector which registers the interaction in the form of an image. The radionuclide most commonly utilised for PET is [18F]-fluoro-2-deoxy-D-glucose [FDG]. *In vivo*, FDG behaves like glucose and provides a means for quantifying glucose metabolism. Unlike glucose, the metabolite of FDG is not a substrate for glycolytic enzymes. Therefore, the radioactive tracer is trapped in the cell, allowing for subsequent imaging. The amount of tracer accumulation reflects the tissue's glucose metabolism. Many types of tumours have higher rates of glycolysis than uninvolved normal tissue.

Tumour grading

Accurate differentiation of high grade from low grade and benign tumours and a close correlation between the FDG-uptake and tumour grading has been reported in the vast majority of studies [45-51] **(IIb/B)**. Additionally, FDG-PET can improve selection of the optimal site for tumour biopsy by determining the most aggressive region. However, FDG-PET is inadequate to discriminate between low-grade malignant lesions and benign tumours. Furthermore, false positive PET findings were reported in aggressive benign tumours and in inflammatory lesions.

In a study by Schulte *et al* [51], soft tissue tumours with a tumour to background ratio >3.0 were defined as malignant and <1.5 as benign. This definition resulted in a sensitivity of 97% and a specificity of 66% for detecting malignant soft tissue tumours.

A meta-analysis of clinical studies on FDG-PET and sarcomas by Bastiaannet *et al* [52] looked at 29 studies that met their inclusion criteria. Pooled sensitivity, specificity and accuracy of PET for the detection of sarcomas were 0.91, 0.85 and 0.88, respectively. The difference between the mean standard uptake value (SUV) in malignant and benign tumours was statistically significant, as was the difference in FDG uptake between low- and high-grade sarcomas.

Conclusions

The radiological evaluation of a suspected soft tissue sarcoma has changed dramatically with the developments of ultrasound, MRI, CT and more recently, PET. Imaging is valuable along the entire treatment pathway from the detection and characterisation of a soft tissue mass to guiding tissue biopsy, staging and surgical planning. Postoperatively, imaging plays a crucial role in the local and distant recurrence surveillance and detection. It is important to understand the relative strengths and, more importantly, limitations of each imaging modality.

Recommendations	Evidence level
◆ MRI is recommended for localised staging and characterisation of extremity soft tissue sarcomas.	IIb/B
◆ Contrast-enhanced CT may be substituted where MRI is not available or is contraindicated.	II/B
◆ MRI can correctly diagnose benign soft tissue masses with characteristic imaging features, but in lesions whose imaging appearances are non-specific, MRI is not reliable for distinguishing benign from malignant.	III/B
◆ PET imaging has proved accurate for differentiating high-grade from low-grade sarcomas, but not low-grade lesions from benign lesions.	IIb/B
◆ Chest CT is recommended for patients with >5cm intermediate or high-grade lesions to detect pulmonary metastases.	IIb/B
◆ Abdominopelvic CT for primary staging is recommended only in specific circumstances.	IV/C
◆ Core biopsy of the tumour under ultrasound guidance provides a high accuracy of histopathological diagnosis. CT-guided biopsy can be reserved for inaccessible sites.	IIb/B
◆ T2-weighted MRI should be performed for detection of local recurrence.	IIb/B
◆ CXR can be used for the surveillance of pulmonary metastases but there is no evidence to direct the frequency or duration.	IIb/B

Chapter 12

References

1. Hajdu SI. Soft tissue sarcomas: classification and natural history. *CA Cancer J Clin* 1981; 31: 271-80.
2. du Boulay CEH. Immunohistochemistry of soft tissue tumours: a review. *J Pathol* 1985; 146: 77-94.
3. Enzinger FM, Weiss SW. General considerations. In: *Soft tissue tumors*, 3rd ed. Enzinger FM, Weiss SW, Eds. St. Louis: Mosby-Year Book, 1995: 1-16.
4. Mettlin C, Priore R, Rao U, Gamble D, Lane W, Murphy GP. Results of the national soft-tissue sarcoma registry: analysis of survival and prognostic factors. *J Surg Oncol* 1982; 19: 224-7.
5. Kransdorf MJ, Jelinek JS, Moser RP, *et al*. Soft tissue masses: diagnosis using MR imaging. *Am J Roentgenol* 1989; 153: 541-7.
6. Berquist TH, Ehman RL, King BF, Hodgman CG, Ilstrup DM. Value of MR imaging in differentiating benign from malignant soft-tissue masses: study of 95 lesions. *Am J Roentgenol* 1990; 155: 1251-5.
7. Crim JR, Seeger LL, Yao L, Chandnani V, Eckardt JJ. Diagnosis of soft-tissue masses with MR imaging: can benign masses be differentiated from malignant ones? *Radiology* 1992; 185: 581-6.
8. Alexander AA, Nazarian LN, Feld RI. Superficial soft-tissue masses suggestive of recurrent malignancy: sonographic localization and biopsy. *Am J Roentgenol* 1997; 169: 1449-51.
9. Yao L, Nelson SD, Seeger LL, Eckardt JJ, Eliber FR. Primary musculoskeletal neoplasms: effectiveness of core-needle biopsy. *Radiology* 1999; 212: 682-6.
10. Lagalla R, Iovane A, Caruso G, Lo Bello M, Derchi LE. Color Doppler ultrasongraphy of soft-tissue masses. *Acta Radiol* 1998; 39: 421-6.
11. Bodner G, Schocke MFH, Rachbauer F, Seppi K, Peer S, Fierlinger A, Sununu T, Jaschke WR. Differentiation of malignant and benign musculoskeletal tumors: combined color and power Doppler US and spectral wave analysis. *Radiology* 2002; 223: 410-6.
12. Ramos IM, Taylor KJ, Kier R, Burns PN, Snower DP, Carter D. Tumor vascular signals in renal masses: detection with Doppler ultrasonography. *Radiology* 1988; 168: 633-7.
13. Recommendations for Cross-sectional Imaging in Cancer Management: Computed Tomography - CT, Magnetic Resonance Imaging - MRI, Positron Emission Tomography. The Royal College of Radiologists, 2006.
14. Beltran J, Chandnani V, McGhee RA, Kursungoglu-Brahme S. Gadopentate dimeglumine-enhanced MR imaging of the musculoskeletal system. *Am J Roentgenol* 1991; 156: 457-66.
15. Verstraete KL, De Deene Y, Roels H, Dierick A, Uyttedaele D, Kunnen M. Benign and malignant musculoskeletal lesions: dynamic contrast-enhanced MR imaging-parametric 'first pass' images depict tissue vascularisation and perfusion. *Radiology* 1994; 192: 835-49.
16. McDonald DJ, Limb-salvage surgery for treatment of sarcomas of the extremities. *Am J Roentgenol* 1994; 163: 509-13.
17. Myhre-Jensen O. A consecutive 7-year series of 1331 benign soft tissue tumours: clinicopathological-data comparison with sarcomas. *Acta Orthop Scand* 1981; 52: 287-93.

Chapter 12

18. Rydholm A. Management of patients with soft tissue tumors: strategy developed at a regional oncology center. *Acta Orthop Scand Suppl* 1983; 203: 13-77.

19. Peabody TD, Simon MA. Principles of staging of soft-tissue sarcomas. *Clin Orthop* 1993; 289: 19-31.

20. Dalinka MK, Zlatkin MD, Chao P, Kricum ME, Kressel HY. The use of magnetic resonance imaging in the evaluation of bone and soft tissue tumors. *Radiol Clin North Am* 1990; 28: 461-70.

21. Wertzel L, Levin E, Murphey M. A comparison of MR imaging and CT in the evaluation of musculoskeletal masses. *Radiographics* 1987; 7(5): 851-74.

22. Demas BE, Heelan RT, Lane J, Marcove R, Hajdu S, Brennan MF. Soft-tissue sarcomas of the extremities: comparison of MR and CT in determining the extent of disease. *Am J Roentgenol* 1988; 150: 615-20.

23. CT and MR imaging in the local staging of primary malignant musculoskeletal neoplasms: report of the Radiology Diagnostic Oncology Group. *Radiology* 1997; 202: 237-46.

24. Moulton J, Blebea J, Dunco D, Braley S, Bisset G, Emery K. MR imaging of soft-tissue masses: diagnostic efficacy and value of distinguishing between benign and malignant lesions. *Am J Roentgenol* 1995; 164: 1191-9.

25. DeSchepper A, Ramon F, Degryse H. Statistical analysis of MRI parameters predicting malignancy in 141 soft tissue masses. *Fortschr Röntgenster* 1992; 156: 587-91.

26. Kransdorf MJ, Jelinek JS, Moser RP, *et al.* Soft-tissue masses: diagnosis using MRI imaging. *Am J Roentgenol* 1989; 153: 541-7.

27. Dupuy DE, Rosenberg AE, Punyaratabandhu T, Tan MH, Mankin HJ. Accuracy of CT-guided needle biopsy of musculoskeletal neoplasms. *Am J Roentgenol* 1998; 171: 759-62.

28. Torriani M, Etchebehre M, Amstalden EMI. Sonographically-guided core needle biopsy of bone and soft tissue tumors. *J Ultrasound Med* 2002; 21: 194-7.

29. Clark MA, Thomas JM. Portsite recurrence after laparoscopy for staging of retroperitoneal sarcoma. *Surg Laparosc Endosc Percutan Tech* 2003; 13: 290-1.

30. Fleming JB, Cantor SB, Varma DG, Holst D, Feig BW, Hunt KK, Patel SR, *et al.* Utility of chest computed tomography for staging in patients with T1 extremity soft tissue sarcomas. *Cancer* 2001; 92(4): 863-8.

31. Porter GA, Cantor SB, Ahmad SA, Lenert JT, Ballo MT, Hunt KK, Feig BW, *et al.* Cost-effectiveness of staging computed tomography of the chest in patients with T2 soft tissue sarcomas. *Cancer* 2002; 94(1): 197-204.

32. Soft Tissue Sarcoma. Clinical practice guidelines in oncology. National Comprehensive Cancer Network, v.3, 2006.

33. Kole AC, Plaat BE, Hoekstra HJ, Vaalburg W, Molenaar WM. FDG and L-[1-11C]-tyrosine imaging of soft-tissue tumors before and after therapy. *J Nucl Med* 1999; 40: 381-6.

34. Schuetze SM, Rubin BP, Vernon C, Hawkins DS, Bruckner JD, Conrad EU, 3rd, Eary JF. Use of positron emission tomography in localized extremity soft tissue sarcoma treated with neoadjuvant chemotherapy. *Cancer* 2005; 103(2): 339-48.

35. van Rijswijk CS, Geirnaerdt MJ, Hogendoorn PC, Peterse JL, van Coevorden F, Taminiau AH, Tollenaar RA, Kroon BB, Bloem JL. Dynamic contrast-enhanced MR imaging in monitoring response to isolated limb perfusion in high-grade soft tissue sarcoma: initial results. *Eur Radiol* 2003; 13(8): 1849-58.

36. Whooley BP, Gibbs JF, Mooney MM, McGrath BE, Kraybill WG. Primary extremity sarcoma: what is the appropriate follow-up? *Ann Surg Oncol* 2000; 7: 9-14.

37. Vanel D, Shapeero LG, De Baere T, Gilles R, Tardivon A, Genin J, Guinebretiere JM. MR imaging in the follow-up of malignant and aggressive soft-tissue tumors: results of 511 examinations. *Radiology* 1994; 190: 263-8.

38. Choi H, Varma DG, Fornage BD, Kim EE, Johnston DA. Soft-tissue sarcoma: MR imaging vs sonography for detection of local recurrence after surgery. *Am J Roentgenol* 1991; 157(2): 353-8.

39. Arya S, Nagarkatti DG, Dudhat SB, Nadkarni KS, Joshi MS, Shinde SR. Soft tissue sarcomas: ultrasonographic evaluation of local recurrences. *Clin Radiol* 2000; 55(3): 193-7.

40. Kole AC, Nieweg OE, van Ginkel RJ, Pruim J, Hoekstra HJ, Paans AM, Vaalburg W, Koops HS. Detection of local recurrence of soft tissue sarcoma with positron emission tomography using [18F] fluorodeoxyglucose. *Ann Surg Oncol* 1997; 4: 57-63

41. Lucas JD, O'Doherty MJ, Wong JC, Bingham JB, McKee PH, Fletcher CD, Smith MA. Evaluation of fluorodeoxyglucose positron emission tomography in the management of soft tissue sarcomas. *J Bone Joint Surg* 1998; 80: 441-7.

42. Shwarzbach M, Willeke F, Dimitrakopoulou-Strauss A, Strauss LG, Zhang YM, Mechtersheimer G, Hinz U, Lehnert T, Herfarth C. Functional imaging and detection of local recurrence in soft tissue sarcomas by positron emission tomography. *Anticancer Res* 1999; 19: 1343-9.

43. Hain SF, O'Doherty MJ, Lucas JD, Smith MA. Fluorodeoxyglucose PET in the evaluation of amputations for soft tissue sarcoma. *Nucl Med Commun* 1999; 20: 845-8.

44. Garcia R, Kim EE, Wong FC, Korkmaz M, Wong WH, Yang DJ, Podoloff DA. Comparison of fluorine-18-FDG PET and technetium-99m-MIBI SPECT in evaluation of musculoskeletal sarcomas. *J Nucl Med* 1996; 37: 1476-9.

45. Adler LP, Blair HF, Markley JT, Wiliams RP, Joyce MJ, Leisure G, al-Kaisi N, Miraldi F. Noninvasive grading of musculoskeletal tumors using PET. *J Nucl Med* 1991; 32: 1508-12.

46. Kern KA, Brunetti A, Norton JA, Chang AE, Malawer M, Lack E, Finn RD, Rosenberg SA, Larson SM. Metabolic imaging of human extremity musculoskeletal tumors by PET. *J Nucl Med* 1988; 29: 181-6.

47. Eary JF, Conrad EU, Bruckner JD, Folpe A, Hunt KJ, Mankoff DA, Howlett AT. Quantitative [F-18]fluorodeoxyglucose positron emission tomography in pre-treatment and grading of sarcoma. *Clin Cancer Res* 1998; 4: 1215-20.

48. Lodge MA, Lucas JD, Marsden PK, Cronin BF, O'Doherty MJ, Smith MA. A PET study of 18FDG uptake in soft tissue masses. *Eur J Nucl Med* 1999; 26: 22-30.

49. Lucas JD, O'Doherty MJ, Cronin BF, Marsden PK, Lodge MA, McKee PH, Smith MA. Prospective evaluation of soft tissue masses and sarcomas using fluorodeoxyglucose positron emission tomography. *Br J Surg* 1999; 86: 550-6.

50. Nieweg OE, Pruim J, van Ginkel RJ, Hoekstra HJ, Paans AM, Molenaar WM, Koops HS, Vaalburg W. Fluorine-18-fluorodeoxyglucose PET imaging of soft-tissue sarcoma. *J Nucl Med* 1996; 37: 257-61.

51. Schulte M, Brecht-Krauss D, Heymer B, Guhlmann A, Hartwig E, Sarkar MR, Diederichs CG, Schultheiss M, Kotzerke J, Reske SN. Fluorodeoxyglucose positron emission tomography of soft tissue tumours: is a non-invasive determination of biological activity possible? *Eur J Nucl Med* 1999; 26: 599-605.

52. Bastiaannet E, Groen H, Jager PL, Cobben DC, van der Graaf WT, Vaalburg W, Hoekstra HJ. The value of FDG-PET in the detection, grading and response to therapy of soft tissue and bone sarcomas; a systematic review and meta-analysis. *Cancer Treat Rev* 2004; 30(1): 83-101.

Chapter 13

Hypospadias correction: one or two stages?

Norbert Kang MB BS MD FRCS (Plast.)
Consultant Plastic Surgeon

Marc Pacifico BSc MB BS MD MRCS
Specialist Registrar, Plastic Surgery

ROYAL FREE HOSPITAL, LONDON, UK AND RAFT INSTITUTE FOR
PLASTIC SURGERY RESEARCH, MOUNT VERNON HOSPITAL, NORTHWOOD, MIDDLESEX, UK

Introduction

The authors believe that the long-running debate on the merits of one-stage versus two-stage hypospadias repairs is finally at an end [1] **(IV/C)**. Simply put, the majority of primary cases of hypospadias (two thirds) are suitable for a one-stage repair. This reflects the proportion of cases which are distal/anterior (with little or no chordee) compared with those which are more proximal; 65% being distal, 15% being mid-shaft and 20% being proximal [2] **(III/B)**. For all other forms of hypospadias (especially salvage cases), the best results are probably obtained with some form of two-stage repair which corrects any chordee at the first stage and paves the way for tubularisation of the ventral surface of the penis at the second stage [1] **(IV/C)**. In this chapter, we will review the evidence to support this view and present an algorithm which should help trainees and surgeons developing an interest in hypospadias to select the appropriate procedure(s) from the wonderful variety that has evolved to deal with this challenging condition.

Before doing so, a warning: when counselling the parents of a newborn child with hypospadias for the first time, it is important to remember that hypospadias is not a life-threatening condition. Sometimes, it is the least of a spectrum of disorders that affect the child. Give parents the time and space to consider the options; this can (and should) include doing nothing until the child is old enough to consider having surgery for themselves. This may avoid the (thankfully infrequent) occurrence of an adult hypospadias cripple who wishes that his parents had never agreed to surgery of any kind. Remember, most cases of hypospadias are mild and men with this type of hypospadias do very well without surgery or are blissfully unaware that they even have a deformity [3] **(III/B)**.

Methodology

A Medline search was performed using the following search terms: 'hypospadias', 'reviews', 'results', 'series', 'complications', 'GRAP repairs', 'islanded flap repairs', 'MAGPI repairs', 'Mathieu repairs', 'one-stage repairs', 'Snodgrass repairs', 'Thiersch-Duplay repairs', 'TIP repairs', 'two-stage repairs'.

The ideal hypospadias repair

With this in mind, the ideal procedure for hypospadias achieves the following aims with one operative procedure (in decreasing order of importance):

- Urethral meatus at the tip of the glans penis.
- Straight erection.
- Slit-like meatus.
- Cone-shaped glans.
- 'Cork-screw' stream, i.e. so that there is no spraying.
- No strictures or stenoses.
- No fistulae.
- No residual hooding.
- No hair growing on the inside of the urethra.
- No need for repeated dilatation of the urethra.
- No dilatation of the urethra with time.
- Avoidance of balanitis xerotica obliterans (BXO).

Achieving a terminal meatus

The need to achieve a terminal meatus as the principal goal of any operative procedure cannot be overstated. Too often, surgical techniques (and surgeons) compromise on the results and accept some degree of 'ventralisation' of the meatus (i.e. migration of the meatus from its ideal position to a point closer to the original site of the meatus). This is a particular criticism of procedures involving the 'advancement' of tissues, especially the MAGPI (meatal advancement and glansplasty included) [4, 5] (III/B) or UGPI (urethral advancement and glansplasty included) [6]. In most cases, the urethra is not actually 'advanced'. Rather, the glans is flexed giving the illusion the urethra has been lengthened. However, it is a potential problem even with the currently popular TIP (tubularised incised plate or Snodgrass-type) repairs. In order to avoid problems of meatal stenosis with the TIP procedure, some surgeons avoid incising the urethral plate too deeply [7] (IIa/B). This can make it difficult to wrap the glans around the catheter, unless the meatus is allowed to open slightly more ventrally rather than at the tip of the glans.

Achieving a straight erection

Achieving a straight erection is another fundamental goal of surgery. However, procedures to correct chordee are only necessary in 15% of cases [8] (IV/C). The authors believe that the methods chosen to correct chordee should be determined by the degree of ventral curvature present and/or the length of the penis (assessed at rest but especially after an erection test). Where chordee is minimal and the penis is relatively long, a Nesbit procedure [9] to plicate Buck's fascia or the tunica albuginea on the opposite (dorsal) side is usually enough to correct the curvature. Where the chordee is more significant and/or the penis is short, then a Nesbit procedure would result in a significantly shortened penis. Since most patients with hypospadias already have a short penis, further shortening to correct chordee is unacceptable [10, 11] (III/B). In these cases, a two-stage approach has the lowest complication rate with chordee being corrected at the first stage while preparing the way for tubularisation of the ventral surface at the second stage.

Creating a slit-like meatus

Creating a slit-like meatus ensures that the urinary stream 'corkscrews' as the profile of the urethra changes from a tube proximally to a slit distally. This has the same effect as the rifling in a gun barrel and plays a part in ensuring that the urinary stream does not spray and can be directed. Creating a slit-like meatus also ensures that the hypospadias repair comes as close as possible to resembling a normal penis in appearance. However, it is more or less difficult to achieve a slit-like meatus with certain operative procedures. Specifically, the unmodified versions of the MAGPI [4, 5] (III/B), flip-flap (Mathieu) [12-14] (Ib/A), islanded Duckett's and vascularised onlay procedures generally fail in this regard [14] (III/B). These procedures tend to create a round meatus which is (nowadays) cosmetically and functionally unacceptable when good alternatives are available. TIP, Snodgraft and two-stage procedures produce a slit-like meatus because a glans/dorsal split is an integral part of these operations [15, 16] (III/B). When the V-shaped split is closed ventrally, it heals as a vertical slit not a round tube [14] (III/B).

Avoiding strictures and stenoses

To avoid strictures and stenoses, there are several important principles about the soft tissues that need to be kept in mind:

- Poorly vascularised tissues become ischaemic and contract when (and if) they eventually heal.
- Flaps which use dartos fascia as the pedicle are not axial pattern flaps and are therefore subject to the 1:1 length:breadth ratio if they are to survive intact [17] **(III/B)**.
- Random pattern flaps (e.g. flip-flap) are also subject to the 1:1 length:breadth ratio for survival [17] **(III/B)**.
- Tissues sutured together under tension will become progressively more ischaemic as postoperative oedema develops.
- Circular scars (e.g. at the junction of the native and neo-urethra) will heal by constriction unless a conscious effort is made to avoid this (e.g. by making the junction oblique).
- Any large, raw, areas in the urethral plate which are left to heal by secondary intention will also contract [7, 18, 19] **(IIa/B)**.

The solutions are increasingly clear. Specifically, avoid using islanded flaps or other procedures which use random pattern flaps (e.g. the flip-flap procedure). Although the dartos fascial layer nourishing an islanded flap is well vascularised, the pedicle does not follow an axial pattern and may be unable to nourish a large skin island, especially when oedema develops postoperatively resulting in compression of the pedicle. Problems with vascularity probably explain the high fistula rates, strictures and other problems reported in many series of islanded flaps [20-24] **(III/B)**. The complications associated with islanded flaps increase as the meatus becomes more proximal, probably because the flaps used to reconstruct such a length of neo-urethra eventually exceed the 1:1 length:breadth ratio which can be sustained by the random pattern supply. Indeed, the authors believe that in many cases, such large skin islands survive as skin grafts. Much the same is probably true of the flip-flap procedure or other procedures using random pattern skin flaps. Ensuring that the tissues (when tubed) are of sufficient dimension to allow them to be sutured together without tension is difficult when the tissues are in short supply. However, failure to do so

compromises the blood supply to the suture line which will then fail along with the repair [25] **(III/B)**. Where possible, avoid creating a circular suture line along the reconstructed urethra. This simply creates the opportunity for a circular scar to form which will contract, creating a stricture in the neo-urethra. Finally, when using a procedure which includes longitudinal incision of the urethral plate (e.g. TIP), resurface any wide, raw areas with a graft to prevent healing by contraction [7, 18, 19] **(III/B)**. How wide an area? Surprisingly, there are relatively few data to guide us. What data there are suggest that if the urethral plate to be tubed is <8mm in width, then the risk of stenosis or fistula increases [25] **(III/B)**. However, incising the urethral plate longitudinally to allow the tissues to be tubed around a catheter more easily does not necessarily increase the final diameter of the neo-urethra [25, 26], implying that the raw areas do not stay open as much, as suggested by Snodgrass and others [27-30] **(IIa/B)**. The implication is that (up to a point) the raw area created by longitudinal incision of the urethral plate (i.e. after TIP repair) heals by contraction, as expected with any wound left to heal by secondary intention [19] **(IIa/B)**.

Avoiding fistula formation

Fistula formation can be avoided by:

- Using operative techniques which do not rely on tissues with questionable vascularity. Therefore, avoid using vascularised island flaps or the flip-flap procedure.
- Avoiding excessive tension on the suture lines, because this leads to ischaemia and breakdown of the suture line. Therefore, ensure that any tissues which are tubularised are of sufficient dimension.
- Using a suture technique (when tubing the tissues over the catheter) where the suture does not pass through the epithelium as this creates a potential fistula track.
- Using a 'waterproofing' layer of vascularised tissue (dartos fascia) which can be placed over the suture line of any repair to the urethra. This avoids the creation of overlapping suture lines which can connect and form a fistula. Using a dartos fascial flap for waterproofing is such a good way of preventing fistula formation that it

should be an essential part of any operative procedure to deal with hypospadias [31, 32] **(III/B)**.

The ideal tissue for a neo-urethra

The ideal tissue for creating a neo-urethra is:

* Hairless.
* Easily accessed.
* Present in large quantities.
* Readily vascularised.
* Resists the effects of continuous exposure to urine.

No such tissue exists, although the day is fast approaching when tissue engineering may offer an off-the-shelf equivalent to urothelium [33]. In the absence of such developments, the best alternative at present is the prepuce, either as a graft or as a vascularised island. The next best source of graft material is intra-oral mucosa (either buccal or lower lip). Both preputial skin and oral mucosa are usually present in sufficient quantities for a full repair of most primary hypospadias cases. However, preputial grafts do not tolerate the effects of continuous wetting as well as oral mucosa. Therefore, a small percentage go on to develop BXO [34]. This almost never happens with oral mucosa. Post-auricular skin can also be used as a graft but this is vastly inferior to the prepuce or oral mucosa [35] **(III/B)**. The best epithelium is bladder lining since this is transitional epithelium and most suited to continuous exposure to urine [36] **(III/B)**. However, it is difficult to obtain, requiring a transabdominal (but retroperitoneal) approach for harvest. Other tissues that have been described include the peritoneum [37], intestinal mucosa [38] and even vein graft [39].

Preventing dilatation of the neo-urethra

To prevent dilatation of the neo-urethra with time, the ideal repair mimics the structure of the normal urethra and is supported on all sides by erectile tissue. This also helps with emptying of the neo-urethra, as the erectile tissue is elastic and causes the neo-urethra to collapse after micturition. TIP,

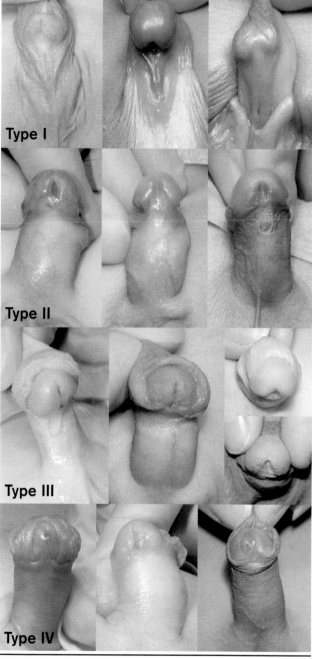

Figure 1. Examples of the four different types of hypospadias commonly encountered

Snodgraft and two-stage repairs achieve this aim because the epithelium lining the neo-urethra becomes closely adherent to the underlying erectile tissue. The grafts used to resurface the ventral surface of the penis are firmly held down by scar tissue onto the underlying erectile tissue and therefore

Table 1. Four types of hypospadias (from a surgical perspective).

Type	Description
I	Nothing there, i.e. proximal meatus, no glans groove, poorly developed urethral plate, variable degree of chordee
II	Something there but poorly formed, i.e. distal or midshaft meatus, glans groove present but shallow, urethral plate present but narrow, variable degree of chordee
III	Something there and well formed, i.e. distal meatus, glans groove well formed and deep, urethral plate present and wide, absent or minimal chordee
IV	More or less all there, i.e. sub-terminal meatus, with incomplete prepuce, and absent or minimal chordee

resist dilatation over time. In contrast, vascularised island flaps (either tubed or onlay) fail completely in this regard. The neo-urethra remains unsupported and may develop into a mega-urethra with time [40] **(III/B)**.

Selecting the right operation

The list of requirements for an ideal hypospadias procedure is clearly long. How then does the neophyte surgeon/trainee select the right operation(s) for their patient? The answer may be a classification system that describes the morphology of the different types of hypospadias which are commonly encountered. The classification system views the different types of hypospadias from the perspective of the surgeon trying to decide what needs to be done to achieve the perfect repair. This is summarised in Table 1 and illustrated in Figure 1. Using this system, an algorithm is devised to incorporate the length of the penis and the degree of chordee present (Figure 2).

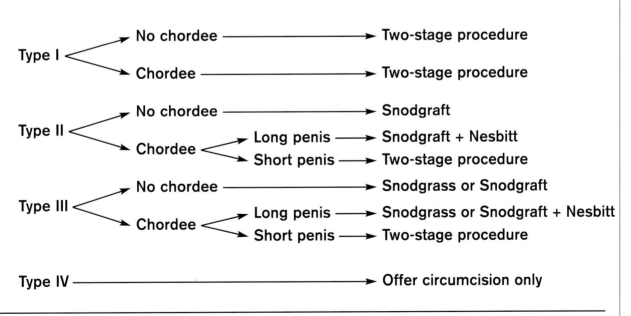

Figure 2. Algorithm for selection of procedure according to degree of deformity.

Using the algorithm

To demonstrate the use of the algorithm it may be helpful to use it in an illustrative case (Figure 3). Typically, this is a patient with an anterior (distal) hypospadias (e.g. with a subcoronal or coronal meatus). Close inspection on the operating table indicates a patient with a Type II penis. An erection test shows no evidence for chordee. Therefore, a Snodgraft (or similar one-stage procedure) is appropriate. The sequence of images shows the steps involved in performing this procedure. The steps are essentially the same as for a TIP procedure (Snodgrass procedure) with one important exception. When the urethral plate/glans is split it creates a large raw area (Figure 3C). If the width of the raw area exceeds 8mm, then a preputial (or other epithelium) graft must be used to line the defect. If this is not done, then healing will occur by

contracture resulting in stenosis or stricture of the meatus.

The sequence of images in Figure 3 show the steps involved in performing the Snodgraft procedure. The authors believe that great emphasis must be placed on the need to check and recheck that the depth of the dorsal incision is sufficient to allow the tissues to be tubed over a catheter without tension. However, it also means that a graft is more (rather than less) often required than would be suggested by those who believe that the TIP procedure is the solution to all degrees of hypospadias [19] **(III/B)**.

The algorithm in Figure 2 advises that for all other patients, a two-stage procedure provides a reliable and reproducible means for correcting primary hypospadias cases. It also provides a reliable and predictable method for salvaging cases regardless of

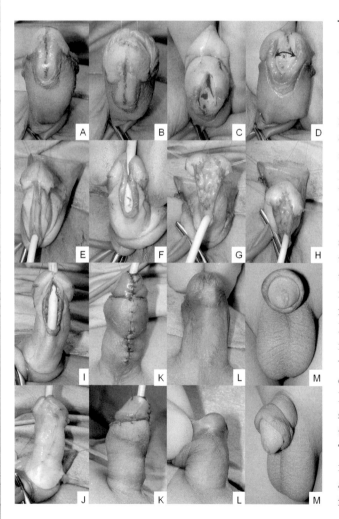

Figure 3. A patient with a Type II penis and no chordee. Surgical steps for a Snodgraft repair: a & b) Markings showing the position of the longitudinal split in the urethral plate and glans. c & d) The urethral plate is incised deeply. d) The width of the raw area is measured (curved arrow). If it exceeds 8mm then a preputial graft is used to line the raw surface converting this operation into a Snodgraft procedure. If the width of the raw area is <8mm, then a TIP procedure is performed allowing the raw area to heal by 'spontaneous' re-epithelialisation. e & f) The depth of the dorsal incision is checked. It should be deep enough to allow the tissues to be tubularised around a catheter without tension. If the dorsal incision is not deep enough then the incision is deepened as required. The width of the raw area is checked again. If it exceeds the 8mm limit then a graft is used. g & h) The preputial graft is secured with multiple quilting sutures of 7/0 vicryl rapide. i) The tissues are tubed around the catheter. j) A waterproofing layer of dartos fascia is laid over the repair and secured with 7/0 vicryl sutures. The surgeon is advised to release the tourniquet at this point to secure haemostasis. k) The completed repair. l) Pre-operative appearance. m) Postoperative appearance at one year. Although a circumcision was performed, a new 'prepuce' is forming.

Table 2. Table summarising results of studies using MAGPI, TIP, or GRAP procedures for one-stage repairs of primary hypospadias.

Authors & year	Type of procedure	Number of patients	Follow-up period	Initial site of meatus	Fistula rate	Stricture & stenosis rate	Redo rate	Overall complication rate
Duckett and Snyder [2] (1991)	MAGPI	1111	2 weeks - 2 years	Distal	0.45%	0%	1.2%	1.2%
Snodgrass [15] (1994)	TIP	16	22 months	Distal	0%	0%	0%	0%
Snodgrass et al [43] (1996)	TIP	137	1-3 years	Distal	3.6%	2%	3.6%	7%
Johnson and Coleman [42] (1998)	GRAP	35	3-6 years	Distal	0%	0%	0%	0%
Borer et al [31] (2001)	TIP	181	6-38 months	Distal	5%	0.7%	2.8%	5%
Jayanthi [46] (2003)	TIP	110	2-42 months	Distal	0.9%	0%	0.9%	0.9%
Riccabona et al [49] (2003)	TIP	188	5-71 months	Distal + proximal	5.3%	0%	Not stated	6.9%
Nuininga et al [47] (2005)	MAGPI	37	1-23 years	Distal	8%	2.7%	Not stated	22%
Cheng et al [32] (2002)	TIP	514	4 -66 months	All sites	0.5%	0.4%	1%	1%
Gray and Boston [41] (2003)	GRAP	205	>10 years	All sites	7%	Not stated	6%	7%

Chapter 13

the initial surgery performed to correct the hypospadias. In other words, it is the 'default' procedure for any degree of severity of hypospadias. The main disadvantage of a two-stage procedure is the need to perform a second operation. In other words, it builds in a 'complication'. Most patients and most surgeons want to perform as few procedures as possible. Therefore, a one-stage procedure that reliably produces results which are as close to the ideal as possible is highly desirable, e.g. a TIP (Snodgrass) or Snodgraft procedure.

Other one-stage procedures exist which are also able to produce excellent results according to the criteria outlined earlier, e.g. GRAP repairs [41, 42]. It is purely the authors' personal preference to use a TIP or Snodgraft procedure as the one-stage procedure of choice for the majority of repairs. However, since the majority of patients with hypospadias present with either a Type II or III deformity (>60%), a one-stage procedure using one or other of these techniques should be successful.

Comparing the different techniques

In summary, the discussion so far has centred around what procedure(s) should be performed to achieve the ideal hypospadias repair in terms of function and appearance. The data presented suggest that the best cosmetic results are currently obtained with procedures which include longitudinal incision of the urethral plate as part of the procedure, i.e. following the principle of Snodgrass [15, 31, 32, 43] **(III/B)**. The data also show that the most reliable procedures (in terms of the lowest complication rates) are those which involve tubularisation of the ventral tissues (i.e. following the principle of Thiersch-Duplay) combined with a waterproofing manoeuvre, e.g. dartos fascial flap [10, 16, 32, 42, 44, 45] **(III/B)**. The marked differences in complication rates with the different procedures are highlighted when comparing the data in Tables 2, 3 and 4.

Table 3. Table summarising results of studies using islanded flaps (either onlay or tubularised) for one-stage repair of primary hypospadias.

Authors & year	Type of procedure	Number of patients	Follow-up period	Initial site of meatus	Fistula rate	Stricture & stenosis rate	Redo rate	Overall complication rate
Kumar & Harris [50] (1994)	Onlay & tubed	35	10 years	Not stated	14%	10%	Not stated	33%
Koyanagi et al [51] (1994)	Onlay & tubed	120	10 years	All sites	24%	17.5%	35%	42%
Wiener et al [20] (1997)	Onlay & tubed	132	8-13 years	All sites	15%	10%	~20%	34%
Nuininga et al [47] (2005)	Matthieu/Duckett /Devine-Horton	126	>10 years	All sites	23%	20%	43%	54%
Gershbaum et al [10] (2002)	Tubed	40	5-15 years	Penoscrotal	42%	5%	Not stated	61%
Patel et al [48] (2004)	Tubed	3049	>10 years	Penoscrotal/ scrotal	7%	13%	33%	33%

Table 4. Table summarising the results of studies in which the ventral tissues are tubularised in two stages to repair a primary hypospadias.

Authors & year	Type of procedure	Number of patients	Follow-up period	Initial site of meatus	Fistula rate	Stricture & stenosis rate	Redo rate	Overall complication rate
Bracka [16] (1995)	2-stage with full thickness graft	391	0.5-10 years	All sites	3%	2%	9%	14%
Asopa [52] (1998)	Byars flaps	12	<5 years	Not stated	Not stated	Not stated	Not stated	16.6%
Johnson & Coleman [42] (1998)	2-stage with full thickness graft	57	3-6 years	All sites	5.3%	3.5%	Not stated	>8.8%
Price et al [45] (2003)	2-stage with full thickness graft	112	3.4 years	All sites	8.9%	2.7%	11.6%	11.7%
Retik et al [44] (1994)	2-stage with flaps	58	1-8 years	Scrotal + perineal	5%	0%	Not stated	7%
Gershbaum et al [10] (2002)	2-stage with full thickness graft	11	5-15 years	Penoscrotal	9%	0%	Not stated	18%

If these data are correct, the continuing debate on whether to perform a one-stage versus two-stage repair becomes irrelevant. What is more relevant is the exact procedure performed (and why) rather than whether it is carried out in one or two stages. The data presented so far clearly show that for distal hypospadias, the complication rates for a wide range of different procedures is similar (Table 2). Therefore, the choice of procedure must be made on the basis of other issues, specifically cosmesis. In this regard, TIP (and other procedures which include this manoeuvre) clearly produces the best cosmetic results [32, 43, 46]

Chapter 13

(III/B). Unmodified MAGPI and other one-stage procedures (especially the flip-flap and islanded procedures) can also be used to repair a distal hypospadias with a relatively low complication rate [2, 47] **(III/B)**. However, as previously discussed, these procedures fail to achieve an adequate cosmetic result in the majority of cases and should therefore be consigned to history [10, 32] **(III/B)**.

For more proximal cases, the complication rates increase for all types of procedures - both one-stage and two-stage (Tables 3 and 4). This reflects the greater complexity of the surgery required to achieve a successful repair in these cases. Nevertheless, the data still show clear differences in the complication rates comparing the different techniques available (Tables 3 and 4). Specifically, two-stage repairs (whether using grafts or Byars flaps to resurface the ventral side of the penis) have very much lower complication rates compared with islanded flaps (whether onlay, islanded or double-faced) regardless of whether the indication for surgery was a proximal or distal hypospadias [10, 16, 48] **(III/B)**. On this basis, the cautious surgeon will elect to perform a two-stage procedure rather than a one-stage procedure. Other major advantages of a two-stage approach include the greater ease with which a glansplasty can be incorporated (resulting in improved cosmesis) and the greater ease with which the surgery can be learnt.

Since the majority of hypospadias cases are distal, the majority of cases can be dealt with using a one-stage procedure. This more than makes up for the 'added complication' of having to perform a two-stage procedure in a minority of cases. Such an approach to the management of hypospadias should secure the lowest complication rates and the best cosmetic results for the patient.

Conclusions

One-stage and two-stage procedures both have a place in the armamentarium of the hypospadias surgeon. There is no 'conflict' between the two approaches; indeed both are complementary. The complete hypospadias surgeon will individualise the treatment of his/her patient and use the appropriate (either one- or two-stage) procedure to deal with the particular needs of the case. Surgeons who think that it is possible to use a single operation (whether one- or two-stage) to deal with every case of hypospadias are doing a disservice to their patients.

Chapter 13

Chapter 13

Recommendations	Evidence level

♦ The majority of hypospadias cases are distal (60%) and can therefore be managed with a one-stage operative procedure. — Ib/A

♦ The remaining (more proximal) cases of hypospadias are best managed with a two-stage procedure because these produce the lowest complication rates and the best cosmetic results. — III/B

♦ The complication rates of islanded flap or flip-flap procedures are so high that these procedures should no longer be performed, especially by the occasional surgeon. — III/B

♦ The complication rates for most one-stage procedures (except flip-flap and islanded flap procedures) are relatively low. Therefore, the best choice of one-stage procedure is determined by the cosmetic result of the repair. — III/B

♦ Amongst one-stage procedures, the best cosmetic results are produced by those that aim to produce a slit-like meatus, e.g. GRAP or TIP repairs. — III/B

♦ The cosmetic results of unmodified MAGPI, UGPI, flip-flap and islanded flap procedures are so poor that they should no longer be performed by any surgeon. — III/B

♦ A dartos fascia flap should be used to 'waterproof' every repair except (of course) islanded flaps which rely on the dartos fascia for their vascular supply. — III/B

♦ If a TIP procedure is performed, a dorsal inlay graft should be used to line the dorsal wall if incision of the urethral plate produces a raw area which is >8mm in width, otherwise the surgeon must 'ventralise' the meatus or risk a meatal/neo-urethral stenosis. — IIa/B

References

1. Manzoni G, Bracka A, Palminteri E, Marrocco G. Hypospadias surgery: when, what and by whom? *BJU Int* 2004; 94: 1188-5.

2. Duckett JW, Snyder HM, 3rd. The MAGPI hypospadias repair in 1111 patients. *Ann Surg* 1991; 213: 620-5.

3. Fichtner J, Filipas D, Mottrie AM, Voges GE, Hohenfellner R. Analysis of meatal location in 500 men: wide variation questions need for meatal advancement in all pediatric anterior hypospadias cases. *J Urol* 1995; 154: 833-4.

4. Hastie KJ, Deshpande SS, Moisey CU. Long-term follow-up of the MAGPI operation for distal hypospadias. *Br J Urol* 1989; 63: 320-2.

5. Issa MM, Gearhart JP. The failed MAGPI: management and prevention. *Br J Urol* 1989; 64: 169-71.

6. Harrison DH, Grobbelaar AO. Urethral advancement and glanuloplasty (UGPI): a modification of the MAGPI procedure for distal hypospadias. *Br J Plast Surg* 1997; 50: 206-11.

7. Lorenz C, Schmedding A, Leutner A, Kolb H. Prolonged stenting does not prevent obstruction after TIP repair when the glans was deeply incised. *Eur J Pediatr Surg* 2004; 14: 322-7.

8. Mouriquand PD, Mure PY. Current concepts in hypospadiology. *BJU Int* 2004; 93 Suppl 3: 26-34.

9. Nesbit RM. Congenital curvature of the phallus: report of three cases with description of corrective operation. 1965. *J Urol* 2002; 167: 1187-8.

10. Gershbaum MD, Stock JA, Hanna MK. A case for 2-stage repair of perineoscrotal hypospadias with severe chordee. *J Urol* 2002; 168: 1727-8.

11. Greenfield JM, Lucas S, Levine LA. Factors affecting the loss of length associated with tunica albuginea plication for correction of penile curvature. *J Urol* 2006; 175: 238-41.

12. Oswald J, Korner I, Riccabona M. Comparison of the perimeatal-based flap (Mathieu) and the tubularised incised-plate urethroplasty (Snodgrass) in primary distal hypospadias. *BJU Int* 2000; 85: 725-7.

13. Samuel M, Capps S, Worthy A. Distal hypospadias: which repair? *BJU Int* 2002; 90: 88-91.

14. Ververidis M, Dickson AP, Gough DC. An objective assessment of the results of hypospadias surgery. *BJU Int* 2005; 96: 135-9.

15. Snodgrass W. Tubularised, incised plate urethroplasty for distal hypospadias. *J Urol* 1994; 151: 464-5.

16. Bracka A. A versatile two-stage hypospadias repair. *Br J Plast Surg* 1995; 48: 345-52.

17. Hinman F, Jr. The blood supply to preputial island flaps. *J Urol* 1991; 145: 1232-5.

18. Kolon TF, Gonzales ET, Jr. The dorsal inlay graft for hypospadias repair. *J Urol* 2000; 163: 1941-3.

19. Singh RB, Pavithran NM. Lessons learnt from Snodgrass tip urethroplasty: a study of 75 cases. *Pediatr Surg Int* 2004; 20: 204-6.

20. Wiener JS, Sutherland RW, Roth DR, Gonzales ET, Jr. Comparison of onlay and tubularised island flaps of inner preputial skin for the repair of proximal hypospadias. *J Urol* 1997; 158: 1172-4.

21. Ghali AM. Hypospadias repair by skin flaps: a comparison of onlay preputial island flaps with either Mathieu's meatal-based or Duckett's tubularised preputial flaps. *BJU Int* 1999; 83: 1032-8.

22. Castanon M, Munoz E, Carrasco R, Rodo J, Morales L. Treatment of proximal hypospadias with a tubularised island flap urethroplasty and the onlay technique: a comparative study. *J Pediatr Surg* 2000; 35: 1453-5.

23. Demirbilek S, Kanmaz T, Aydin G, Yucesan S. Outcomes of one-stage techniques for proximal hypospadias repair. *Urology* 2001; 58: 267-70.

24. Emir L, Germiyanoglu C, Erol D. Onlay island flap urethroplasty: a comparative analysis of primary versus re-operative cases. *Urology* 2003; 61: 216-9.

25. Holland AJ, Smith GH. Effect of the depth and width of the urethral plate on tubularised incised plate urethroplasty. *J Urol* 2000; 164: 489-91.

26. Hafez AT, Herz D, Bagli D, Smith CR, McLorie G, Khoury AE. Healing of unstented tubularised incised plate urethroplasty: an experimental study in a rabbit model. *BJU Int* 2003; 91: 84-8.

27. Lopes JF, Schned A, Ellsworth PI, Cendron M. Histological analysis of urethral healing after tubularised incised plate urethroplasty. *J Urol* 2001; 166: 1014-7.

28. Snodgrass WT, Nguyen MT. Current technique of tubularised incised plate hypospadias repair. *Urology* 2002: 60: 157-62.

29. Bleustein CB, Esposito MP, Soslow RA, Felsen D, Poppas DP. Mechanism of healing following the Snodgrass repair. *J Urol* 2001; 165: 277-9.

30. Genc A, Taneli C, Gunsar C, *et al.* Histopathological evaluation of the urethra after the Snodgrass operation: an experimental study in rabbits. *BJU Int* 2002; 90: 950-2.

31. Borer JG, Bauer SB, Peters CA, *et al.* Tubularised incised plate urethroplasty: expanded use in primary and repeat surgery for hypospadias. *J Urol* 2001; 165: 581-5.

32. Cheng EY, Vemulapalli SN, Kropp BP, *et al.* Snodgrass hypospadias repair with vascularised dartos flap: the perfect repair for virgin cases of hypospadias? *J Urol* 2002; 168: 1723-6.

33. Wunsch L, Ehlers EM, Russlies M. Matrix testing for urothelial tissue engineering. *Eur J Pediatr Surg* 2005; 15: 164-9.

34. Kumar MV, Harris DL. Balanitis xerotica obliterans complicating hypospadias repair. *Br J Plast Surg* 1999; 52: 69-71.

35. Webster GD, Brown MW, Koefoot RB, Jr., Sihelnick S. Suboptimal results in full thickness skin graft urethroplasty using an extra-penile skin donor site. *J Urol* 1984; 131: 1082-3.

36. King LR. Bladder mucosal grafts for severe hypospadias: a successful technique. *J Urol* 1994; 152: 2338-40.

37. Shaul DB, Xie HW, Diaz JF, Mahnovski V, Hardy BE. Use of tubularised peritoneal free grafts as urethral substitutes in the rabbit. *J Pediatr Surg* 1996; 31: 225-8.

38. Grossklaus DJ, Shappell SB, Adams MC, Brock JW, 3rd, Pope JCT. Small intestinal submucosa as a urethral coverage layer. *J Urol* 2001; 166: 636-9.

39. Foroutan HR, Khalili A, Geramizadeh B, Rasekhi AR, Tanideh N. Urethral reconstruction using autologous and everted vein graft: an experimental study. *Pediatr Surg Int* 2006; 22: 259-62.

40. Elbakry A. Complications of the preputial island flap-tube urethroplasty. *BJU Int* 1999; 84: 89-94.

41. Gray J, Boston VE. Glanular reconstruction and preputioplasty repair for distal hypospadias: a unique day-case method to avoid urethral stenting and preserve the prepuce. *BJU Int* 2003; 91: 268-70.

42. Johnson D, Coleman DJ. The selective use of a single-stage and a two-stage technique for hypospadias correction in 157 consecutive cases with the aim of normal appearance and function. *Br J Plast Surg* 1998; 51: 195-201.

43. Snodgrass W, Koyle M, Manzoni G, Hurwitz R, Caldamone A, Ehrlich R. Tubularised incised plate hypospadias repair: results of a multicenter experience. *J Urol* 1996; 156: 839-41.

44. Retik AB, Bauer SB, Mandell J, Peters CA, Colodny A, Atala A. Management of severe hypospadias with a 2-stage repair. *J Urol* 1994; 152: 749-51.

45. Price RD, Lambe GF, Jones RP. Two-stage hypospadias repair: audit in a district general hospital. *Br J Plast Surg* 2003; 56: 752-8.

46. Jayanthi VR. The modified Snodgrass hypospadias repair: reducing the risk of fistula and meatal stenosis. *J Urol* 2003; 170: 1603-5.

47. Nuininga JE, RP DEG, Verschuren R, Feitz WF. Long-term outcome of different types of 1-stage hypospadias repair. *J Urol* 2005; 174: 1544-8; discussion 1548.

48. Patel RP, Shukla AR, Snyder HM, 3rd. The island tube and island onlay hypospadias repairs offer excellent long-term outcomes: a 14-year followup. *J Urol* 2004; 172: 1717-9; discussion 1719.

49. Riccabona M, Oswald J, Koen M, Beckers G, Schrey A, Lusuardi L. Comprehensive analysis of six years experience in tubularised incised plate urethroplasty and its extended application in primary and secondary hypospadias repair. *Eur Urol* 2003; 44: 714-9.

50. Kumar MV, Harris DL. A long-term review of hypospadias repaired by split preputial flap technique (Harris). *Br J Plast Surg* 1994; 47: 236-40.

51. Koyanagi T, Nonomura K, Yamashita T, Kanagawa K, Kakizaki H. One-stage repair of hypospadias: is there no simple method universally applicable to all types of hypospadias? [see comments]. *J Urol* 1994; 152: 1232-7.

52. Asopa HS. Newer concepts in the management of hypospadias and its complications. *Ann Roy Coll Surg Engl* 1998; 80: 161-8.

Chapter 13

Appendix: Glossary of terms

Byars flaps

A procedure to resurface the ventral side of the penis using the excess preputial skin on the dorsum of the penis which is brought around to the ventral side as flaps.

Chordee

Refers to ventral curvature of the penis.

Hooding

In hypospadias, the prepuce is usually incomplete ventrally. However, the prepuce is complete dorsally giving the appearance of a 'hood' gathered up behind the glans.

Hypospadias

A congenital abnormality of the external male genitalia characterised by ventral meatal dystopia. This is frequently accompanied by other abnormal features such as hooding of the prepuce and chordee.

Islanded flaps

The inner preputial skin is raised as an island with a vascular pedicle based on the vessels within the dartos fascia. This island of skin can then be used as an onlay (sutured over the urethral plate thus forming the ventral wall of the neo-urethra) or tubed over a catheter (thus forming the entire neo-urethra). A double-faced islanded flap takes the inner and outer layers of the prepuce. The inner layer is then used either as an onlay or tubularised around a catheter. The outer layer is used for ventral skin cover.

GRAP repair

Glanular reconstruction and preputioplasty. This repair is best suited for distal hypospadias and includes a reconstruction of the prepuce.

MAGPI repair

Meatal advancement and glansplasty included. A procedure to 'advance' the urethra by flexing the glans ventrally.

Meatal dystopia

The opening of the urethra (i.e. the meatus) is in the wrong place. For hypospadias, the meatus opens on the ventral surface of the penis. For epispadias, the meatus opens on the dorsal surface of the penis.

Snodgrass repair

A tubularised incised plate (TIP) repair. The urethral plate is incised longitudinally. This allows the ventral structures to be tubed around a catheter without tension. Spontaneous re-epithelialisation of the raw area created on the dorsal wall of the neo-urethra is supposed to occur over the following days/weeks.

Snodgraft repair

Same as a Snodgrass repair but uses a graft to resurface the raw area on the dorsal wall that is created when the urethral plate is incised longitudinally. This avoids the risk of healing by wound contraction with subsequent stricture or stenosis.

Spatulated glans

Because the terminal meatus fails to form in hypospadias, the glans penis is frequently broad and/or square (spatulated) rather than conical in shape. One of the aims of surgery is to restore the normal conical shape to the glans penis.

Thiersch-Duplay

The ventral tissues of the penis are tubularised around a catheter to create the neo-urethra. This can be combined with a TIP manoeuvre which deepens the ventral tissues to allow them to be closed over a catheter. Alternatively, it may be combined with other glansplasty manoeuvres to allow the distal part of the penis to be closed over a catheter.

Chapter 14

Cleft palate closure: the timing and options for surgical repair

Simon van Eeden BSc MChD FFDRCSI FRCSEd (OMFS)
Cleft Fellow
Loshan Kangesu MB BS FRCS (Plast.)
Consultant Plastic Surgeon
Brian Sommerlad MB BS FRCS (Eng) FRCSEd (Hon)
Consultant Plastic Surgeon

GREAT ORMOND STREET HOSPITAL FOR CHILDREN AND ST ANDREWS CENTRE FOR PLASTIC SURGERY, BROOMFIELD HOSPITAL, CHELMSFORD, ESSEX, UK

Introduction

Clefts of the palate may occur as an isolated cleft palate, or as part of a cleft lip and palate. The two patient populations are separate, with the former being more often associated with other conditions, e.g. Pierre Robin sequence, velocardiofacial, Stickler, and Treacher Collins syndrome. Cleft palate repair remains a major challenge because of the technical difficulties of operating in a confined space in children, and because surgical outcomes are measured not just by successful closure of the cleft but more by functional parameters. The aims of palatal closure are to separate the oral and nasal cavities, and to achieve normal speech, hearing, and maxillary growth. Final assessment of speech and mid-facial development may only be carried out when the child reaches adulthood. This makes objective assessment of any one technique, protocol or surgeon difficult to evaluate.

Methodology

A Medline search was employed to gather evidence using the search terms 'cleft palate', 'cleft lip and palate', 'cleft palate repair', 'speech and cleft palate' and 'growth and cleft palate'. The Cochrane Library database was accessed looking at reviews and trials in cleft lip and palate.

Difficulties with outcome evaluation in cleft palate surgery and types of studies

There has been government intervention in the UK to centralise cleft services to create high volume operators within multi-disciplinary teams with a focus on outcome analysis [1]. However, this has not been the case previously, and even in the same unit protocols and techniques have varied between surgeons. Consequently, many reports in peer-reviewed journals relate to small numbers of patients, short-term outcomes and, varying degrees of clefts. The difficulty in presenting the evidence for the ideal operation for cleft palate repair can be summarised by the following three factors. Firstly, the outcomes of cleft palate repair vary depending on patient and surgeon factors.

Patient factors:

- Condition: cleft palate (CP) or cleft lip with or without cleft of the palate (CL +/-P), either unilateral or bilateral).
- Severity: complete or incomplete clefts.
- Presence of associated conditions or anomalies, e.g. deafness, other causes of developmental delay.

Surgeon factors:

- ◆ Skill. There is a long learning curve.
- ◆ Technique. There has been a tendency to follow local teaching and dogma rather than learn from published evidence. Similarly, texts are now seen to be misleading.
- ◆ Protocol. The timing of surgery appears to be critical to speech development.

Secondly, added to these variables is the lack of international standards for measuring outcome. Thirdly, a major obstacle to evidence-based practice is that emerging data suggest that speech and facial growth parameters get worse with age. Hence, final outcomes should not be assessed until the child is 20 years of age [2] **(III/B)**.

Few randomised controlled trials exist because of difficulties in the context of cleft surgery. The Cochrane database only lists one review at the current time. Cohort studies, which attempt to simulate a randomised controlled trial without the randomisation, are regarded as the second choice method. The aim is to collect data on all factors that could influence the outcome, including interventions used. These studies are regarded as observational because the investigator does not influence which patient receives which intervention, may be either prospective or retrospective and may include inter-centre studies. There are several retrospective cohort studies in cleft lip and palate research, but by their nature they have many variables. Inter-centre comparisons may be prospective or retrospective and are useful to increase the number of cases of a particular subtype being investigated. These studies, however, introduce other variables such as differences in surgeons, protocols and data collection that may make interpretation of results difficult. External blinded assessment increases the rigour of these studies. Meta-analysis, which may be prospective or used retrospectively on published studies, may offer definitive answers [3].

Historical control studies are also common in the field of cleft lip and palate surgery, and they compare treatments used in one period with those used in a subsequent period. They may arise naturally from changes in treatment in a single centre and are particularly useful if durable records exist. Once again confounding variables exist, such as the surgeon's skill and ancillary services [3].

This brief insight into research methodology as it pertains to the cleft lip and palate is to inform the reader of the difficulties experienced in providing evidence for and against a certain technique or protocol. Most studies reviewed for this chapter should be ranked as level III evidence.

One of the strongest forms of outcome measure in cleft surgery is, for example, from a series of consecutive, non-syndromic patients with a single cleft type, all operated on by the same surgeon, where the outcome measures were assessed when patients have completed growth by an external assessor in a blinded manner [2-5].

Historical review

Hippocrates (circa 460-355 BC) or his followers were among the first to understand the mechanism of speech [6]. However, it was not until the middle 16th century in 1556 when Franco (1505-1579) recognised congenital clefts of the palate in his famous 1556 text: "cleft lips are sometimes congenital, through a defect of nature … furthermore they are sometimes cleft without a cleft of the jaw or palate, sometimes the cleft is only slight and at times the cleft is long and wide as the lip." In 1561, he wrote further saying "those who have cleft palates are more difficult to cure: and they always speak through the nose." Palatal syphilis with perforation had been first described half a century before and was extremely common. This held back the progress of cleft palate surgery for centuries because many believed that most palatal clefts were due to syphilis. Paré (1561) realised the importance of the uvula for speech, noting that those patients with conditions of the uvula spoke with nasal speech [7].

Obturators to occlude palatal perforations have been used since the 16th century (Lusitanus 1560, Paré 1564). Houllier (circa 1562) is credited with being the first to propose suture of palatal perforations due to syphilis in the late 16th century. The first report of surgery to lengthen the soft palate for a destroyed uvula is accredited to André Myrrhen in 1706. In 1766, Robert reported on the earlier work of Le Monnier, a dentist from Rouen, who successfully operated on a child with a complete palatal cleft from the incisors to the velum. He first placed a few stitches along the two edges of the cleft to approximate them and then freshened these margins with hot cautery. Simple techniques of closure of congenital cleft palate were introduced by von Graefe from Germany in 1816, by Roux from France in 1819, Warren from the USA in 1820 and, Alcock from England in 1821. Dieffenbach in 1826 was the first to describe elevation of soft tissue flaps rather than just paring the edges. In a staged manner he used lateral relaxing osteotomies to facilitate palate closure. From the 1840s a number of surgeons described division of the palatal muscles at their insertion to lessen the tension on the palatal repair. Fergusson's anatomical studies led him to divide the levator veli palatini (LVP) muscles, the posterior and, if necessary, the anterior tonsillar pillars. This prevented lateral pull and disruption of the velar repair. These were all destructive solutions to prevent dehiscence of the palatal repair [7]; now we rely on suture of the palatal muscles to take the tension off the mucosal repair.

Von Langenbeck provided the first major solution to the problem of dehiscence of cleft palate closure with elevation of muco-periosteal flaps which are still used today. Veau criticised the von Langenbeck technique in a series of lectures in 1927 saying that the technique resulted in short immobile palates due to the fibrosis caused by scarring on the nasal aspect of the palate from the wide undermining necessary. Veau recommended closure of the nasal layer, fracture of the hamular process and suture of the palatal muscles using a V-Y 'pushback' technique which was thought to increase palatal length [7]. Similarly, in the UK, pushback flaps according to the technique of Kelsey and Fry were also gaining in popularity [8, 9]. In 1937, a pushback technique more radical than Veau's technique was described independently by Wardill [10] and Kilner [11], both in 1937. All these techniques left raw exposed bone on the hard palate that was seen to heal by epithelial migration. However, the underlying scar tissue was to compromise maxillary growth. The V-Y pushback concept gained widespread popularity

but is now recognised to have caused significant scarring, maxillary retrusion and had no evidence of increasing palatal length from the pushback [12] **(III/B)**. It was Europe's worst export in cleft surgery.

The techniques of delayed closure and the use of a vomerine flap brought controversy to hard palate closure. Gillies and Fry, aware of the maxillary growth retardation following early palatal surgery, suggested delaying hard palate surgery [9] and in the 1940s the concept was popularised by Schweckendiek[13]. With time this was shown to be favourable for growth if the delay was until adolescence, but unfavourable for speech (see later) [14]. An alternative method of closure for the hard palate was to use the superiorly-based muco-perichondrial vomerine flap[15]. This single layer flap is unlined, but soon epithelialises on the oral surface and within three months there is a new bone formed within the two mucosal surfaces. Critics have contended that raising of a vomerine flap is disadvantageous for midface growth [16], but others were able to demonstrate satisfactory growth results [17, 18] **(III/B)**. Furthermore, a study on rare facial clefts where complete disjunction existed between the nasal septum/vomer and the secondary palate, it was shown that facial morphology well within normal ranges was attained [19]. There remain two schools of thought for the hard palate.

The next advance in palate surgery was to address the muscles of the soft palate. The abnormal muscles in the cleft palate were described as being in an antero-posterior direction rather than as a sling by Fergusson and then by Veau [20] (see anatomical consideration). Braithwaite, in 1964 [21] and 1968 [22] and, Kriens in 1969 [23], wrote of repositioning the displaced palatal muscles to establish the levator sling and provide the patient with a functional velum. Furlow in 1986 described the double opposing Z-plasty of the soft palate which reforms the levator sling and also lengthens the soft palate [24]. Cutting and Sommerlad independently described radical dissection and retropositioning of the individual muscles with division of the tensor palati tendon [20, 25]. Sommerlad gains access to the soft palate musculature via marginal incisions alone [20]. The operating microscope allows for more precise dissection and greater comfort for the surgeon, as well as the facility for audio-visual links [26]. Again, these two methods remain in contemporary practice.

Anatomy: theory for constructing the levator sling

The velopharynx needs to close during speech and swallowing, and it does so by the pharynx constricting and, mostly, by the soft palate elevating. A failure of this mechanism causes speech with velopharyngeal incompetence (VPI) that is characterised by a hypernasal tone, emission and turbulence; and nasal regurgitation when swallowing. Opening is also important to facilitate nasal breathing. Snoring and sleep apnoea may be consequent to failure of opening. Cleft palate repair may result in VPI. The rates of VPI after cleft palate closure vary from 10-50%. Secondary surgery, especially with pharyngoplasty may cause obstruction to nasal breathing [27] **(IIa/B)**.

The classical understanding of palate anatomy was advanced by studies on normal cadavers by cleft surgeons [28-31]. These dissections have elucidated the normal anatomy of the velum and pharynx, and may serve as a basis for anatomical reconstruction of the abnormal muscular insertions found in infants with cleft palates. Dissections have shown that the LVP forms a muscle sling that suspends the velum from the cranial base. It is attached superiorly to the postero-medial aspect of the eustachian tube at the junction of its bony and cartilaginous parts. From its origin the levator bundles descend in an antero-medial direction in the space between the superior constrictor and the cranial base to enter the velum by fanning out between the two heads of the palatophayngeus. Fibres from each side fuse with one another in the midline with some decussation within the paramedian zone. The intra-velar part of the levator occupies the middle 40% of the velar length measured from the posterior nasal spine to the tip of the uvula. It is attached anteriorly to the posterior margin of the aponeurosis of the tensor veli palatini (TVP) with some overlap on its oral surface medially. The musculus uvulae when present may be found on the nasal aspect of the velum as a single or paired muscle along the cleft margin.

In comparison with normal anatomy, in the cleft palate the TVP, having passed around the hook of the hamulus, forms a thick triangular insertion into the lateral part of the posterior edge of the hard palate and fails to form the palatal aponeurosis; the LVP, palatopharyngeus and palatoglossus pass more anteriorly to insert into the margins of the cleft, the oral and nasal mucosa and the abnormal palatal aponeurosis. The palatopharyngeus in contrast to the levator veli palatini continues forwards to insert into the posterior border of the hard palate. Although the palatopharyngeus and LVP are separate muscles, near the midline they fuse to form what appears to be one muscle, which Veau called the 'cleft muscle'.

Dissections suggest that the LVP elevates and elongates the velum posteriorly on closure. The distribution of its fibres in the middle 40% of the velum corresponds with the knee observed in velar elevation on lateral videofluoroscopy. This investigation visualises the velum and velopharyngeal defect during speech. Visualisation of the velum during speech demonstrates the importance of the LVP in velar movement. Using magnetic resonance imaging (MRI) it is also possible to visualise and measure changes in the LVP during speech [32, 33] **(IIa/B)**. This cumulative knowledge supports the theoretical basis to establish the LVP sling during palatal repair (Figure 1).

Physiology: theory for early surgery

The neonate with a cleft palate is immediately compromised by the inability to create an intra-oral vacuum to suck, and the subsequent inability of developing an intra-oral pressure for talking. There is also a higher incidence of language delay and some theories suggest an association with the cleft. Feeding is one of the earliest experiences in life and is obviously critical for survival. It is also thought to be important for the development of communication as the connections between external stimuli and the development of cognitive patterns in the brain are set in motion. Disruption of normal feeding is hypothesised to cause abnormal neuromotor oro-sensory patterns to develop [34]. This may result in delayed or deviant pre-speech development which may account for early cognitive and language lags in cleft palate infants. The use of certain feeding techniques and treatment protocols is believed to influence speech development. Kaplan argued that palatal closure around six months, during the pre-linguistic phase of speech development (at about the stage of babbling) will provide the child

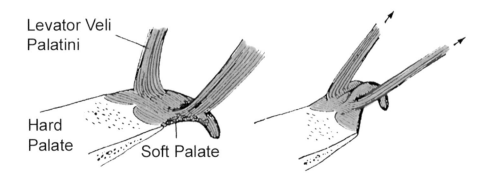

Figure 1. Levator palati muscles at rest and the effect of contraction on the soft palate.

with the best chance for correct sound production when first learnt [35].

It was also argued that pre-surgical orthodontics may help feeding, speech, growth and facilitate surgery by narrowing the cleft. However, studies show that pre-surgical orthodontic plates do not influence feeding [36] **(Ib/A)**. Conclusion about the other parameters is awaited.

Hearing difficulties may further compromise communication in infants with cleft palates. It is well established that there is a high incidence of otitis media in these patients. The associated conductive hearing loss may fluctuate and obviously increase the risk of speech and language problems, but hearing does improve after palate repair. Hearing loss even over a short period of time may have permanent irreversible effects at the level of the brainstem during the active period of child development [37]. In a cohort of 55 cleft lip and palate patients, all 27 infants who had cleft palate closure between 11 and 16 weeks had normal middle ears at the time of surgery and four subseqeuntly required grommets in the first year of life (7%), which is about the same as the normal average. However, of 28 infants closed after 16 weeks and tested at the time of surgery, 16 had abnormal tympanograms. Seven of 11 children operated at 17-18 weeks with normal tympanograms prior to their repair subsequently developed middle ear effusion requiring ventilation tubes within ten months of birth

and three out of six who needed grommets at the time of surgery needed to have further grommets placed. Too-Chung therefore concludes that early palatal closure before four months of age can avoid middle ear complications [38] **(IIa/B)**. Although the technique of palatal closure is not reported in this study it is apparent that it is the timing rather than the technique of closure that is most important.

Our current surgical protocol

The authors advocate early palate surgery at six months. The details are as follows:

- ◆ CP: palate repair at six months. Microscope-aided direct apposition of the nasal muco-periosteal layers is aided by use of bilateral vomerine flaps if required. Muscle dissection and LVP muscle sling construction is undertaken with deliberate set-back to the posterior 1/3 to 1/2 of the velum (Figure 2). Direct closure of the oral muco-periosteal flaps is aided by lateral releasing incisions (Langenbeck) when necessary (in 10% of cases).

- ◆ CL+P-Unilateral: at the time of lip repair at three months, if the cleft is complete, closure of the anterior palate and nasal floor using an unlined superiorly-based vomerine muco-perichondral flap. Closure of the remaining hard and soft

Before

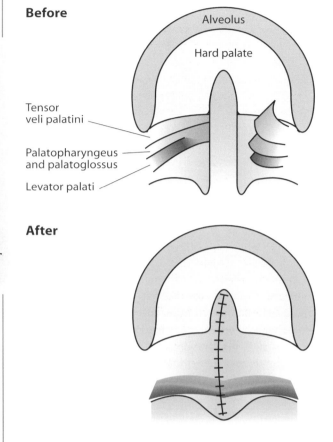

After

Figure 2. Diagram illustrating the principles of muscle sling construction and setback.

palate at 6-8 months with posterior muscle dissection is as described above, with a lateral releasing incision to the oral layer if needed.

♦ CL+P-Bilateral: lip repair at 3-4 months with closure of one hemi-anterior hard palate using a vomerine flap and partial closure of the contralateral hemi-anterior hard palate using a limited vomerine flap (raised up to the pre-vomerine suture). At six months velar closure is as described above. Lateral releasing incisions may again be required.

All patients have their hearing monitored from birth to three months, and if there is otitis media with significant hearing loss (>55dBnHL in the better ear), ventilatory tubes (grommets) are placed at the time of velar surgery. With this protocol approximately a third

of patients with all types of cleft palate require middle ear ventilation [39].

Evidence for current practice

Development of abnormal articulation

Studies of babbling have shown that non-cleft infants exhibit a predominance of anterior sounds in pre-speech production, whereas in cleft infants, babbling is dominated by posterior consonants with fewer frontal sounds. The un-operated cleft infant seems to avoid sounds produced at the palate with articulations in the extremes of the vocal tract (glottal and labial) [34] (Figure 3). Similarly, those infants with a repaired soft palate and un-repaired residual cleft of the hard palate have this abnormal compensatory articulation. Speech therapists describe this as anterior (apico-dental) to posterior (dorso-velar) displacement of consonant sounds. These deviant patterns are thought to develop early and are hard to change [40].

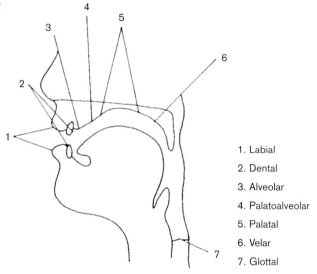

Figure 3. Location of articulatory positions.
Adapted from Wyatt R, Sell D, Russell J, Harding A, Harland K, Albery E. Cleft palate speech dissected: a review of current knowledge and analysis. British Journal of Plastic Surgery 1996; 49: 143-9. Reproduced with permission from Elsevier, © 1996.

Studies from un-operated cleft patients

Studies on children with very late surgery for cleft palate in the developing world provided evidence of poor speech outcome following delayed surgery. Despite inadequate speech assessment and longitudinal follow-up, early studies reported that surgery after 12 years of age fails to improve speech in those patients with an established abnormal pattern [41] **(III/B)**. Sell *et al* carried out a detailed analysis of speech in un-operated teenagers in Sri Lanka [42] **(III/B)**. Speech investigations were carried out before surgery, after surgery but before speech therapy, and after speech therapy. They found that speech in patients with un-repaired clefts was severely disordered, that there is minimal spontaneous improvement when surgery only is provided and that an improvement in controlled speech (i.e. not spontaneous speech) can be attained with speech therapy. Patients with smaller clefts of the posterior third of the hard palate and/or soft palate did improve in spontaneous speech [42, 43]. Earlier surgical and phoniatric intervention at 6-12 was thought to be of benefit [41].

Palate surgery below one year

Evans and Renfrew evaluated the speech results of one surgeon and reported results that suggested that repair at eight months or earlier gives better speech results than those children repaired after eight months of age [44] **(III/B)**. Grobbelaar *et al* provided evidence, in a large retrospective study of five different techniques, that there is a significant difference in speech and less velopharyngeal incompetence when the palate was repaired before six months of age [45] **(III/B)**. Ysunza *et al* carried out a randomised controlled trial on speech and maxillary growth in patients with a unilateral cleft lip and palate (UCLP) operated on at six (35 patients) months versus 12 months (41 patients). They found significantly better phonological development in the group operated at six months; none of the patients in this group developed compensatory articulation. There was no statistically significant difference in maxillary arch development, soft tissue profile and velopharyngeal incompetence between the two groups at four years from surgery. They concluded that early palate repair at six months improves speech outcome and prevents compensatory articulation [46] **(Ib/A)**. Dorf and Curtin

compared the results of speech from surgery before or after age one in a mixed cleft population. They reported glottal and pharyngeal articulatory errors in 86% of patients who had palatal closure after one year, as compared to only 10% when closed before one year of age. Eighty-three percent of UCLP patients and 92% of isolated cleft palate patients developed normal articulation skills, compared with only 13% and 17%, respectively, repaired after one year. However, the age at surgery was very variable (early group - 5 to 12 months, late group - 12 to 27 months) [47]. Jones *et al* in a prospective trial investigated speech in children pre-surgery (11 months) and post-surgery (17 months), and compared the results with speech in non-cleft babies at the same time periods. Although improvements in speech were noted, the children with a cleft palate continued to exhibit smaller consonant inventories and produced less oral stops, which they feel reinforces the idea that early deficits impact later speech development [48] **(IIa/B)**. This, they suggest, is in line with others [49], that palatal repair by 12 months or prior to the acquisition of words may not be early enough if optimal communication is the goal.

A number of other studies have reported improved speech outcome with earlier closure [20, 50, 51], but the optimal age for closure is still contentious. The only randomised trial supports closure at six months (Ysunza's trial mentioned above).

Delayed hard palate closure

The term 'delayed hard palate closure' covers a broad range of protocols where hard palate repair has been delayed from 18 months to 15 years.

Speech

As described in the historical review, following the introduction by Gillies and Fry [9], Schwekendiek popularised delayed, two-stage palate closure where the hard palate defect was obturated with a prosthesis and closed at 12-15 years of age [13]. Peer review reported poor speech with 81% velopharyngeal incompetence and 86% of patients with glottal or pharyngeal articulatory errors. Most of his patients required pharyngeal surgery to improve speech [14] **(III/B)**.

Numerous other reports have documented poor speech from protocols that favoured delayed hard palate closure after the age of 18 months [52-55]. Cosman and Falk [52] **(III/B)**, after reviewing 32 cases with complete palatal clefts treated using an early soft palate and late hard palate repair technique, cautioned against delayed closure. They showed a high incidence of articulatory errors, velopharyngeal incompetence (reported as 37% but predicted to rise to 66%) and only 72% with acceptable speech, despite pharyngeal flaps and speech therapy. Similarly, Agerskov et al [56] reported the speech results for 15 patients treated with early soft palate closure at 6-8 months and hard palate closure at 8-9 years of age. These children had a high incidence of velopharyngeal incompetence, necessitating pharyngeal flap surgery (33%) and, articulatory errors. Twenty percent of children had retracted consonants, which failed to improve despite considerable speech therapy **(III/B)**.

Rohrich et al [55] compared speech outcome in 17 and 18-year-olds following early (10.8 months) vs late repair (48.6 months). They found the delayed group faring significantly worse in articulatory errors, nasal resonance and intelligibility **(III/B)**. Again, the poorer group did not appear to normalise over time.

Studies reporting on delayed closure show that narrowing of the residual cleft does occur [13, 52]. Wider defects have more speech defects [54], but once established the size of the residual cleft only marginally influences the articulatory errors [57] **(IIa/B)**.

Growth

Growth outcome does differ when comparing isolated cleft palate cases with cleft lip and palate cases, with the latter demonstrating substantial growth disturbance. Hence, all the growth concerns and subsequent discussion relates to this latter group where it is also known that lip and alveolar surgery may also contribute to maxillary retardation.

Follow-up of ten patients treated with the Gillies and Fry protocol in which the soft palate was repaired between the ages of two and 21 years and the hard palate was left open showed reasonable occlusion on dental cast analysis and cephalometry [58]. When Schweckendiek delayed hard palate closure until 12-15 years, excellent growth was reported at the price of speech [13] **(III/B)**. The evidence for improved growth following delayed hard palate closure since Schweckendiek's study has been contradictory. Some have found better growth when repair was carried out in the first 12-15 months [55, 59], with worse growth when repair was carried out between four and nine years [55, 59] **(IIb/B)**, and between 8-15 years [60] **(III/B)**. Others could not demonstrate any benefit of delaying palatal surgery to five years compared with a group closed at 12-15 months [61] **(III/B)**. Conversely, the Göteborg unit delayed hard palate closure until children were 8-10 years old. The final outcome in 46 consecutive patients at 19 years was recently published and demonstrated excellent growth as measured by the dento-alveolar relationship. However, this unit has since changed their protocol by lowering the age for hard palate closure to three years of age because of speech concerns [4] **(III/B)**.

In conclusion, delaying hard palate surgery until age eight (Göterborg study) [4], but especially until adolescence, will benefit maxillary growth, but at the cost of speech defects that may not be correctable. Any shorter delay does not benefit growth and still affects speech adversely, giving compelling evidence to close the entire palate in the first year. Delayed palatal closure is, however, still practised in some units in Europe.

Techniques of palate repair

A problem with all speech (and growth) evaluation is the lack of standard evaluation. For speech, centres may report VPI rates or the rates of secondary surgery. The latter are probably more significant from a clinical perspective, but the threshold for surgery will vary. Speech results without muscle dissection have not been optimal. Pharyngoplasty rates following von Langenbeck, Veau-Wardill-Kilner or the two-flap procedures as described by Bardach, or their modifications, have been reported as giving rates in excess of 20% [62-67].

Following the interest by Braithwaite [21, 22] and Kriens [23] in surgery to the velar muscles (intravelar veloplasty), the concept of the functional velum and reconstruction of the velar muscle sling gained support [68-70]. These studies all had methodological limitations, however, which made definite conclusions about outcome benefit impossible [71]. The one attempt to randomise muscle dissection showed no advantage, but subsequent personal communication suggested flaws in study design [71] **(IIb/B)**. Hence, as with so much cleft work, one has to look at single-centre outcome studies.

Furlow in 1986 described the double reverse Z-palatoplasty which aligns the LVP sling while also lengthening the velum [72]. Reports using this technique have also been favourable with normal or near normal speech reported in over 85% of patients [73-75] **(III/B)**.

Sommerlad advanced the muscle dissection by carrying out a more radical procedure aided with a standard operating microscope. This enabled accurate visualisation of the palatal musculature which facilitated radical dissection of the levator veli palatini laterally, identification of the palatopharyngeus and formation of the levator sling [20, 26]. Evaluation of this technique with a minimum follow-up of ten years has shown a secondary velopharyngeal surgery rate of 10.2%, 4.9% and 4.6% for all palatal repairs between 1978-1982 inclusive, 1983-1987 inclusive and 1988-1992, respectively [20]. These outcomes are some of the best so far published. Twenty consecutive patients with complete UCLP were reviewed at age ten and 20 showing a secondary re-operation rate of 5% and 5%, respectively [2] **(III/B)**.

Conclusions

It is clear then that the outcome of palatal surgery can be influenced by many different factors. Unfortunately the water is further muddied by the fact that the quality of evidence in the cleft literature is such that very few definite conclusions can be made. The small case load, the necessary long follow-up times, variations in protocol, data collection and assessment, variation in surgical skill and, a preponderance of retrospective case studies make interpretation of the literature difficult. A recent systematic review of hard palate timing and facial growth found that only 15 studies met the reviews selection criteria [76]. However, we feel that there is sufficient evidence to promote early palate surgery involving muscle dissection, with selective middle ear ventilation. With appropriate training and teamwork this is a safe and effective strategy.

Recommendations	Evidence level
◆ Timing. Perform early palate closure at six months of age.	Ia/B
◆ Technique. Use magnification to carry out a detailed anatomical muscle dissection to accurately and reliably establish the levator veli palatini muscle sling.	III/B
◆ Feeding plates. We do not recommend the use of feeding plates as they have not been shown to improve feeding in patients with cleft palate.	Ib/B

Chapter 14

References

1. Clinical Standards Advisory Group. Report on cleft lip and or/palate. London: The Stationery Office, 1998.

2. Sommerlad BC, Hay N, Mayne A, *et al*. A 20 year follow-up of unilateral cleft lip and palate patients. Proceedings of the Craniofacial Society of Great Britain and Ireland, 2007.

3. Roberts CT, Semb G, Shaw W. Strategies for the advancement of surgical methods in cleft lip and palate. *Cleft Palate Craniofac J* 1991; 28: 141-9.

4. McComb HK, Coghlan BA. Primary repair of the unilateral cleft lip nose. Completion of a longitudinal study. *Cleft Palate Craniofac J* 1996; 33: 23-31.

5. Lilja J, Mars M, Elander L, *et al*. Analysis of dental arch relationships in Swedish unilateral cleft lip and palate subjects: 20-year longitudinal consecutive series treated with delayed hard palate closure. *Cleft Palate Craniofac J* 2006; 43: 606-11.

6. Weinburger BW. *An introduction to the history of dentistry*. St Louis: Mosby, 1948: 117.

7. Rogers BO. History of cleft lip and palate treatment. In: *Cleft Lip and Palate: Surgical, Dental and Speech Aspects*. Grabb WC, Rosenstein SW, Bzoch KR, Eds. Boston: Little Brown, 1971: 143-65.

8. Fry WK. The dental aspect of the treatment of congenital cleft palates. *Proc R Soc Med (Sect Odont)* 1921; 14: 57-60.

9. Gillies HD, Fry WK. A new principle in the surgical treatment of 'congenital cleft palate' and its mechanical counterpart. *Br Med J* 1921; 1: 335.

10. Wardill WEM. Technique of operation for cleft lip and palate. *Br J Surg* 1937; 25: 117.

11. Kilner TP. Cleft lip and palate repair technique. In: *Postgraduate Surgery*, Vol 3. Maingot R, Ed. London: Medical Publishers, 1937: 3696.

12. Muir IFK. Maxillary development in cleft palate patients with special reference to the effects of the operation. *Ann Roy Coll Surg Engl* 1986; 68: 62-7.

13. Schweckendiek W. Primay veloplasty: long-term results without maxillary deformity: a twenty-five year report. *Cleft Palate J* 1978; 15: 268-74.

14. Bardach J, Morris HL, Olin WH. Late results of primary veloplasty: the Marburg project. *Plast Reconstr Surg* 1984; 73: 207-15.

15. Grabb WC. General aspects of cleft palate surgery. In: *Cleft Lip and Palate: Surgical, Dental and Speech Aspects*. Grabb WC, Rosenstein SW, Bzoch KR, Eds. Boston: Little Brown, 1971: 389.

16. Delaire J, Precious D. Avoidance of use of vomerine mucosa in primary surgical management of velopalatine clefts. *Oral Surgery Oral Medicine and Oral Pathology* 1985; 60: 589-97.

17. Semb G. A study of facial growth in patients with unilateral cleft lip and palate treated by the Oslo CLP team. *Cleft Palate Craniofac J* 1991; 28: 1-21.

18. Bütow KW. Caudally based single-layer septum-vomer flap for cleft palate closure. *J Cranio-Max-Fac Surg* 1987; 15: 10-3.

19. Bergland O, Borchgrevink H. The role of the nasal septum in midfacial growth in man elucidated by maxillary development in certain types of facial clefts. *Scand J Plast Reconstr Surg* 1974; 8: 42-8.

20. Sommerlad BC. A technique for palate repair. *Plast Reconstr Surg* 2003; 112: 1542-8.

21. Braithwaite F. Cleft palate repair. In: *Modern Trends in Plastic Surgery* I. Gibson T, Ed. London: Butterworth, 1964: 30-49

22. Braithwaite F, Maurice D. The importance of the levator palati muscle in cleft palate closure. *Br J Plast Surg* 1968; 21: 60-2.

23. Kriens OB. An anatomical approach to veloplasty. *Plast Reconstr Surg* 1969; 43: 29-41.

24. Furlow LT. Cleft palate repair by double opposing Z-plasty. *Plast Reconstr Surg* 1986; 78: 724-73.

25. Cutting CB, Rosenbaum J, Rovati L. The technique of muscle repair in the cleft soft palate. *Oper Tech Plast Recon Surg* 1995; 2: 215-22.

26. Sommerlad BC. The use of the operating microscope in cleft palate repair and pharyngoplasty. *Plast Reconstr Surg* 2003; 112: 1540-1.

27. Liao Y-F, Chuang M-L, Chen PKT, Chen N-H, Yun C, Huang C-S. Incidence and severity of obstructive sleep apnea following pharyngeal flap surgery in patients with cleft palate. *Cleft Palate Craniofac J* 2002; 39: 312-6.

28. Boorman JG, Sommerlad BC. Musculus uvulae and levator palati: their anatomical and functional relationship in velopharyngeal closure. *Br J Plast Surg* 1985; 38: 333-8.

29. Boorman JG, Sommerlad BC. Levator palati and palatal dimples. Their anatomy, relationship and clinical significance. *Br J Plast Surg* 1985; 38: 326-32.

30. Huang MHS, Lee ST, Rajendran K. Anatomic basis of cleft palate and velopharyngeal surgery: implications from a fresh cadaveric study. *Plast Reconstr Surg* 1998; 101: 613-27.

31. Mehendale FC. Surgical anatomy of the levator veli palatini: a previously undescribed tendinous insertion of the anterolateral fibres. *Plast Reconstr Surg* 2004; 114: 307-15.

32. Ettema SL, Kuehn DP, Perlman AL, Alperin N. Magnetic resonance imaging of the levator veli palatini muscle during speech. *Cleft Palate Craniofac J* 2002; 39: 130-44.

33. Kane AA, Butman JA, Mullick R, Skopec M, Choyke P. A new method for the study of velopharyngeal function using gated magnetic resonance imaging. *Plast Reconstr Surg* 2002; 109: 472-81.

34. Russel VJ, Harding A. Speech development and early intervention In: *Management of cleft lip and palate*. Watson ACH, Sell D, Grunwell P, Eds. London: Whurr, 2001: 191-209.

35. Kaplan, EN. Cleft palate repair at three months? *Ann Plast Surg* 1981; 7: 179-90.

36. Masarei AG, Wade A, Mars M, Sommerlad BC, Sell D. A randomized controlled trial investigating the effect of presurgical orthopedics on feeding in infants with cleft lip and/or palate. *Cleft Palate Craniofac J* 2007; 44: 182-93.

37. Webster DB, Webster M. Neonatal sound deprivation affects brain stem auditory nuclei. *Arch Otolaryngol* 1977; 103: 392-6.

38. Too-Chung MA. The assessment of middle ear function and hearing by tympanometry in children before and after early cleft palate repair. *Br J Plast Surg* 1983: 36: 295-9.

39. Andrews PJ, Chorbachi R, Sirimanna T, Sommerlad B, Hartley BE. Evaluation of hearing thresholds in 3 month-old children with a cleft palate: the basis for a selective policy for ventilation tube insertion at the time of palatal repair. *Clin Otolaryngol Allied Sci* 2004; 29: 10-7.

40. Lohmander-Agerskov A. Speech outcome after cleft palate surgery with the Göteborg regimen including delayed hard palate closure. *Scand J Plast Reconstr Surg Hand Surg* 1998; 32: 63-80.

41. Ortiz-Monasterio F, Olmedo A, Trigos I, Yudovich M, Velasquez M, Fuento del Campo A. Final results from the delayed treatment of patients with clefts of the lip and palate. *Scand J Plast Reconstr Surg Hand Surg* 1974; 8: 109-15.

42. Sell D, Grunwell P. Speech studies and the unoperated cleft palate subject. *Eur J Disord Commun* 1994; 29: 151-6.

43. Sell DA, Grunwell P. Speech results following late palatal surgery in previously unoperated Sri Lankan adolescents with cleft palate. *Cleft Palate J* 1990; 27: 162-8.

44. Evans D, Renfrew C. The timing of primary cleft palate repair. *Scand J Plast Reconstr Surg* 1974; 8: 153-5.

45. Grobbelaar AO, *et al*. Speech results after repair of the cleft soft palate. *Plast Reconstr Surg* 1995; 95: 1150-4.

46. Ysunza A, Pamplona C, Mendoza M, García-Velasco, Aguilar P, Guerero E. Speech outcome and maxillary growth in patients with unilateral complete cleft lip/palate operated on 6 versus 12 months of age. *Plast Reconstr Surg* 1998; 102: 675-9.

47. Dorf D, Curtin JW. Early cleft palate repair and speech outcome. *Plast Reconstr Surg* 1982; 70: 74-9.

48. Jones CE, Chapman KL, Hardin-Jones MA. Speech development in children with cleft palate before and after palatal surgery. *Cleft Palate Craniofac J* 2003; 40: 19-31.

49. Hardin-Jones M, Chapman KL, Wright J, Halter KA, Schulte J, Dean JA, Havlik RJ, Goldstein J. The impact of early palatal obturation on consonant development in babies with unrepaired cleft palate. *Cleft Palate Craniofac J* 2002; 39: 157-63.

50. O'Gara MM, Logemann JA, Rademaker AW. Phonetic features by babies with unilateral cleft lip and palate. *Cleft Palate Craniofac J* 1994; 31: 446-51.

51. Copeland M. The effects of very early palate repair on speech. *Br J Plast Surg* 1990; 43: 676-82.

52. Cosman B, Falk AS. Delayed hard palate repair and speech deficiencies: a cautionary report. *Cleft Palate J* 1980; 17: 27-33.

53. Witzel MA, Salyer KE, Ross RB. Delayed hard palate closure: the philosophy revisited. *Cleft Palate J* 1984; 21: 263-9.

54. Noordhoff MS, Kuo J, Wang F, Huang H, Witzel MA. Development of articulation before delayed hard palate closure in children with cleft palate: a cross-sectional study. *Plast Reconstr Surg* 1987; 80: 518-23.

55. Rohrich RJ, Roswell AR, Johns DF, *et al*. Timing of hard palate closure: a critical long-term analysis. *Plast Reconstr Surg* 1996; 98: 236-46.

56. Lohmander-Agerskov A, Söderpalm E, Friede H, Lilja J. A longitudinal study of speech in 15 children with cleft lip and palate treated by late repair of the hard palate. *Scand J Plast Reconstr Hand Surg* 1995; 29: 21-31.

57. Lohmander-Agerskov A, Friede H, Söderpalm E, Lilja J. Residual clefts in the hard palate: correlation between cleft size and speech. *Cleft Palate Craniofac J* 1997; 34: 122-8.

58. Walter JD, Hale V. A study of long-term results achieved by Gillies Fry procedure. *Br J Plast Surg* 1987: 40: 384-90.

59. Ross RB. Treatment variables affecting growth in unilateral cleft lip and palate. Part 5: timing of palate repair. *Cleft Palate J* 1987b; 24: 54-63.

60. Koberg W, Koblin J. Speech development and maxillary growth in relationship to technique and timing of palatoplasty. *J Maxillofac Surg* 1973; 1: 44-50

61. Robertson NRE, Jolleys A. The timing of hard palate repair. *Scand J Plast Reconstr Surg* 1974; 8: 49-51.

62. Enemark H, Bolund S, Jørgensen I. Evaluation of unilateral cleft lip and palate treatment: long-term results. *Cleft Palate Craniofac J* 1990; 27: 355-61.

63. Schnitt DE, Agir H, David DJ. From birth to maturity: a group of patients who have completed protocol management. Part 1 unilateral cleft lip and palate. *Plast Reconstr Surg* 2004; 113: 805-17.

64. Morris HC, Bardach J, Ardinger H, Jones D, Kelly K, Olin WH, Wheeler J. Multidisciplinary treatment results for patients with isolated cleft palate. *Plast Reconstr Surg* 1993; 92: 842-51.

65. Becker M, Svensson H, Sarnäs KV, Jakobsson S. Von Langebeck or Wardill procedures for primary palatal repair in patients with isolated cleft palate - speech results. *Scand J Plast Reconstr Surg Hand Surg* 2000; 34: 27-32.

66. Witzel MA, Clarke JA, Lindsay WK, Thompson HG. Comparison of results of pushback or von Langenbeck repair of isolated cleft of the hard and soft palate. *Plast Reconstr Surg* 1979; 64: 347-52.

67. Haapanen MC, Rintala AE. Comparison of quality of speech after Veau-Wardill-Kilner pushback operation and the Cronin modification in the primary treatment of cleft palate. *Scand J Plast Reconstr Surg Hand Surg* 1993; 27: 113-8.

68. Trier WC, Dreyer TM. Primary von Langenbeck palatoplasty with levator reconstruction: rationale and technique. *Cleft Palate J* 1984; 21: 254-62.

69. Brown AS, Cohen MA, Randall P. Levator muscle reconstruction: does it make a difference? *Plast Reconstr Surg* 1983; 72: 1-6.

70. Coston GN, *et al*. Levator muscle reconstruction resulting in velopharyngeal competence - a preliminary report. *Plast Reconstr Surg* 1986; 72: 7-8 .

71. Marsh JL, Grames LM, Holtman B. Intravelar veloplasty; a prospective study. *Cleft Palate J* 1989; 26: 46-50.

72. Furlow LT. Cleft palate repair by double opposing Z-plasty. *Plast Reconstr Surg* 1986; 78: 724-36.

73. Kirschner RE, Wang P, Jawad AF. Cleft palate repair by modified Furlow double opposing Z-plasty: the Childrens Hospital of Philadelphia experience. *Plast Reconstr Surg* 1999; 104: 1998-2014.

Chapter 14

74. La Rossa D, Jackson OH, Kirschner RE, *et al*. The Childrens Hospital of Philadelphia modification of the double opposing Z-plasty: long-term speech and growth results. *Clin Plast Surg* 2004; 31: 243-9.

75. Gunter G, Wisser JR, Cohen MA, Brown AS. Palatoplasty: Furlow's double reversing Z-plasty versus intravelar veloplasty. *Cleft Palate Craniofac J* 1998; 35: 546-9.

76. Liao Y-F, Mars M. Hard palate timing and facial growth in cleft lip and palate: a systematic review. *Cleft Palate Craniofac J* 2006; 43: 563-70.

Chapter 15

Post-traumatic wrist instability

Rob Gilbert MB BS BMed Sci (Hons) MRCS (Glasg)
Specialist Registrar, Trauma and Orthopaedic Surgery

Neil Ashwood BSc (Hons) MB BS FRCS (Tr & Orth)
Consultant Orthopaedic Surgeon

QUEEN'S HOSPITAL, BURTON ON TRENT, UK

Introduction

Carpal instability is defined as the loss of normal alignment of the carpal bones as a result of carpal injury or disease. The instability may arise after an acute single traumatic insult or may be secondary to chronic attenuation of supporting ligaments after a traumatic event or due to an underlying disease process, e.g. rheumatoid arthritis or pseudogout.

Methodology

A Medline search identifying all relevant references was undertaken using the search words 'instability', 'wrist' and 'carpus' and other terms used in the classification and treatment of this condition. Evidence was obtained from at least one well designed quasi-experimental study in drawing together this chapter. These are listed in the references and many substantive texts have an outline of this complicated topic. This chapter aims to provide the reader with an overview and points the reader to various papers to enable further reading.

Incidence

The incidence of carpal instability is unknown. Jones [1] looked at 100 consecutive patients with wrist sprains and found that by using dynamic radiography (clenched fist views), 19 patients had an increased scapholunate gap. It may be that what is diagnosed as a simple sprain, is actually carpal instability in a significant number of patients. Tang [2] reviewed 134 distal radial fractures and found radiological evidence of carpal instability in 30% of cases. Due to their concomitant injury this group of patients may also be under-diagnosed. Dobyns et al [3] found that 10% of all carpal injuries resulted in instability **(III/B)**.

Anatomy

Carpal instability results from injury to the ligamentous or bony constraints of the wrist. It is, therefore, necessary to have an intimate understanding of the anatomy of the wrist joint and carpus, and the structures that support them.

The geometry and kinetics of the carpal bones have been described using various theoretical models, including the column theory [4], oval-ring theory [5] and the row theory [6]. Of the various concepts, the row theory has been the most popular and best explains carpal dynamics.

The row theory divides the wrist into a proximal row (scaphoid, lunate, and triquetrum) and distal row (trapezium, trapezoid, capitate and hamate) of carpal bones, separated by the midcarpal joint. The row theory is based on the principle that the proximal and distal rows work as two separate functional units. Intrinsic ligaments connect the bones in each row and extrinsic ligaments span the midcarpal joint. The scaphoid functions as a link or bridge between the two rows to stabilise an otherwise unstable construct.

Ligamentous stability [7, 8]

Multiple ligaments help to stabilise the wrist between the forearm and hand (Figure 1). They can be divided into intrinsic ligaments, which connect individual carpal bones and extrinsic ligaments, which span the radiocarpal joint.

The intrinsic ligaments are strong ligaments that both originate and insert within the carpus. The two most important intrinsic ligaments are the scapholunate (SLIL) and the lunotriquetral ligaments (LTIL). They are located either side of the lunate and hold it in a balanced position.

The scapholunate ligament is a C-shaped ligament that can be divided into three proximal, dorsal and palmar components. The proximal component consists of fibrocartilage and has minimal mechanical strength. The dorsal and palmar components have true ligamentous characteristics.

The lunotriquetral ligament is also C-shaped and has three components: a dorsal ligament, a palmar ligament and a fibrocartilaginous membrane that interconnects the two and closes the joint proximally.

The scaphocapitate and the dorsal intercarpal ligament cross from the proximal to the distal carpal row. The scaphocapitate ligament crosses the volar midcarpal joint and attaches from the distal pole of scaphoid to the body of the capitate. The dorsal

intercarpal ligament originates from the triquetrum, attaches to the dorsal ridge of the scaphoid before inserting into the distal third of the dorsum of the scaphoid and to the scaphoid-trapezium ligament.

The extrinsic ligaments span the radiocarpal joint. The volar extrinsic ligaments are thicker and more functionally important than the dorsal extrinsic ligaments. From radial to ulnar they are the radioscaphocapitate, radioscapholunate, short radiolunate, long radiolunate, ulnolunate and ulnotriquetrum ligaments.

An important extrinsic ligament is the dorsal radiocarpal ligament, which originates on the radius and has minor attachments to the lunate; however, it mostly attaches to the triquetrum.

Osseous stability

The geometry of the bones of the wrist gives it additional stability. The distal radial articular surface has a double obliquity, 11° in the lateral view and 23° when viewed postero-anteriorly. In addition to this, the posterior lip of the distal radius and the radial styloid have a buttressing effect on the carpus. The carpal articular surface has a smaller diameter of curvature than the distal radius, therefore conferring further stability.

Aetiology

Carpal instability results from an injury to one or more of the ligamentous or bony constraints of the wrist. The type of instability that ensues depends upon the magnitude and direction of force, rate and point of impact on the wrist. A simple fall onto an outstretched hand can produce a spectrum of wrist sprains, distal radial and carpal fractures, as well as ligamentous damage causing instability.

Diagnosis

Carpal injuries may be acute or chronic. Carpal instability may present with obvious injury with clear radiographic evidence to confirm the diagnosis or it

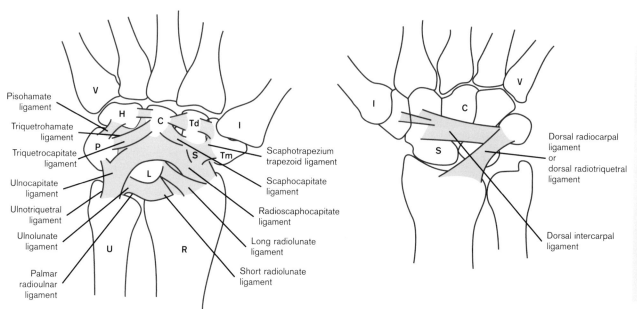

Figure 1. Extrinsic dorsal and volar ligaments of the wrist. R=radius, U=ulna, S=scaphoid, H=hamate, C=capitate, Tm=triquetrum, Td=trapezoid, L=lunate, P=pisiform, I=1st metacarpal, V=5th metacarpal.

may present more subtly some time after the initial insult.

Patients may have pain; if so, its location can be key to diagnosis. They may have weakness or a feeling of the wrist giving way. They may also describe snapping or clicking sensations upon loading the wrist.

Physical examination

All bony landmarks and ligaments of the wrist are palpated. Point tenderness over specific carpal ligaments, such as the SLIL or LTIL, may indicate injury to those structures. Pain at the extremities of movement may also suggest instability.

Specific tests

A number of dynamic manoeuvres have been described to diagnose specific carpal instabilities.

Watson's test (scapholunate instability test) [9] *(Figure 2)*

With the patient's forearm pronated and their hand in ulnar deviation and slight extension, the scaphoid is prevented from moving into palmar flexion by the thumb of the examiner pressing on the scaphoid tuberosity. The patient's hand is radially deviated and flexed. The examiner's thumb attempts to block normal scaphoid flexion. If the SLIL is incompetent, the proximal scaphoid subluxes dorsally over the rim of the radius (rotatory subluxation of the scaphoid). A positive result is when a painful 'clunk' is elicited as the scaphoid reduces back into the scaphoid fossa of the distal radius as the thumb pressure is released.

Examination of the patient's contralateral uninjured wrist is mandatory, as Easterling and Wolfe [10] have shown a significant number of false positive results in healthy/asymptomatic wrists.

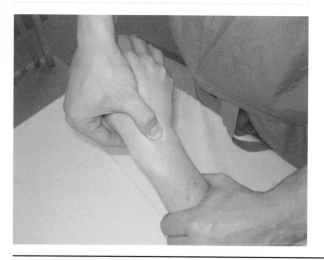

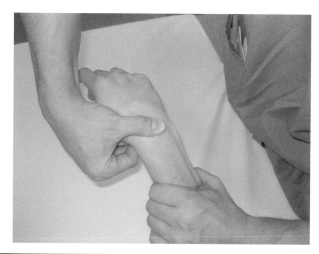

Figure 2. Watson's test (scapholunate instability test).

Kleinman's shear test (lunotriquetral instability) [11] (Figure 3)

The patient's wrist is held in neutral. The examiner's contralateral hand is placed over the dorsal lunate, while the ipilateral thumb loads the pisotriquetral joint with a dorsally directed force. A positive result for lunotriquetral instability is when the manoeuvre causes pain.

Reagan's test (lunotriquetral instability) [12] (Figure 4)

Again with the patient's wrist in neutral, the examiner's contralateral thumb and index finger grasp the triquetrum and lunate. The lunate and the triquetrum are stressed in dorsal and volar directions. This creates a shear force at the lunotriquetral joint and, if painful, indicates a positive result.

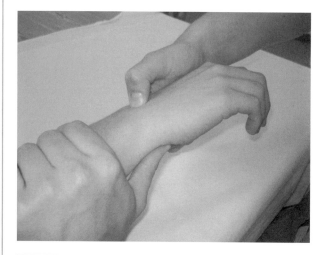

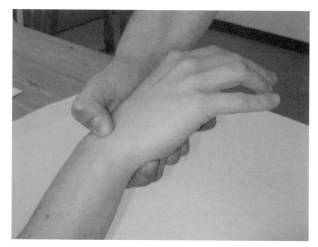

Figure 3. Kleinman's shear test (lunotriquetral instability).

Figure 4. Reagan's test (lunotriquetral instability).

Linscheid's compression test (lunotriquetral instability) [13]

The examiner uses his thumb to apply load to the ulnar border of the triquetrum in a radial direction. This causes a compressive force across the lunotriquetral joint and pain signifies a positive result.

Lichtman's pivot shift test (midcarpal instability) [5]

The examiner applies a combination of ulnar deviation, axial compression and pronation to the patient's wrist. A painful click signifies a positive result.

Imaging studies

Standard radiographs should include a postero-anterior (PA) view in neutral and lateral views of the symptomatic and asymptomatic wrists. These will show any static instability patterns.

Dynamic radiographs can also be obtained in order to diagnose dynamic instability, including clenched fist PA, maximum radial deviation PA, maximum ulnar deviation PA, maximum flexion lateral view and maximum extension lateral views.

Other tests include fluoroscopy, wrist arthrography, CT scanning, MRI and ultrasonography.

Arthrography has been used extensively to diagnose tears of the scapholunate and lunotriquetral ligaments. Triple injection techniques are important in evaluating the flow of contrast between radiocarpal, midcarpal and distal radio-ulnar joints. When abnormal flow is seen, a ligamentous tear is suspected. A disadvantage of arthrography is that it only allows for assessment of the intrinsic ligaments of the wrist and not the extrinsic. Arthrography also has a relatively high false positive rate, especially in patients older than 40 years [14]. It is, therefore, worth comparing images from the contralateral wrist. Communication between different compartments of the wrist may not necessarily be the direct result of trauma, but may represent age-related degenerative changes [15].

MRI has become a more popular mode of evaluating the wrist as imaging technology has improved.

Fluoroscopy is useful for the work-up of dynamic instability patterns (IV/C).

Wrist arthroscopy remains the gold standard for the diagnosis of ligament injuries in the wrist [16-18]. It allows direct evaluation of the location, type and degree of ligament disruption. It also allows surgical management to take place concurrently (IIa/B).

Patterns of injury

No single classification system can easily describe all the various carpal injuries. Specific patterns of injury can be used to guide treatment and predict outcomes.

Lunate and perilunate disruption

Mayfield et al [19] investigated the pathomechanics of carpal instability using a cadaveric trauma model. They observed a progressive injury pattern when the wrist was loaded in extension, ulnar deviation and carpal supination resulting in progressive perilunar instability. Mayfield described four stages of sequential ligamentous failure:

- ◆ Stage I. Scapholunate diastasis.
- ◆ Stage II. Dorsal subluxation of the capitate relative to the lunate due to a tearing capitolunate ligament.
- ◆ Stage III. Perilunate dislocation. As the load increases the lunotriquetral ligament is injured.
- ◆ Stage IV. Dislocation of the lunate.

Dorsal perilunate and volar lunate dislocation

This pattern of injury is often missed at initial presentation. Rawlings [20] found that only 17 of 30 cases (57%) were diagnosed on the day of admission, and Campbell et al [21] reported that 66% of their cases (22 out of 33 patients) were treated within two weeks of diagnosis.

Chapter 15

Volar perilunate and dorsal lunate dislocation

Dorsal dislocations of the lunate are rare and have been recorded in a handful of isolated reports [22]. Volar perilunar dislocation is only slightly more common [23].

Lesser arc and greater arc patterns

Perilunar injury can involve ligamentous failure, carpal fracture or a combination of both. When injury is purely ligamentous, it is referred to as a lesser arc pattern. A greater arc pattern involves a carpal fracture.

The most common greater arc injury is the trans-scaphoid perilunar fracture dislocation of the carpus.

Axial disruption patterns

Axial or longitudinal injuries have been classified according to their lines of cleavage through the carpus. As a result, the carpus is separated longitudinally and usually displaced with the respective metacarpals.

Patterns of instability

Instability patterns may develop following an injury or may be non-traumatic (e.g. rheumatoid arthritis). Carpal injury may go unnoticed until it has progressed to more severe symptoms with advanced instability. It is for this reason that there is overlap between acute injury and chronic instability.

Scapholunate instability (Figure 5)

Scapholunate instability is the most common form of carpal instability and is the main cause of post-traumatic wrist osteoarthritis. We will first consider scapholunate instability prior to the onset of osteoarthritis.

Chapter 15

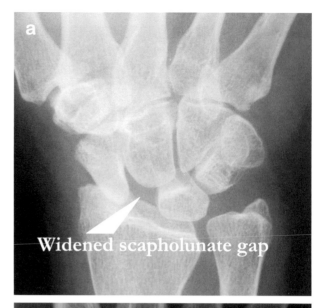

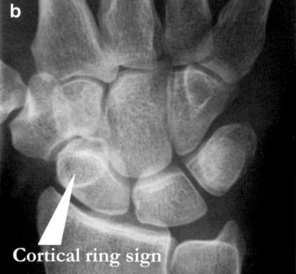

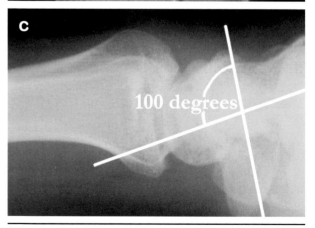

Figure 5. Radiographic features of scapholunate instability. a) Shows a widened scapholunate gap; b) Demonstrates the cortical ring sign; c) Demonstrates an increased scapholunate angle.

Clinical symptoms

Pain is often localised to the dorsal and radial aspects of the wrist. Palpation elicits pain at the scapholunate joint, which should be examined with the wrist in flexion. Watson's test is often positive and ballotting the scapholunate in an anteroposterior direction and vice versa often shows more movement than the uninjured side.

Radiology

A PA radiograph of the wrist may demonstrate a scapholunate gap >3mm (Terry Thomas sign), or a 'cortical ring' sign. The cortical ring sign is due to the scaphoid being rotated on its axis and therefore appears shortened with a circle superimposed on its distal part.

Lateral radiographs can be used to calculate the scapholunate angle, which normally ranges from 30° to 60° (average = 47°). An angle >60° represents a dorsal intercalated segmental instability (DISI) pattern of scapholunate instability (Figure 6).

DISI refers to a pattern in which the scaphoid and the lunate become disconnected or dissociated, as a result of a scapholunate ligament tear. As the lunate is disconnected from the its scaphoid attachment, it rotates dorsally under the influence of the triquetrum (via the lunotriquetral ligament). The unsupported scaphoid rotates/collapses into flexion. In addition, the capitolunate angle (normally up to 15°) and the radiolunate angle (normally up to 15°) are also increased.

Dynamic radiography

Radiographs in flexion, extension, radial and ulnar deviation may demonstrate the reduced rotatory movement of the scaphoid in radio-ulnar deviation and of the lunate in flexion-extension.

A scapholunate gap, which was not previously seen on static radiographs, may appear under dynamic conditions. 'Stress views' (clenched fist views) may also reveal a gap not seen on plain PA views.

Arthrography

A midcarpal injection of contrast is performed, followed by distal radiolunar joint injection. Contrast leaking between compartments is suggestive of a tear in the ligaments; however, arthrography has a relatively high false positive rate as previously discussed.

A CT scan following arthrography using 1mm cuts gives precise information about the site and length of ligament tears, the suitability for ligament stump repair or reinsertion, and the condition of the cartilage.

Treatment

The treatment of scapholunate dissociation is more successfully achieved if initiated early. The aim of treatment is to restore the anatomical alignment of the carpus, to restore the normal orientation of the scaphoid and to recover a normal congruency of the proximal pole of the scaphoid with the scaphoid fossa of the distal radius. Early treatment will hopefully

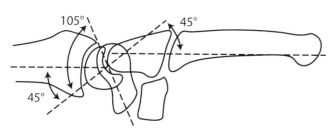

Figure 6. Dorsal intercalated segmental instability. The scapholunate angle is high (105°), the capitolunate angle is high (45°) and the radiolunate angle is high (45°).

Chapter 15

decrease the risk of developing secondary osteoarthritis. It is possible to find total cartilage wear of the scaphoid proximal pole six months after injury and in other cases this may take many years.

In the acute setting, Palmer, Dobyns and Linscheid [24] reported good results from immobilisation for eight weeks in plaster if initiated within four weeks of injury and if anatomical reduction was maintained. Anatomical alignment by closed reduction alone is often best supplemented with percutaneous K-wire fixation [25] **(III/B)**. Wolfe [10] and Watson [26] also recommended initial splinting or casting for partial scapholunate ligament injury. However, cast immobilisation alone does not reduce or prevent scapholunate diastasis in a complete scapholunate ligament injury [10].

Should anatomical reduction not be adequately achieved by closed methods, open reduction via a dorsal approach between the third and fourth compartments should be employed. Reduction is achieved under direct vision by manipulation of the scaphoid using the surgeon's thumb pressure (volarly) and a K-wire to de-rotate the flexed scaphoid. K-wires are then passed from the scaphoid into the lunate and capitate in order to maintain reduction. The scapholunate ligament should be repaired back to bone with suture anchors or through drill holes **(IV/C)**.

If insufficient ligament is present, the repair is augmented with a dorsal capsule used to stabilise and suspend the scaphoid (Blatt dorsal capsulodesis) [27].

Palmer *et al* [24] reported on 17 patients treated within one month of injury by closed reduction, open reduction alone or combined with direct suture of torn ligaments or ligament reconstruction. Nine patients (53%) had no pain; six (35%) had only slight pain. Grip strength was 53-80% of normal and the average range of movement was decreased from normal by almost 50%. Patient satisfaction was reported as good in nine (53%) patients, fair in five patients (29%) and poor in three (18%).

If the diagnosis is delayed for three months or more, repair of the intraosseous ligaments becomes much more difficult. If the patient's disability is minor, with retentions of more than 80% of range of motion

and grip strength, no treatment is required [3] **(IV/C)**. If there is significant disability then a number of surgical procedures are available. These can be divided into soft tissue repairs and limited arthrodeses.

Soft tissue repairs are ligament repair, ligament reattachment, ligamentoplasty and capsulodesis. As mentioned above, if diagnosis is delayed then there is frequently little ligament found to repair or reattach.

In patients with an irreparable scapholunate ligament but with a reducible scapholunate interval (and prior to the onset of degenerative changes), then both indirect and direct ligamentoplasty have been advocated **(IIb/B)**.

Indirect ligament reconstruction is based on stabilising the scaphoid in order to prevent the rotatory subluxation that often occurs in scapholunate instability. Some also attempt to close the scapholunate diastasis. A popular indirect ligamentoplasty is the Blatt dorsal capsulodesis. As discussed above this procedure uses a flap of dorsal capsule to stabilise the scaphoid. The flap is attached to the distal radius and therefore can lead to limited wrist flexion (average 20%).

More recent techniques of indirect ligamentoplasty have been developed to avoid limited flexion by avoiding tethering of the scaphoid to the distal radius [28, 29]. Berger [30] described detaching a strip of dorsal intercarpal ligament from the triquetrum and using it to tether the distal pole of the scaphoid to the lunate. Slater *et al* [29] described the use of the portion of distal intercarpal ligament that attaches to the distal scaphoid and trapezoid, and reinserting it to the distal pole of the scaphoid tuberosity. These authors believe that this technique not only serves to limit scaphoid flexion but also reduces the scapholunate diastasis more effectively than a Blatt capsulodesis.

Direct ligamentoplasty is indicated when the scapholunate ligament is not directly reparable, when the scapholunate dissociation is reducible and when no evidence of degenerative osteoarthritis is observed. Direct ligamentoplasty uses techniques that aim to recreate the scapholunate ligament. These involve either a tendon to reconstruct the scapholunate ligament or a bone-ligament-bone construct, similar in principle to anterior cruciate ligament reconstruction [24, 31-34].

Brunelli and Brunelli have developed a promising technique of ligamentoplasty for stabilising the distal scaphoid. They describe using a strip of flexor carpi radialis (FCR) and passing it through the scaphoid; the tendon is also sutured across the scapholunate interval. Early results are promising with 33 out of 38 patients remaining pain-free and five complaining of only minor pain under stressful conditions [35].

Indifferent results from ligament reconstruction have persuaded many surgeons to perform limited carpal arthrodeses. It should be remembered that these procedures alter the mechanics of the carpus and that load transfer from hand to forearm is modified.

There are several types of limited carpal arthrodesis:

♦ Scapholunate (SL) [36].
♦ Scaphotrapezial-trapezoidal (STT) [37-40].
♦ Scaphocapitate (SC) [41].
♦ Scapholuno-capitate [42].

Limited carpal arthrodesis is indicated if the scaphoid is not easily reducible, especially in manual workers **(IV/C)**. Viegas *et al* found that the scaphocapitolunate and scapholunate fusions distributed the load more uniformly across both the scaphoid and lunate fossae than did the scaphotrapezial-trapezoidal or scaphocapitate fusions [43].

When arthritic changes, scapholunate advanced collapse (SLAC) (Figure 7) or a wide irreducible scapholunate diastasis exists, treatment options are guided towards a salvage procedure **(IIb/B)**. These involve a radial styloidectomy (for limited styloscaphoid arthritis), proximal row carpectomy, capitolunate arthrodesis or scaphoid excision and fusion of the lunate, triquetrum, capitate and hamate (four-corner fusion). Once pancarpal arthritis involves the lunate fossa, the total wrist fusion is often the best surgical option.

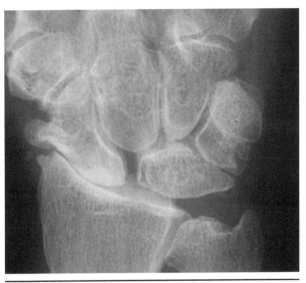

Figure 7. Scapholunate advanced collapse (SLAC) of the wrist.

Lunotriquetral instability

Less common than scapholunate instability, lunotriquetral instability occurs as the result of incompetence of the lunotriquetral ligament. It results in functional impairment but rarely leads to osteoarthritis.

This pattern of instability often follows falls onto the outstretched hand on the hypothenar eminence. Pain is often felt at the lunotriquetral junction and on examination a 'click' in pronation and ulnar deviation, as well as in pro-supination, suggests lunotriquetral instability. A positive Kleinman's shear test, Reagan's test and Linscheid's compression test (as previously discussed) all indicate lunotriquetral instability.

Plain radiographs are often normal; however, a volar intercalated segmental instability (VISI) pattern (Figure 8) may be observed. In this case, the lateral radiograph shows a decreased scapholunate angle (<30°), as well as increased capitolunate and radiolunate angles. On the PA radiograph, a gap of more than 2mm between the lunate and the triquetrum is abnormal. Disruption of Gilula's arcs is the most significant sign on PA views. This may only be seen on dynamic series.

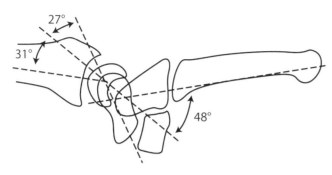

Figure 8. Volar intercalated segmental instability. The scapholunate angle is low (27°).

The treatment options for lunotriquetral instability depend upon both the type of injury and time to presentation.

For acute injuries, Reagan, Linscheid and Dobyns [12] recommended a period of immobilisation. Ruby [44] recommended arthroscopic evaluation and percutaneous pinning **(III/B)**.

For patients in whom non-operative treatment fails, lunotriquetral dissociation direct repair with or without augmentation has been advocated **(IV/C)**. Open reattachment of the lunotriquetral ligament to its site of avulsion (usually the triquetrum) has achieved good results [12]. Augmentation is most commonly in the form of a capsulodesis which aims to prevent excessive flexion of the proximal carpal row by imbricating the radiotriquetral ligament [44].

Presentation is commonly late after the initial injury. In these circumstances a staging system has been developed to guide treatment of these injuries:

- Stage I represents isolated tears of the lunotriquetral ligament without midcarpal (VISI) involvement. Stage I injuries can be treated non-operatively with splinting, anti-inflammatory medication and local injections **(IV/C)**.
- Stage II injuries have disruption of the lunotriquetral ligament and are associated with a dynamic VISI pattern.

- Stage III injuries are more severe and are characterised by a static VISI pattern.

Treatment for stage II and III disease includes soft tissue reconstruction, limited arthrodesis, or four-corner fusion **(III/B)**.

Shin *et al* [45] have described a ligament reconstruction using a distal strip of the extensor carpi ulnaris tendon. Reconstruction of the dorsal ligament capsule using half of the extensor carpi ulnaris has been recommended by Stanley [46] if a posterior triangular fibrocartilage complex is found on arthroscopy and in the absence of midcarpal instability.

As some patients with symptomatic lunotriquetral instability have ulnar impaction syndrome, Ruby [44] recommends ulnar shortening alone in patients with chronic tears, especially if they are ulnar positive. It is felt that by shortening the ulna, the volar ulnotriquetral and ulnolunate ligaments tighten which indirectly improves lunotriquetral instability.

Pin *et al* [47], in a series of lunotriquetral fusions using a compression screw, achieved union in all 11 patients; however, three patients (27%) suffered persistent pain. Most of the range of motion was preserved in 11 patients but only 59% of grip strength was achieved, compared with the uninjured side.

Kirschenbaum, Coyle and Leddy [48] reported better results with lunotriquetral fusion. In a series of 14 patients, one had persistent pain and average grip strength was 94% compared with the unoperated side. Non-union occurred in two patients, one of whom underwent revision fusion, the other was asymptomatic. In this series, 80-85% range of movement was preserved compared with the unoperated wrist.

Other studies have not found such successful results with lunotriquetral fusion. Non-union rates as high as 57% and persistent pain in 52% have been published [49].

Triquetrohamate fusion has been recommended by Stanley [46] and lunotriquetrohamate by Bednar [50].

Midcarpal instability

Patients with midcarpal instability often present with a painful 'clunk' in the wrist on ulnar deviation and pronation. It may follow a traumatic event or the patient may have had a persistent 'clunk' in the wrist, which has become painful.

Midcarpal instability occurs as a result of loss of the normal couple between the proximal and distal carpal rows. Normally as the wrist deviates ulnarly, the distal row translates from dorsal to volar and the proximal row moves from flexion to extension. With midcarpal instability, the triquetrohamate and capitolunate ligaments volarly, and the radiotriquetral ligament dorsally, become incompetant due to trauma, laxity or attenuation. This results in the proximal row flexing as the distal row remains excessively volarly translated, until maximum ulnar deviation is reached. At maximum ulnar deviation the proximal row abruptly reduces back into extension and the distal row reduces dorsally causing a 'clunk'. The surgeon can recreate this clunk by ulnar deviation, compression and pronation of the wrist.

Plain radiographs are often unremarkable but cinefluoroscopy can demonstrate the instability. Both postero-anterior and lateral projections should be taken as the patient moves the wrist from radial to ulnar deviation in an attempt to reproduce the clunk.

Johnson and Carrera [51] identified attenuation of the radiocapitate ligament as the primary cause of midcarpal instability; therefore, they advocated tightening this ligament in patients with a positive fluoroscopic dorsal-displacement stress test. The radiocapitate ligament was tightened by tethering its middle part to the radiotriquetral ligament to close the space of Poirier.

Lichtman et al [52] reviewed 13 patients (15 procedures) over an eight-year period, who underwent surgery for midcarpal instability. They found better results with midcarpal arthrodesis than soft tissue reconstruction (six out of nine procedures failed) **(III/B)**.

Axial disruption (Figure 9)

Axial disruption injuries are rare. They present following high energy trauma to the hand and wrist. The carpus is separated longitudinally, usually with the metacarpals. Garcia-Elias et al [53] described a classification based on the direction of the instability: axial-ulnar or axial-radial disruption. The two categories could be further subdivided according to the pattern of disruption through the carpus.

Axial-ulnar:

- Transhamate/peripisiform.
- Perihamate/peripisiform.
- Perihamate/transtriquetrum.

Axial-radial:

- Peritrapazoid/peritrapezium.
- Peritrapezium.
- Transtrapezium.

Axial-ulnar is the commoner pattern of axial disruption. An ulnar column is created that is displaced proximal and ulnar, often at or around the hamate.

Axial-radial dislocation occurs when the ulnar carpus remains aligned but the radial carpus is displaced. Usually, the trapezium is dislocated along with the first metacarpal, or a combined trapezoid-trapezium dislocation can occur with the first, second, and third metacarpals. A combined axial-radial-ulnar dislocation has also been reported.

The prognosis of these types of injuries is determined more by the extent of the soft tissue injury than the carpal derangement **(IV/C)**.

Conclusions

Carpal instability is a complex subject that is under-diagnosed. It should remain a differential diagnosis for patients presenting with chronic wrist pain, especially with a history of previous wrist sprain.

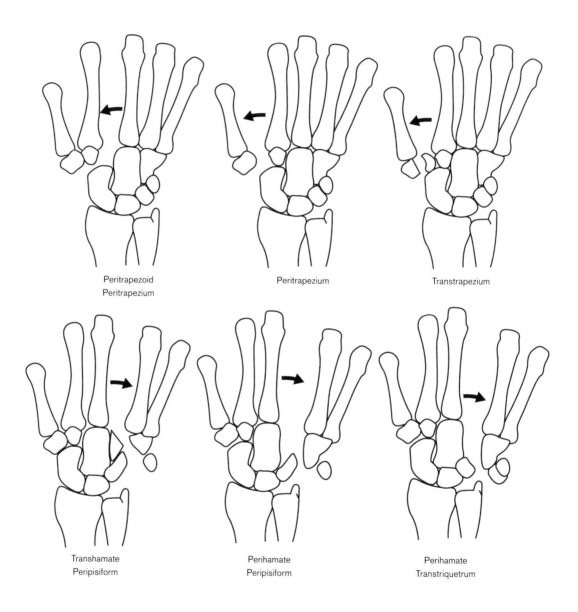

Peritrapezoid
Peritrapezium

Peritrapezium

Transtrapezium

Transhamate
Peripisiform

Perihamate
Peripisiform

Perihamate
Transtriquetrum

Figure 9. Patterns of axial carpal instability.

The diagnosis of carpal instability can often be difficult and its treatment may require specialist skills; however, the clinician should always begin with a thorough history followed by a systematic clinical examination.

Imaging should commence with both plain and stress radiographs. If further information is required to confirm the diagnosis, then fluoroscopy, wrist arthrography, CT scanning, MRI, ultrasonography and arthroscopy have all be advocated.

Following acute injury, treatment should aim to restore normal carpal alignment and hold this position with plaster immobilisation, commonly supplemented by K-wires. Should anatomical alignment not be achieved by closed methods, an open reduction should be employed and any disrupted ligaments repaired.

Presentation is commonly delayed, making ligamentous primary repair difficult. In these circumstances a soft tissue reconstruction (ligamentoplasty or capuslodesis) may be required. Remember, if the patient's disability is minor, with retention of more than 80% of range of motion and grip strength, no treatment is required.

Should the carpus be irreducible or arthritic changes present, then arthrodesis would be the treatment of choice.

Recommendations	Evidence level
◆ Carpal instability is probably under-diagnosed.	III/B
◆ Start with the simplest, non-invasive imaging investigations (PA and lateral radiographs). If this does not yield the diagnosis, obtain dynamic radiographic views. If the diagnosis remains elusive following dynamic radiography, wrist arthrography, CT or MRI scanning may be helpful. MRI is becoming increasingly popular.	IV/C
◆ Wrist arthroscopy remains the gold standard for the diagnosis of ligament injuries of the wrist.	IIa/B

Scapholunate instability

◆ Acute scapholunate injury (within four weeks of injury) should be anatomically reduced and held with plaster immobilisation supplemented with K-wire fixation.	III/B
◆ Should closed anatomical reduction of acute scapholunate dissociation not be achieved, open reduction via a dorsal approach between the 3rd and 4th compartments should be employed, plus K-wire fixation and direct scapholunate ligament repair or reconstruction.	IV/C
◆ If diagnosis is delayed (≥3months from injury) and the patient's disability is minor, no treatment is needed.	IV/C
◆ In chronic injury, if the scapholunate ligament is irreparable, with a reducible scapholunate interval and prior to onset degenerative changes, indirect or direct ligament reconstruction can be employed.	IIb/B
◆ Limited carpal arthrodeses are indicated if the scaphoid is not easily reducible.	IV/C
◆ When arthritic changes, schapholunate advanced collapse or a wide irreducible scapholunate diastasis exists, treatment options are guided towards salvage procedures.	IIb/B

Lunotriquetral instability

◆ Acute injuries should be treated with immobilisation +/- K-wire fixation.	III/B
◆ When closed treatment fails, lunotriquetral dissociation direct repair, with or without augmentation, has been advocated.	IV/C
◆ Stage I injuries can be treated non-operatively.	IV/C
◆ Treatment for stages II and III include soft tissue reconstruction, limited arthrodesis or four-corner fusion.	III/B

Midcarpal instability

◆ Better results have been found following midcarpal arthrodesis than soft tissue reconstruction.	III/B

Axial instability

◆ Prognosis following axial disruption is determined more by the extent of the soft tissue injury than the carpal derangement.	IV/C

References

1. Jones WA. Beware the sprained wrist. *J Bone Joint Surg (Br)* 1998; 70(2): 293-7.

2. Tang JB. Carpal instability associated with fractures of the distal radius. Incidence, influencing factors and pathomechanics. *Chin Med J (Engl)* 1992; 105(9): 758-65.

3. Dobyns JH, Linschied RL, Chao EYS. Traumatic instability of the wrist. American Academy of Orthopaedic Surgeons Instructional Course Lectures, 1975; 182-99.

4. Navaro A. Anales de Instituto de Clinica Quirurgica y Cirgia Experimental. Montevideo: Imprenta Artistica de Dornaleche Hnos, 1935.

5. Lichtman DM, Schneider JR, Swafford AR, Mack GR. Ulnar midcarpal instability - clinical and laboratory analysis. *J Hand Surg (Am)* 1981; 6(5): 515-23.

6. Gilford WW, Bolton RH, Lambrinudi C. The mechanism of the wrist joint with special reference to fractures of the scaphoid. *Guy's Hospital Report* 1943; 92: 52-9.

7. Taleisnik, J. The ligaments of the wrist. *J Hand Surg (Am)* 1976; 1: 110-8.

8. Berger RA, Blair WF, Crowninshield RD, Flatt AE. The scapholunate ligament. *J Hand Surg (Am)* 1982; 7(1): 87-91.

9. Watson HK, Ashmead D, Maklouf MV. Examination of the scaphoid. *J Hand Surg (Am)* 1988; 70: 1262-8.

10. Easterling KJ, Wolfe SW. Scaphoid shift in the uninjured wrist. *J Hand Surg (Am)* 1994; 19(4): 604-6.

11. Kleinman WB. The lunotriquetral shuck test. *Am Soc Surg Hand Corr News* 1985; 51.

12. Reagan DS, Linscheid RL, Dobyns JH. Lunotriquetral sprains. *J Hand Surg (Am)* 1984; 9-A: 502-14.

13. Linscheid RL. Scapholunate ligamentous instabilities (dissociations, subdislocations and dislocations). *Ann Chir Main* 1984; 3(4): 323-30.

14. Herbert TJ, Faithful RG, McCann DJ, Ireland J. Bilateral arthrography of the wrist. *J Hand Surg (Br)* 1990; 15(2): 233-5.

15. Viegas SF, Ballantyne G. Attritional lesions of the wrist joint. *J Hand Surg (Am)* 1987; 12(6): 1025-9.

16. Cooney WP. Evaluation of chronic wrist pain by arthrography, arthroscopy and arthrotomy. *J Hand Surg (Am)* 1993; 18(5) 815-22.

17. Kelly EP, Stanley JK. Arthroscopy of the wrist. *J Hand Surg (Br)* 1990; 15(2): 236-42.

18. Roth KH, Haddad RG. Radiocarpal arthroscopy and arthrography in the diagnosis of ulnar wrist pain. *Arthroscopy* 1986; 2(4): 234-43.

19. Mayfield JK. Mechanism of carpal injuries. *Clin Orthop* 1980; 45-54.

20. Rawlings D. The management of dislocation of the carpal lunate. *Injury* 1981; 12: 312-30.

21. Campbell RD, Lance EM, Yeoh CB. Lunate and perilunate dislocations. *J Bone Joint Surg (Br)* 1964; 46: 55-72.

22. Bilos ZJ, Hui PW. Dorsal dislocation of the lunate with carpal collapse. *J Bone Joint Surg (Am)* 1981; 63: 1484-6.

23. Taleisnik J. *The wrist.* Edinburgh: Churchill Livingstone, 1985.

24. Palmer AK, Dobyns JH, Linsheid RL. Management of post-traumatic instability of the wrist secondary to ligament rupture. *J Hand Surg (Am)* 1978; 3(6): 507-32.

25. O'Brien ET. Acute fractures and dislocation of the carpus. *Orthop Clin North Am* 1984; 15: 237-57.

26. Watson HK, Wienzweig J, Zeppieri J. The natural progression of scaphoid instability. *Hand Clin* 1997; 13(1): 39-49.

27. Blatt G. Capsulodesis in reconstructive hand surgery. Dorsal capsulodesis for the unstable scaphoid and volar capsulodesis following excision of the distal ulna. *Hand Clin* 1987; 3(1): 81-102.

28. Dagum AB, Hurst LC, Finzel KC. Scapholunate dissociation: an experimental kinematic study of two types of indirect soft tissue repairs. *J Hand Surg (Am)* 1997; 22(4): 714-9.

29. Slater RR, Szabo RM, Bay BK, Laubach J. Dorsal intercarpal ligament capsulodesis for scapholunate dissociation: biomechanical analysis in a cadaver model. *J Hand Surg (Am)* 1999; 24(2): 232-9.

30. Berger RA, Bishop AT, Bettinger PC. New dorsal capsulotomy for the surgical exposure of the wrist. *Ann Plast Surg* 1995; 35(1): 54-9.

31. Almquist EE, Bach AW, Sack JT, *et al.* Four-bone ligament reconstruction for treatment of chronic complete scapholunate separation. *J Hand Surg (Am)* 1991; 16(2): 322-7.

32. Brunelli GA, Brunelli GR. A new technique to correct carpal instability with scaphoid rotatory subluxation: a preliminary report. *J Hand Surg (Am)* 1995; 20(3 pt 2): S82-5.

33. Hofstede DJ, Ritt MJ, Bos KE. Tarsal autografts for reconstruction of the scapholunate interosseous ligament: a biomechanical study. *J Hand Surg (Am)* 1999; 24(5): 967-76.

34. Wolf JM, Weiss AP. Bone-retinaculum-bone reconstruction of scapholunate ligament injuries. *Orthop Clin North Am* 2001; 32(2): 241-6.

35. Brunelli GA, Brunelli GA. Carpal instability with scapho-lunate dissociation treated using the flexor carpi radialis and scaphoid-trapezoid ligament repair: foundations, technique and results of preliminary series. *Rev Chir Orthop Reparatrice Appar Mot* 2003; 89(2): 152-7.

36. Hom S, Ruby LK. Attempted scapholunate arthrodesis for chronic scapholunate dissociation. *J Hand Surg (Am)* 1991; 16(2): 334-9.

37. Eckenrode JF, Louis DS, Green TL. Schaphoid-trapezium-trapezoid fusion in the treatment of chronic scapholunate instability. *J Hand Surg (Am)* 1986; 11(4): 497-502.

38. Kleinman WB, Carroll C. Scapho-trapezio-trapezoid arthrodesis for treatment of chronic static and dynamic scapho-lunate instability: a 10-year perspective on pitfalls and complications. *J Hand Surg (Am)* 1990; 15(3): 408-14.

39. Peterson HA, Lipscomb PR. Intercarpal arthrodesis. *Arch Surg* 1967; 95(1): 127-34.

40. Watson HK, Hempton RF. Limited wrist arthrodesis. The triscaphoid joint. *J Hand Surg (Am)* 1980; 5(4): 320-7.

41. Pisano SM, Peimer CA, Wheeler DR, Sherwin F. Scaphocapitate intercarpal arthrodesis. *J Hand Surg (Am)* 1991; 16(2): 328-33.

Chapter 15

42. Rotman MB, Mansake PR, Pruitt DL, Szerzinski J. Scaphocapitolunate and lunotriquetral injuries of the wrist. *J Hand Surg (Am)* 1996; 21(3): 412-7.

43. Viegas SF, Patterson RM, Pertson PD, *et al.* Evaluation of the biomechanical efficacy of limited intercarpal fusions for the treatment of scapho-lunate dissociation. *J Hand Surg (Am)* 1990; 15(1): 120-8.

44. Ruby JH. Carpal instability. *Instr Course Lect* 1996; 45: 3-13.

45. Shin AY, Weinstein LP, Berger RA, Bishop AT. Treatment of isolated injuries of the lunotriquetral ligament. A comparison of arthrodesis, ligament reconstruction and ligament repair. *J Bone Joint Surg (Br)* 2001; 83(7): 1023-8.

46. Stanley JK, Trail IA. Carpal instability. *J Bone Joint Surg (Br)* 1994; 76(5).

47. Pin PG, Young VL, Gilula LA, Weeks PM. Management of chronic lunotriquetral ligament tears. *J Hand Surg (Am)* 1989; 14(1): 77-83.

48. Kirschenbaum D, Coyle MP, Leddy JP. Chronic lunotriquetral instability: diagnosis and treatment. *J Hand Surg (Am)* 1993; 18: 1107-12.

49. Shin AY, Battaglia MJ, Bishop AT. Lunotriquetral instability: diagnosis and treatment. *J Am Acad Orthop Surg* 2000; 8(3): 170-9.

50. Bednar JM, Osterman AL. Carpal instability: evaluation and treatment. *J Am Acad Orthop Surg* 1993; 1(1): 10-7.

51. Johnson RP, Carrera GF. Chronic capitolunate instability. *J Bone Joint Surg (Am)* 1986; 68(8): 1164-76.

52. Lichtman DM, Bruckner JD, Culp RW, Alexander CE. Palmer midcarpal instability: results of surgical reconstruction. *J Hand Surg (Am)* 1993; 18(2): 307-15.

53. Garcia-Elias M, Dobyns JH, Cooney WP, Linscheid RL. Traumatic axial dislocations of the carpus. *J Hand Surg (Am)*; 14(3): 446-57.

Chapter 16

Wrist arthroscopy: its role in diagnosis and treatment

Cronan Kerin BSc MRCS (Eng)

Specialist Registrar, Trauma and Orthopaedic Surgery

Neil Ashwood BSc (Hons) FRCS (Tr & Orth)

Consultant Orthopaedic Surgeon

QUEEN'S HOSPITAL, BURTON ON TRENT, UK

Introduction

Most acute sprains of the wrist with normal radiographic findings resolve after non-surgical treatment. However, the evaluation of the patient who does not improve after such treatment is controversial. Historically, tricompartmental wrist arthrography has been the gold standard for the detection of intra-articular pathology [1, 2]. Visualisation by means of arthroscopy has revolutionised orthopaedics by allowing direct diagnosis and treatment of intra-articular pathology.

Wrist arthroscopy has evolved from the successful application of arthroscopy in larger joints. The wrist comprises eight carpal bones, multiple articular surfaces with extrinsic and intrinsic ligaments, and a triangular fibrocartilage complex (TFCC), all within a 5cm interval. The surgeon who uses wrist arthroscopy is able to directly visualise cartilage, synovial tissue, and ligaments under bright illumination and magnification.

Wrist arthroscopy can be used to diagnose and simultaneously treat wrist injuries. This along with

magnetic resonance imaging (MRI) has changed the way wrist pathology is treated [3-5] **(IIa/B)**. Arthroscopy was used by Adolfsson to examine 144 patients who had post-traumatic wrist pain and normal findings on standard imaging [6]. Ligamentous changes were observed in 75 patients, TFCC lesions including lunotriquetral instability in 61 patients, and degrees of scapholunate instability in 14 patients.

This chapter aims to give a broad overview of the role of arthroscopy in the management of post-traumatic and degenerative conditions of the wrist.

Methodology

A Medline search to identify all relevant references was undertaken using the search words 'arthroscopy', 'wrist' and 'techniques'. Evidence was obtained from at least one well designed quasi-experimental study in drawing together this overview. This chapter outlines the versatility and practical use of the technique in modern practice and points the reader to various papers to enable further reading.

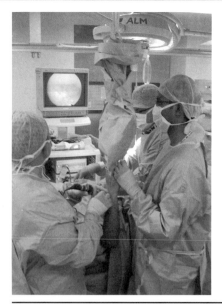
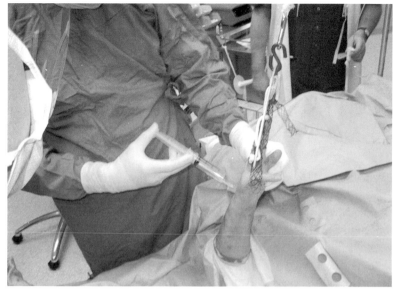

Figure 1. Arthroscopic set up.

Indications

As new techniques and instrumentation evolve the indications and applications for wrist arthroscopy continue to expand. Diagnostically, wrist arthroscopy can allow for assessment of interosseous ligament tears, evaluation of the TFCC, inspection for chondral defects in the carpal and midcarpal spaces, and evaluation of chronic wrist pain of unknown aetiology.

Indications for operative intervention include treatment of intra-articular fractures of the distal radius and scaphoid, wrist lavage, synovectomy (rheumatoid arthritis), ganglionectomy, distal ulnar shortening, loose body detection and removal, debridement of degenerative arthritis, debridement and repair of the TFCC, resection arthroplasty (proximal row carpectomy), management of septic arthritis (arthroscopic incision and drainage), and stabilisation of interosseous ligaments.

Procedure

Positioning and preparation

The appropriate small-bore arthroscope must be available. It is usually 2.7 or 2.9mm in diameter and generally has a 30° or 70° visualising angle. A small probe designed for wrist arthroscopy is helpful in allowing tissues to be examined through manipulation. A small-joint shaver with various tips is essential for debridement of torn or avulsed tissue. Additionally, various angled punches or grabbers are useful for debridement or removal of tissue.

Knowledge of the normal anatomy and accurate portal placement prior to the procedure is the most important aspect of a successful wrist arthroscopy procedure [7, 8]. Inappropriate portal placement can injure the articular cartilage or the TFCC.

The joint is distracted with finger traps to the index, middle and ring fingers, using a tower system. Counter traction is applied to the arm, which allows the elbow to be flexed at 90°. In this position there is a gravity-assisted inflow. Distraction is not always required for routine wrist arthroscopy (Figure 1). Huracek and Troeger [9] **(IIb/B)** describe a technique for arthroscopy of the wrist that is carried out without traction and with the arm lying horizontally on the operating table.

Pitfalls

It is important to mark out the dorsal wrist veins before exsanguination and elevating the tourniquet, as transection of a vein will require a larger portal skin incision to achieve haemostasis.

All portals should be drawn on the skin (Figure 2). The bases of the index, long, and ring finger metacarpals are marked. The extensor carpi ulnaris (ECU) tendon becomes prominent after traction and should be marked. The dorsal lip of the radius should be identified. Provided the wrist is not swollen from acute injury, the extensor pollicis longus (EPL) and extensor digitorum communis (EDC) tendons can be palpated and marked.

Wrist portals

Portals are named according to the interspace through which they course with respect to the extensor compartments (Figure 3). The portal

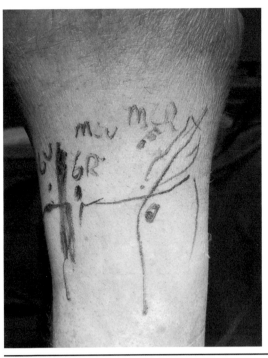

Figure 2. The portals are drawn with the associated landmarks on the extensor surface of the wrist.

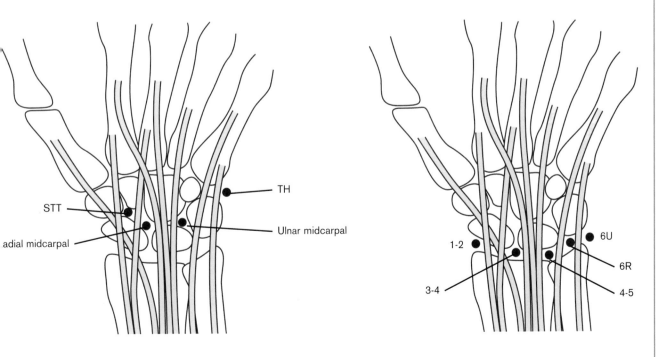

Figure 3. Positioning of wrist arthroscopy portals in relation to extensor tendon compartments. (STT = scaphotrapezio-trapezoid and TH = triquetrohamate).

incisions should be longitudinal to the extensor tendons so they are not transected accidentally if the blade is passed too deeply. To assist with ideal placement, a needle is placed intra-articularly in the proposed location of the portal prior to the skin incision. Avoid injury to the underlying sensory branches by careful use of the tip of a No. 11 blade. The cannula with the blunt trocar should be placed at a 30-40° angle pointing proximally to allow the cannula to enter in line with the articular surfaces. The various portals are described as follows:

- Arthroscopic portal. The most commonly used is the 3-4 portal. This is introduced between the extensor carpi radialis longus (ECRL) and EPL tendons, 1cm distal to the Lister's tubercle. This is also in line with the radial border of the middle finger. The scope is then inserted parallel to the dorsal radial slope.

- Instrumentation portal. The most commonly used is the 4-5 portal, introduced between the EDC and extensor digiti minimi (EDM) tendons. The arthroscope may be inserted through this portal in order to visualise a TFCC tear.

- Mid-carpal portal. This lies in the scaphocapitate interval. The scope is inserted radial to the third ray, distal to the proximal row, just radial to the EDC tendon to the index finger.

- 1-2 wrist portal. This may serve as the portal for the inflow cannula. The 1-2 wrist portal lies between the extensor carpi radialis brevis (ECRB) and abductor pollicis longus (APL) tendons. The radial artery courses along the volar aspect of this interval. This portal should be inserted near the proximal and dorsal portion of the snuffbox adjacent to the EPL and ECRL tendons, in order to avoid injury to the artery. The joint should be inflated with irrigation solution prior to the introduction of the trocar. This can be accomplished by placement of a separate inflow portal or by introduction of 3-5ml of irrigation solution into the radiocarpal space. As fluid enters the joint, the dorsal capsule between the 3-4 portal bulges. Pressurised controlled pumps can assist in maintaining a constant pressure or flow to prevent fluid extravasation. Alternatively, gravity-fed inflow irrigation through an arthroscopic sheath or via a separately placed

16- or 18-gauge cannula can be used. Inflow can be controlled using a pinch pump of the infusion line or by having an assistant regulate the inflow by using a 50ml syringe.

- Outflow cannula. Many operators do not use an outflow cannula. It is suggested that one should use a 14-gauge angiocatheter placed just ulnar to the ECU tendon (6U portal). The 6R and 6U portals are named based on their positions relative to the ECU tendon, with the 6R being radial and the 6U being ulnar. Be aware of the dorsal ulnar cutaneous branch, which is close by.

- Alternative portals. For specific indications, alternative arthroscopic portals can be used [10] **(IIb/B)**. One example of this is the scaphotrapezio-trapezoid-radial (STT-radial) portal which is situated immediately radial to the APL (abductor pollicis longus) at the STT level. Carro [11] described its use for the arthroscopic debridement of isolated STT arthritis. Alternatively, the portal can be placed on the ulnar side of the EPL tendon as described in a cadaveric study by the senior author; this is safer for the radial artery, but the superficial branch of the radial nerve and the ECRL tendon are still at risk. With the STT-radial portal, the radial artery and superficial branch of the radial nerve are both at risk. The radial artery is often tortuous within the anatomical snuffbox. Another example is a palmar-based portal to facilitate the visualisation of the dorsal rim of the STT joint which was first described by Bare in 2003 [12]. In the senior author's experience, this portal is best situated 3mm ulnar to the abductor pollicis tendon, 6mm radial to the scaphoid tubercle and midway between the radial styloid and the base of the thumb metacarpal.

Examination

The wrist should be examined in a systematic pattern, beginning with the radial side of the wrist where the proximal aspect of the scaphoid and radial styloid process can be examined for synovitis or osteoarthritic changes. With ulnar translation of the wrist, the volar extrinsic ligaments can be seen.

The radiocarpal joint is then followed along the lunate fossa of the distal radius to the junction of the distal part of the radius and the articular disk of the TFCC. A probe is drawn across the disk. The disk should be fairly taut, similar to a trampoline, and ballottement of the disk by the probe is performed (Figure 4). This is known as the trampoline test. If the disk is found to be floppy and floating without tension, a tear in the peripheral or central portion of the TFCC must be suspected. The ulnar styloid recess can be mistaken for a peripheral tear, but this is a normal anatomic finding.

The lunotriquetral interosseous ligaments and ulnocarpal ligaments are best observed by placing the arthroscope in the 4-5 or 6U portal. The ulnolunate and ulnotriquetral ligaments are observed as capsular thickenings in the volar aspect of the ulnar capsule.

After evaluating the radiocarpal joint, the midcarpal joint is examined. The arthroscope usually is placed in the radial midcarpal space. In small wrists, the arthroscope may be placed more easily in the ulnar midcarpal portal. After the midcarpal space is entered, the concave curvature of the capitate head is noted distally.

With a proximal view, the scapholunate joint (radially) and the lunotriquetral joint (ulnarly) can be identified. Both joints should be probed to ensure that no instability exists. The STT joint can be observed by passing the arthroscope radially. If the arthroscope is moved completely ulnarly, the capitate-hamate joint also can be observed. If midcarpal instability is present, the amount of capsule on the volar aspect between the hamate and triquetrum is greater than normal.

Complications

The benefits of wrist arthroscopy must be balanced against the possible complications, which can occur with any surgical procedure. Complications of arthroscopy are rare, and the wrist is no exception. In the wrist, potential complications have been reported and include the following:

- Infections.
- Neuromas.
- Tendon injuries.
- Complex regional pain syndromes.

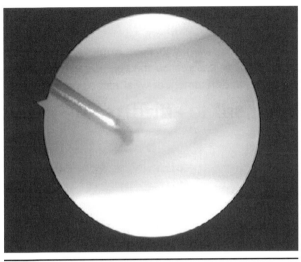

Figure 4. Assessing the TFCC, demonstrating a fenestration.

- Dorsal skin slough.
- Tourniquet neurapraxia.
- Compartment syndromes.
- Finger joint injury or skin slough from finger traps.

Adequate precautions while performing arthroscopy can prevent the majority of these complications. Complications of wrist arthroscopy are rare and usually can be prevented through proper technique.

Rehabilitation

Postoperatively, patients are advised to keep their wrist elevated as much as possible for the first few days. A sling may be needed for comfort. The dressing is kept on for three days and must not get wet. After three days, the bandages may be removed and the wounds covered with clean dressings. The wounds should be kept dry until the first visit after surgery.

Postoperative bleeding is not unusual and the patient should be reassured about this. The use of ice for the first 48 hours postoperatively is recommended.

Rehabilitation begins on the day of surgery. Initially the patient should flex and extend their fingers and shoulder to help reduce swelling. Movement of the elbow should begin on the first postoperative day unless splinted.

the development of small joint arthroplasty (SJA) included migration along the medullary canal, erosion, contracture and ultimately breakage, rendering these initiatives far from satisfactory [13]. Implant failure observed in these early designs can in part be attributed to the large torque forces transmitted through the joints, especially during end-to-side pinching with the thumb [14].

In the early 1960s, Swanson developed a unique concept, a foundation for many of the arthroplasties performed globally [15]. A silicone spacer was inserted into rheumatoid MCP and interphalangeal (IP) joints around which a fibrous capsule developed, that would then determine the biomechanics of the new joint. In contrast to rigid and fixed implants, the unfixed flexible hinge could adjust to the required axis of rotation with little resistance and allow distribution of force over a broader area. This design has been updated and revised over the years but the concept remains the same. Despite widespread acceptance of the Swanson silicone implant as the prosthesis of choice, a number of reported complications such as silicone synovitis, lateral instability and implant fracture [16] led surgeons to search for more anatomically and bio-mechanically sound alternatives. In 1979, Linscheid and Dobyns developed a PIP joint prosthesis with an anatomic centre of rotation that preserved bone stock, the joint capsule and the collateral ligaments - surface replacement arthroplasty (SRA) [17]. From this prototype, several new generation cement-less, press-fit implants have been developed for both the PIP and the MCP joints [18].

In contrast to the fingers, where the surgical options for the treatment of arthritis are limited mainly to arthrodesis and arthroplasty, several procedures have been advocated to treat disease in the thumb TMC joint [19]. Arthroplasty of the basal joint encompasses numerous approaches.

These include:

- Trapeziectomy followed by silicone spacer insertion [20].
- Interposition arthroplasty using a tendon graft [21] or alloplastic material [22].
- The complete replacement of the TMC joint with an anatomic prosthesis [23, 24].

Methodology

Searches using Medline/PubMed, Cochrane, National Institute for Clinical Excellence, Healthstar and Cinahl, with signatory key terms, were performed. Additional articles were identified from the references obtained.

The trapeziometacarpal joint

The TMC joint is a biconcave-convex, articular saddle-type joint permitting three types of motion: retroposition and opposition, adduction and abduction, and circumduction [25]. The second most common site affected by OA, disability can produce profound impact on hand function [26]. Surgical treatment options generally for Eaton-Glickel stage II-IV disease include basal osteotomy, arthrodesis, trapezial excision with or without ligament reconstruction/tendon interposition and an alloplastic arthroplasty [27]. The plethora of procedures indicates a lack of consensus about a truly reliable procedure. Arthrodesis in selected patients can be functionally satisfactory [28] **(IIb/B)** but sacrifices motion. All joint replacements have a finite life and controversy continues over which technique offers the best outcome to patients with OA of the TMC joint beyond stage II.

Silicone implant arthroplasty following complete excision of the trapezium

Swanson reviewed trapeziectomy and silicone implant arthroplasty in 150 patients over 20 years ago [29]. He noted that key pinch and grip strength were increased by factors of 2.5 and 2.7, respectively. Opposition was increased by 38%. Over three quarters of patients improved in their ability to perform activities of daily living. Several subsequent studies by other authors appeared to substantiate these positive results [30-32], but as longer-term results came to light, certain complications such as instability, deformation, synovitis and implant failure provided increasing cause for concern [33]. This came to a head in 1986 when Pellegrini and Burton reported their experience using silastic arthroplasty for the treatment of 32 OA

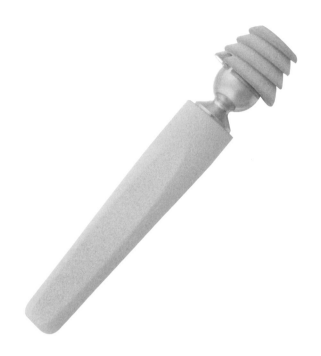

Figure 1. The 'Elektra' trapeziometacarpal joint unconstrained prosthesis made from titanium and chrome-cobalt steel.

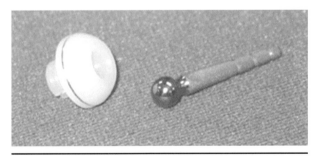

Figure 2. The Braun-Cutter trapeziometacarpal joint prosthesis consists of an ultra-high-molecular-weight polyethylene component which is cemented to the prepared trapezium, and a titanium alloy stem component with integral head which is inserted into the shaft of the first metacarpal.

thumbs [16]. Patients in this study were followed up for an average of four years, but within this short time an alarming 25% had experienced implant failure, mostly with a proliferative synovitis associated with silicone particulate deposition seen at the time of revision. These results, along with similar findings reported by

Crosby [34] a year later, led many surgeons to abandon the use of the Swanson implant for treatment of TMC joint OA. Outcomes using other silicone prostheses, including those developed by Niebauer in 1978 [35] and Eaton in 1979 [36], have been less extensively reported, but in the studies that are available they show no superiority over the Swanson design [37-39] **(IIa/B)**.

Alloplastic interpositional arthroplasty

Alloplastic interpositional arthroplasty, in which the trapezium is only partially excised to facilitate insertion of a silicone prosthesis, was introduced by Kessler in 1973 [22]. This was essentially an SRA, whereby the implant resurfaced the base of the first metacarpal leaving the trapezium undisturbed. This was followed in 1977 by Ashworth *et al* [26] who used a modified neurosurgical Burr hole to resurface the trapezium. Despite initially encouraging results, further studies have reported a high incidence of synovitis, dislocation and fracture [40, 41] **(III/B)**. Proponents of SRA argue that it can stimulate normal joint kinematics and disperse axial load over a wider area to reduce focal stress on trabecular bone [41]. Positioning of a two-component SRA, such as the SR TMC Avanta, is technically demanding, requires image intensification to check the trial components (once the trapezium and metacarpal base are prepared) and insertion of bone cement, with a narrow margin for error. Interestingly, warnings come with the prosthesis that strenuous loading or excessive mobility may lead to accelerated wear and eventual failure, and the patient should be made aware of this. What constitutes an excessive demand remains obscure. Potential adverse events with this technique include cement extrusion into the palmar digital nerves and metal sensitivity reaction [42]. The use of different materials in an attempt to reduce the frequency of these complications has proved unsatisfactory and as a result surface replacement arthroplasty is rarely advocated in the TMC joint [43].

Total joint arthroplasty

TMC joint prostheses (Figures 1 and 2) are available in arthroplasty with a number of designs for total joint replacement [8, 23, 24]. These were often cemented ball and socket prostheses with various modifications to

Chapter 17

enhance fixation or motion (de la Caffiniere [23], Steffee [8], Mayo [44] and others [45]). The aim was to diminish the need for ligament reconstruction and replace the joint with a mechanical bearing surface for frictionless movement. In their original paper, de la Caffiniere and Aucouturier [23] described results using their prosthesis in 34 thumbs affected by OA, RA and trauma. Average follow-up was two years. There were five cases of radiographic loosening but the functional results remained good and there were no revisions. Subsequently, different authors have had varying degrees of success using similar cemented [46] and uncemented [45] total joint replacements. Common problems associated with these designs include dislocation of the prostheses caused by loosening of either the metacarpal stem and/or the polyethylene socket over time, heterotopic bone formation, 'trumpeting' of the metacarpal base and late extension MCPJ contracture **(III/B)**. A recent study by Badia and Sambandam [46] has shown that satisfactory outcomes can be achieved in carefully selected patients with OA restricted to the TMC joint **(IIb/B)**.

The metacarpophalangeal joint

The MCPJ is a condyloid, diarthrodial joint which allows three types of movement: flexion-extension, abduction-adduction and rotation. As in the PIPJ, options for arthroplasty offer three basic designs [47]: hinged prostheses, flexible silicone prostheses (Figure 3) and newer third generation minimally constrained prostheses.

Whilst many studies have been published on arthroplasty in the MCPJ [47-59], only a small proportion of these discuss replacement of osteoarthritic joints [47-52], as inflammatory/rheumatoid disease is more typically seen than degenerative change. Goldfarb and Stern in 2003 [52] published the largest long-term follow-up on SJA in the MCPJ. Two hundred and eight silicone arthroplasties were evaluated with an average follow-up of 14 years. Surgery improved the average postoperative arc of motion by 6°, resulting in a postoperative mean pain-free active motion arc of 36°. Implant fracture rate was high (67%) and determined radiologically, although this

did not correlate strongly with adverse clinical findings. Authors of shorter-term studies [53, 54] have reported average active range of movement between 29-44° and improved hand function in 65-75% of patients. Reported implant fracture rates in studies with less than ten years average follow-up varies between 0-28% [55, 56].

The use of the Sutter silicone implant as an alternative to the Swanson prosthesis gained popularity in the late 1980s and early 1990s [47]. This declined after the publication of several studies reporting high fracture rates of the newer design at short-term follow-up [57]. More recent retrospective [58] and prospective studies [59] comparing the Swanson with Sutter prostheses have found little difference between them in terms of objective and subjective outcome measures, although fracture rates are consistently higher in the latter **(IIb/B)**.

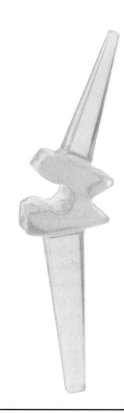

Figure 3. Metacarpophalangeal joint silicastic prosthesis.

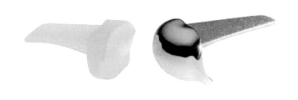

Figure 4. The Avanta surface replacement MCPJ joint arthroplasty consists of distal ultra-high-molecular-weight polyethylene and proximal cobalt chromium alloy components which are cemented into the medullary cavities.

Certain authors have suggested that whilst the patient population is far smaller, arthroplasty is more likely to be successful in MCPJs affected by OA than RA, as joints affected by OA are likely to have a greater bone stock than their rheumatoid counterparts allowing more stable fixation of the prosthesis and less implant subsidence [47] **(III/B)**.

In 2005 Rettig et al [50] reported the results of silicone implant arthroplasty in 13 MCP joints affected by OA. Over a period of 12 years, four different types of prosthesis were inserted. Patients were followed up for an average of 40 months. Active flexion, grip and lateral pinch strength, as well as time to complete Jebson-Taylor tasks, were evaluated to provide objective measures of outcome. Eighty percent of patients reported excellent levels of functional improvement and pain relief. Average active flexion was 59° and seven of the 12 patients completed Jebson-Taylor tasks within normal time constraints. Grip and lateral pinch strength were less than age-matched normative data. One joint required revision surgery after the original Sutter implant fractured. These results are comparable with those reported by Lundborg et al in 1993 [48] in their series using 68 titanium MCPJ replacements in which only three joints were affected by OA.

Surface replacement arthroplasty (Figure 4) for the MCPJ has been increasing in popularity since gaining approval from the FDA in 2001. As a result, several studies reporting short-term outcomes have recently been published. In 2006, Parker et al [47] evaluated the outcomes of SRA, using pyrolytic carbon implants, in 21 MCPJs affected by OA. Mean follow-up was 14 months. Strength and movement were both significantly improved after surgery. Forty-three percent of cases had some radiographic evidence of subluxation and there was one dislocation. Earlier reports using unconstrained SRA have shown similar results, with the majority of joints retaining between 50-60° of active pain-free motion and an objective and subjective improvement in overall hand function [51] **(III/B)**.

The use of SJA at the MCPJ appears to provide benefit to patients affected by rheumatoid and osteoarthritis in terms of both objective and subjective outcome measures **(IIb/B)**. The promising short-term results reported using minimally constrained prostheses will have to be replicated in the longer term before they can be accepted as a superior alternative to the flexible silicone implants still in common use.

The proximal interphalangeal joint

Although less frequently involved than the DIP, the degenerative change at the PIP level results in far greater functional impairment [14]. The PIP joint is a bicondylar, diarthrodial, hinge-like joint that normally has a 0-115° range of motion. When considering surgery at this site three important factors must be taken into account [60]:

- Grip strength is predominantly provided by the ulnar digits and movement at the PIPJ is vital for this action. Pinch strength is provided by the radial digits and is dependent on the stability of the PIPJ in the index and, to a lesser degree, the middle finger.
- The radial digits are subject to large torques generated by the thumb during lateral pinch. This often results in the mechanical failure of implants in these fingers.
- Whilst arthrodesis of the index PIP joint is well tolerated, the quadregia effect from the incomplete separation of the origin of the profunda to the ulnar three fingers may limit motion in the digits adjacent to the fused finger.

Chapter 17

Some hand surgeons therefore advocate arthroplasty for middle, ring and little finger PIP joint OA, and fusion of the index PIP joint.

Although originally described for use in the MCP joint in 1964, Swanson modified the prosthesis within two years to accommodate the smaller canal size in the proximal and middle phalanges [15]. He reviewed 424 PIP joint arthroplasties in 1985 [61]. Around one third were for OA. Within this sub-group of patients, mean maximum flexion was 67° (over 2/3 had a greater than 40° arc of motion) and 98% reported complete pain relief. Overall complications such as implant fracture and dislocation were few within the entire group and when they did occur they were restricted to patients with substantial pre-operative swan neck and Boutonniere deformities secondary to RA.

Pellegrini and Burton [60] in 1990 reviewed their ten years' experience of treating osteoarthritic PIP joints. Fifty-three procedures were performed; around half involved PIP replacement with silicone implants. Seven were replaced with biometric cemented hinged prostheses. Ten joints were fused.

All the biometric cemented prostheses ended in clinical failure, attributed to significant rotational movement at the PIP which is not a simple hinge. The failures described in this series and others prompted the authors to conclude that there is no place for cemented hinged prostheses in PIP joint arthroplasty. Conversely, arthrodesis of PIP joints in radially-based digits provided durable and functional improvement, restoring pinch strength to a level equal to the contralateral hand.

More recently, Takigawa et al in 2004 [62] reviewed the outcomes of 70 silicone implants used to treat a variety of arthritic conditions in the PIP joint. Fourteen of the cases had OA. The authors noted no change in grip or pinch strength before and after arthroplasty and the mean active flexion arc was only 36°, which is considerably less than figures reported in similar series.

Many other authors have described the use of Swanson implants in treating PIP joints affected by rheumatoid [63], psoriatic [64] and post-traumatic arthritis [65].

While the results of these reports lie outside the scope of this chapter, the outcomes from some of these studies have influenced the development of new types of prostheses which can be used to replace osteoarthritic joints. Problems including a limited range of motion, instability, fracture, and bone resorption, seen especially when silicone prostheses are used for RA [6], have led to the introduction of several anatomical, semi-constrained prostheses made from a variety of different materials [17, 66, 67]. Surface replacement arthroplasty (SRA) using these new generation prostheses preserves the collateral ligaments which, with the extensor tendons, balance flexion and rotational forces. In theory this increases the stability of the arthroplasty in a way that cannot be achieved by silastic spacers alone [17].

Linscheid et al in 1997 [68] published the largest series to date on SRA of the PIP joints. Cemented prostheses, made from a combination of cobalt-chromium and ultra-high-molecular-weight polyethylene, were used for joints involved with OA, RA and trauma (Figure 5). The mean postoperative active flexion arc was 47°. Complication rates were significant, most notably in the RA group, in which 20% of patients required revision surgery. More encouraging results have been reported since this time using pyrolytic carbon [66] and ceramic [67] implants. In 2007, Bravo [69] et al described outcomes of 50 PIP replacements using the pyrolytic carbon implants with a minimum of two years' follow-

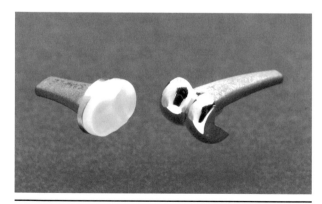

Figure 5. The Avanta surface replacement PIPJ joint arthroplasty consists of distal ultra-high-molecular-weight polyethylene and proximal cobalt chromium alloy components which are cemented into the medullary cavities.

up. Fourteen joints were affected by OA. There was an average of 7° improvement in range of movement making the postoperative mean arc of active flexion 49°. Pinch and grip strength were also improved and these results were shown to be statistically significant in the osteoarthritic group. Arthroplasty of the index finger, included in the review of data for this subgroup, demonstrated significantly improved pinch strength, but also a degree of stability and range of movement that was comparable with the PIPJ replacements in the other digits. The authors proposed that this may be the first indication that arthroplasty may be a viable alternative to fusion in the index finger PIP joint **(III/B)**.

Preservation of the integrity of the collateral ligaments is important when inserting new generation implants, and a palmar, rather than the traditional dorsal, approach may be more successful. However, studies to date that have made comparisons between surgical approaches have only been conducted using Swanson implants [7, 70] and have failed to find any superiority of one technique over the other **(III/B)**.

The distal interphalangeal joint

The DIP joint is the joint most commonly affected by OA [71]. The technical challenges of arthroplasty, the minimal functional deficit arising from impairment of this joint and the proven durability and successful pain relief afforded by fusion have led some authors to rule out the use of joint replacement at this site [72]. Others suggest that whilst the majority of elderly patients tolerate the conversion of a digit into a 'sublimis finger', patients with multiple joint involvements and/or those requiring greater dexterity for fine manipulative activities may find the loss of terminal flexion significantly disabling [73].

Snow et al published the first report of arthroplasty of the DIP joint in 1977 [74] replacing seven OA joints with Swanson silicone implants. This resulted in pain-free joints with between 40-45° of active motion. However, there are relatively few published clinical reports on the use of this intervention. The largest series of 31 patients (11-year follow-up), was reported almost 20 years ago [75] with digits demonstrating a mean extension lag at the DIP joint of 13° but an active range of flexion (33°) and pain

improvement in all, with satisfactory pinch strength and stability. The most recent publication [76], a case report, confirmed a similar arc of flexion, again using a Swanson prosthesis. Overall, the quantity of evidence supporting the use of arthroplasty in the DIP joint remains extremely sparse.

Revisional procedures

Revision rates for SJA vary substantially depending on the joint involved, the surgical technique used and the composition of the inserted prosthesis (Tables 1-6).

Salvage procedures for Swanson MCPJ replacement are relatively straightforward, although fatigue, simple fracture or fragmentation of the prosthesis does not usually necessitate a revision of the arthroplasty **(III/B)**. Revision of other SJA techniques, particularly cemented components, is inevitably more complex. No studies to date have investigated significant numbers of salvage procedures for symptomatic complications of SJA and therefore it is difficult to establish what the optimal management for such cases should be.

Conclusions

Since the introduction of small joint arthroplasty in the 1950s, many authors have reported use of this technique in the treatment of OA affecting various joints of the hand. A variety of different prostheses and surgical techniques have been used. However, in the current era of evidence-based medicine, which is dependent on randomised controlled trials, systematic reviews and meta-analyses, there is a distinct paucity of data regarding the indications for and choice of methods in SJA. Reviews are often narratives. Few display robust methodological quality based on the six criteria recommended by Oxman et al [77].

Recommendations for management may be based on results of retrospective cohort studies of a single technique, with non-standardised staging between groups of patients, failure to randomise, lack of pre-operative measurements, inadequate or differing follow-up times between groups and failure to apply appropriate statistical tests. It is also difficult to perform statistical pooling of data from comparative studies because of clinical heterogeneity with respect to study population and surgical intervention, especially if techniques are modified. Sadly, outcomes may also be described subjectively with variable definitions of an 'acceptable' result. The heterogeneity in published reports extends also to the staging systems used as a guide to treatment. The correlation between radiographic changes and clinical findings is not always strong. In addition, intra-rater and inter-rater reliability of the classification systems used to report the radiographs display further sources for error. The Eaton Classification system has been reported to vary from 0.529 to 0.657 [78].

In the future, could arthroscopic evaluation and histology improve baseline staging of joint pathology? Currently, grading and staging systems of histopathological change have also been questioned over reproducibility and validity with difficulty translating focal pathological changes into a score that encompasses the overall joint pathologic response. Using the Mankin Histological Histochemical Grading System (HHGS), a focal area of cartilage may demonstrate a pathological composite characterised by cellular changes, erosion, and tidemark vessel abnormalities yielding a score of 14 points, (maximal score). In another situation, pathological changes may be more superficial (Mankin score 5), but involving an extended topographic area. Trying to equate the two scenarios and plan a potential treatment strategy for the management of degenerative disease can be imprecise when decisions are based on scoring systems which may be methodologically flawed. Inevitably in human studies histological scores

necessitate examination of tissue available at biopsy or surgery and again this makes it difficult to correlate management with grade and stage *in vivo* [79].

Inadequate or inconsistent staging with comparative groups displaying variability in disease severity coupled with poor outcome measures makes it difficult to form a consensus or evidence-based view. Current assessment protocols for both objective and subjective outcomes can lead to selective and limited reporting of certain parameters, such as range of movement or grip strength. These factors and possibly the inclusion of only English studies in the search, makes it difficult from systematic reviews to indicate the potential superiority of a single arthroplasty technique over another in the small joints of the hand. Clinicians must attempt to use standardised measures of pre-operative severity, intra-operative technique and postoperative outcome. Enough multi-centre randomised controlled trials with condition-specific questionnaires, such as the Michigan Hand Outcomes Questionnaire, the Disabilities of the Arm, Shoulder and Hand Questionnaire and the Neck and Upper Limb Functional Status Index could facilitate a meta-analysis, which may allow comparison of the outcomes of different surgical procedures. This may identify the supporting evidence to treat patients using the appropriate small joint arthroplasty rather than one based on the preference of the surgeon.

Acknowledgement

The authors would like to thank Small Bone Innovations and Northstar Orthopaedics for supplying the images within this chapter.

Table 1. Studies evaluating outcomes of silicone implant arthroplasty after trapeziectomy in TMC joints affected by OA. *Continued overleaf.*

Authors	Sample and follow-up	Procedure	Pinch strength	Grip strength	Abduction	Opposition	Radiological changes and complications
Swanson 1972 [20]	Total 46 OA 29 3.75 years	Trapeziectomy and Swanson implant insertion	2.3Kg in women 6.8Kg in men	4.4Kg in women 9.1Kg in men	48.3°	6.9cm	17% Subluxation 2 revisions in RA group
Haffajee 1977 [80]	Total 100 OA ? Unspecified	Trapeziectomy and Swanson implant insertion	42%, >4.4Kg 30%, 3.3-4.4Kg 20%, 2.2-3.3Kg 8%, <2.2Kg	47% , >0.5Kp/cm^2 30% , 0.2- 0.5Kp/cm^2 52%, <0.2Kp/cm^2	52%, >40° 33%, 20-40° 15%, <20°	Not reported	No fractures of prosthesis No resorption 19% dislocated 2% fractured metacarpal shafts
Ferlic *et al* 1977 [39]	Total 11 OA 11 20 months	Trapeziectomy and Niebauer implant insertion	3.9Kg	23.2Kg	30°	Not reported	No fractures No resorption 18% subluxation No dislocations
Poppen and Niebauer 1978 [35]	Total 17 OA 12 4 years	Trapeziectomy and Niebauer implant insertion	Equal or greater than unoperated side in 52% of thumbs	Equal or greater than unoperated side in 94% of thumbs	35°	Not reported	35% subluxation 12% dislocation 18% revised
Eaton 1979 [36]	Total 50 OA 45 21 months	Trapeziectomy and Eaton silicone implant insertion	5.7Kg in women 7.8Kg in men	Not reported	Not reported	Not reported	4% subluxation 6% dislocation 4% revised
Crawford 1980 [40]	Total 37 OA ? Unspecified	Trapeziectomy and Swanson implant insertion	Not reported	Not reported	Not reported	Not reported	4% dislocation
Rajan *et al* 1982 [38]	Total 16 OA 14 13 months	Trapeziectomy and Niebauer implant insertion	Not reported	Not reported	25%, 55-60° 43%, 40-54° 32%, <20°	Not reported	12% subluxation
Swanson 1985 [29]	Total 150 OA 150 3.5 years	Trapeziectomy and Swanson implant insertion	2.5 times improvement	2.7 times improvement	78% of contra-lateral hand	38% improvement	2.6% destructive osseous change No dislocations No revisions
Kvarnes and Reikeras 1985 [81]	Total 52 OA 52	Comparison between arthrodesis, trapeziectomy alone and trapeziectomy and Swanson prosthesis	Arthrodesis 5.1Kp Trapeziectomy 2.8Kp Swanson 3.1Kp	Arthrodesis 16.1Kp Trapeziectomy 11.4Kp Swanson 11.1 Kp	Not reported	Not reported	Arthrodesis 2% fibrous union Trapeziectomy Nil Swanson 31% dislocation associated with pain

Chapter 17

Table 1. Studies evaluating outcomes of silicone implant arthroplasty after trapeziectomy in TMC joints affected by OA. *Continued overleaf.*

Authors	Sample and follow-up	Procedure	Pinch strength	Grip strength	Abduction	Opposition	Radiological changes and complications
Pellegrini and Burton 1986 [16]	Total 32 OA 32 Swanson 6 years Eaton 3.8 years	Trapeziectomy and Swanson/ Eaton implant insertion	Swanson 3.7Kg in women Eaton 4Kg in men 3.7Kg in women	Swanson 18.8Kg in women Eaton 22Kg in men 13.4Kg in women	Not reported	64% able to oppose thumb to base of small finger	Swanson 59% subluxation 25% loss of vertical height 37% revision - all associated with synovitis Eaton 27% subluxation 50% loss of vertical height 0% revision
Hofammann et al 1987 [32]	Total 20 OA 20 7.8 years	Trapeziectomy/ partial resection and silicone implant insertion	1.8Kgs	19.6Kgs	Not reported	Not reported	20% subluxation 15% dislocation 50% destructive osseous change 5% fractured
Hay et al 1988 [30]	Total 64 OA 51 4.4 years	Trapeziectomy and Swanson implant insertion	7.5Kg in men 4.2Kg in women	38Kg in men 19.6Kg in women	38°	80% able to oppose thumb to base of small finger	22% subluxation 10% dislocation 18% bone resorption
Freeman and Honner 1992 [31]	Total 43 OA 43 5.5 years	Trapeziectomy and Swanson implant insertion	77% compared to opposite hand	102% compared to opposite hand	Not reported	All patients able to oppose thumb to base of small finger	5% dislocation 14% stem fractures 7% removed due to synovitis
Sotereanos et al 1993 [37]	Total 30 OA 29 9 years	Trapeziectomy and Niebauer implant insertion	2.7Kg	13.8Kg	42°	Not reported	83% subluxation 10% revised
Van Cappelle et al 2001 [82]	Total 45 OA 45 13.8 years	Trapeziectomy and Swanson implant insertion	Not reported	Not reported	32°	80% able to oppose thumb to base of small finger	7% loss of sensory function of superficial radial nerve 11% synovitis 40% dislocation 1 fractured implant 26% revision
Bezwada et al 2002 [83]	Total 62 OA 49 16.4 years	Trapeziectomy and modified Swanson implant insertion	Pre-op 2.4Kg 5 years 3.8Kg 15 years 3.3Kg	Pre-op 13.2Kg 5 years 19.1 Kg 15 years 16.2Kg	Not reported	84% thumb to little finger opposition compared with 34% pre-operatively	3% CRPS 19% subluxation 6% revision

CRPS = chronic regional pain syndrome

Table 1. Studies evaluating outcomes of silicone implant arthroplasty after trapeziectomy in TMC joints affected by OA. *Continued.*

Authors	Sample and follow-up	Procedure	Pinch strength	Grip strength	Abduction	Opposition	Radiological changes and complications
Tagil and Kopylov 2002 [84]	Total 26 OA 26 43 months	RCT Trapeziectomy and Swanson implant insertion 13 APL interposition arthroplasty 13	Swanson group 0.34Kp/cm^2 APL group 0.35Kp/cm^2	Swanson group 0.56Kp/cm^2 APL group 0.54Kp/cm^2	Swanson group 34° APL group 36°	Not reported	Swanson group Cyst formation 33% loss of vertical height 15% dislocation 1 revision APL group 67% loss of vertical height
Lovell et al 2003 [85]	Total 104 OA 104 62 months	Retrospective comparison of Swanson vs. sling excision arthroplasties Results based on patient questionnaires assessing pain and ability to perform various tasks Results based on the VAS showed statistically significant greater pain relief and improved ability to perform ADLs in the Swanson group Thumb strength, motion and ability to perform other tasks all greater in Swanson group although not statistically significant 14% of Swanson implants removed					
MacDermid et al 2003 [86]	Total 30 OA 30	Trapeziectomy and Swanson implant insertion	4.7Kg	18.2Kg	45°	Not reported	48% clinical instability 90% lytic changes 10% dislocation 10% fractured 10% revision
Taylor et al 2005 [19]	Total 83 OA 83 Min. 1 year	Comparison between arthrodesis, trapeziectomy alone and trapeziectomy and Swanson prosthesis	Arthrodesis 10Kg Trapeziectomy 10Kg Swanson 11Kg	Not reported	Not reported	Not reported	Arthrodesis 19% revision 11% nerve damage Trapeziectomy Nil Swanson 14% revision 9% nerve damage

VAS = Visual analogue scale

Table 2. Studies evaluating outcomes of alloplastic interpositional/resection arthroplasty in TMC joints affected by OA.

Authors	Sample and follow-up	Procedure	Pinch strength	Grip strength	Abduction	Opposition	Radiological changes and complications
Kessler 1973 [22]	Total 18 OA 18 2-5 years	Interpositional arthroplasty with the Kessler prosthesis	Not reported	Not reported	Not reported	39% able to oppose thumb to base of small finger	None reported
Ashworth et al 1977 [26]	Total 42 OA 31 31 months	Interpositional arthroplasty with the Ashworth prosthesis	Not reporteed	95% had improved grip strength and abduction postoperatively		Not repoorted	5% revision due to fracture of prosthesis
Crawford 1977 [40]	Total 9 OA 9	Interpositional arthroplasty with the Kessler prosthesis	All implants failed due to chronic synovitis and during revision surgery 3 patients were found to have badly torn prostheses				
Swanson et al 1997 [87]	Total 105 OA 96 5 years	Resection arthroplasty with a titanium prosthesis	5.4Kg	23.6Kg	Not reported	89% able to oppose thumb to base of small finger	0% revisions No cystic or heterotopic bone formation No wear
Perez-Ubeda et al 2003 [41]	Total 20 OA 20 33 months	Surface replacement arthroplasty with the cemented SR prosthesis	4.3Kg	16.3Kg	35°	Not reported	86% loosening 20% revision
Minami et al 2005 [43]	Total 12 OA 12	Interpositional arthroplasty with the Ashworth prosthesis	3.2Kg	9.5Kg	38.8°	Not reported	41% dislocation 16% implant fracture
Naidu et al 2006 [88]	Total 50 OA 50 Minimum 2 years	Resection arthroplasty with a titanium prosthesis	5.1Kg	12.2Kg	Not reported	Not reported	4% dislocation 25% failure rate

Chapter 17

Table 3. Studies evaluating outcomes of total joint arthroplasty in TMC joints affected by OA.

Authors	Sample and follow-up	Procedure	Pinch strength	Grip strength	Abduction	Opposition	Radiological changes and complications
de la Caffiniere and Aucouturier 1979 [23]	Total 24 OA 15 24 months	Total joint arthroplasty using the de la Caffiniere prosthesis	Not reported	Not reported	Not reported	Not reported	21% loosening
Alnot and Saint Laurent 1984 [89]	Total 17 OA 11 3 years	Total joint arthroplasty using the Bichat prosthesis	$0.3-0.4Kp/cm^2$ No mean given	$0.6-0.8Kp/cm^2$ No mean given	43°	100% able to oppose thumb to base of small finger	18% revision - 66% due to loosening of trapezial component after fracture of lateral wall
Ferrari and Steffee 1986 [8]	Total 45 OA 37 2 - 6.5 years	Total joint arthroplasty using the Steffee prosthesis	OA group 5Kg	OA group 24Kg	41°	100% able to oppose thumb to base of small finger	OA group 5% septic loosening 3% dislocation 3% revision
Cooney et al 1987 [44]	Total 62 OA 49 4.6 years	Total joint arthroplasty using the Mayo prosthesis	OA group 5.2Kg	OA group 10.9Kg	42 °	7cm	19% frank loosening and were removed 30% heterotopic ossification
Boeckstyns et al 1989 [90]	Total 31 OA 29 48 months	Total joint arthroplasty using the de la Caffiniere prosthesis	51KPa	49KPa	41°	87% had full opposition	13% revision
Sondergaard et al 1991 [91]	Total 22 OA 20 9 years	Total joint arthroplasty using the de la Caffiniere prosthesis	38KPa	Not reported	35°	86% had full opposition	14% aseptic loosening 14% revision
Braun et al 1991 [24]	Total 50 OA 26 Not specified	Total joint arthroplasty using the Braun-Cutter prosthesis	Not reported	Not reported	Not reported	Not reported	10% loosening 8% revision
Nicholas and Calderwood 1992 [92]	Total 20 OA 20 64 months	Total joint arthroplasty using the de la Caffiniere prosthesis	Not reported	Not reported	39°	Not reported	5% trapezial collapse 5% dislocation
Wachtl and Sennwald 1996 [45]	Total 26 OA 26 25 months	Total joint arthroplasty using the Ledoux prosthesis	9.6Kg	19.3Kg	32°	Not reported	59% survival at 16 months
Chakrabarti et al 1997 [93]	Total 93 OA 87 11 years	Total joint arthroplasty using the de la Caffiniere prosthesis	22Kg	168% of non-operated side	Mean Kapandji score 9 (thumb to palmar distal crease of little finger)	Not reported	12% revision, commonest cause was loosening of trapezial component
Badia and Sambandam 2006 [46]	Total 26 OA 26	Total joint arthroplasty using the Braun-Cutter prosthesis	5.5Kg	Not reported	60°	100% able to oppose thumb to base of small finger	4% revision 0% loosening

Table 4. Studies evaluating outcomes of arthroplasty in MCPJs affected by OA.

Authors	Sample and follow-up	Prosthesis	Significant results and conclusions
Lundborg et al 1993 [48]	Total 68 OA 3 2.5 years	Titanium stemmed silicone spacers	OA group: Mean active ROM 53° Extension lag 4° Other outcomes not specified by group
Cook et al 1999 [49]	Total 151 OA 4 11.7 years	Pyrolytic carbon (SRA)	Outcomes not specific for OA
Rettig et al 2005 [50]	Total 12 OA 12 40 months	Swanson silicone 9 Sutter 2 Other 1	Average pinch strength 3.8Kg Average grip strength 21.6Kg 7/12 performed Jebson Taylor tasks in normal time Average active flexion 59° 2 revisions - 1 in Sutter for fracture of implant - 1 in Swanson group Minimal bone resorption in Swanson group
Parker et al 2006 [47]	Total 21 OA 21 14 months	Pyrolytic carbon (SRA)	Average pinch strength 3.2Kg Average grip strength 28.1Kg 5% dislocation 5% extensor tendon rupture No migration of prosthesis 87% subjective function of normal

Chapter 17

Table 5. **Studies evaluating outcomes of arthroplasty in PIPJs affected by OA.** *Continued overleaf.*

Authors	Sample and follow-up	Prosthesis	Surgical approach	Significant results and conclusions
Swanson 1985 [61]	Total 424 OA 153 Minimum 1 year	Swanson silicone	Dorsal	OA group: 68% had >40′ active flexion arc Mean absolute max. flexion 67° 100% pain relief 5 implants fractured
Burton and Pellegrini 1990 [60]	Total 53 OA 43 3.8 years	Swanson silicone 26 Cemented hinge 7	Dorsal	All cemented prosthesis failed Swanson implants in OA group: Mean active flexion arc 56° Mean absolute max. flexion 59.2° 26% >10° deflection arc on stress 100% improved pain relief None needed revision
Lin *et al* 1995 [7]	Total 69 OA 38 3.4 years	Swanson silicone	Palmar	OA group: Mean active flexion arc 58° 5 implant fractures - no group specified 97% complete pain relief OA group fared better than RA and post-traumatic groups
Linscheid *et al* 1997 [68]	Total 66 OA 37 4.5 years	CoCr proximal component Ultra-high-molecular-weight polyethylene distal component Cemented device (SRA)	Dorsal 43 Lateral 13 Palmar 10	OA group: 60% had >45°active flexion arc All joints stable to lateral stress Mean active flexion arc 47° 12 needed revision surgery OA group fared better than RA and post-traumatic groups
Herren and Simmen 2000 [70]	Total 59 OA 36 25 months	Swanson silicone	Dorsal 21 Palmar 38	OA group: Mean active flexion arc 49° No difference in ROM or stability between dorsal and palmar approaches
Burton et al 2002 [94]	Total 12 OA 12 36.8 months	Volar plate arthroplasty	Volar	Mean active flexion arc 47° Increased grip and pinch strength postoperatively Average lateral opening with stress 2.5° No complications
Takigawa *et al* 2004 [62]	Total 70 OA 14 6.5 years	Swanson silicone	Dorsal	OA group: No change in pre vs. postoperative active ROM, pinch strength and grip strength Mean active flexion arc 36°

20. Swanson AB. Disabling arthritis at the base of the thumb: treatment by resection of the trapezium and flexible implant arthroplasty. *J Bone Joint Surg* 1972; 54A: 456-71.

21. Tomaino MM, Pellegrini VD, Burton RI. Arthroplasty of the basal joint of the thumb. Long-term follow-up after ligament reconstruction with tendon interposition. *J Bone Joint Surg* 1995; 77A: 346-55.

22. Kessler I, Axer A. Arthroplasty of the first carpometacarpal joint with a silicone implant. *Plast Reconstr Surg* 1971; 47(3): 252-7.

23. de la Caffiniere JY, Aucouturier P. Trapezio-metacarpal arthroplasty by total prosthesis. *Hand* 1979; 11(1): 41-6.

24. Braun RM. Total joint replacement at the base of the thumb: Preliminary report. *J Hand Surg* 1982; 7A: 245-50.

25. Kauer JMG. Functional anatomy of the carpometacarpal joint of the thumb. *Clin Orthop Relat Res* 1985; 220: 7-13.

26. Ashworth CR, *et al.* Silicone-rubber interposition arthroplasty of the carpometacarpal joint of the thumb. *J Hand Surg* 1977; 2A(5): 345-57.

27. Martou G, Veltri K, Thoma A. Surgical treatment of osteoarthritis of the thumb: a systematic review. *Plast Reconstr Surg* 2004; 114(2): 421-32.

28. Leach RE, Bolton PE. Arthritis of the carpometacarpal joint of the thumb. Results of arthrodesis. *J Bone Joint Surg* 1968; 50A: 1171-7.

29. Swanson AB, De Groot Swanson G. Arthroplasty of the basal thumb joint. *Clin Orthop Relat Res* 1985; 195: 151-60.

30. Hay EL, Bomberg BC, Burke C, Meisenheimer C. Long-term results of silicone trapezial arthroplast. *Journal of Arthroplasty* 1988; 3(3): 215-23.

31. Freeman GR, Honner R. Silicastic replacement of the trapezium. *J Hand Surg* 1992; 17B: 458-62.

32. Hofammann DY, Ferlic DC, Clayton ML. Arthroplasty of the basal joint of the thumb using a silicone prosthesis. *J Bone Joint Surg* 1987; 69A(7): 993-7.

33. Peimer CA. Long-term complications of trapeziometacarpal silicone arthroplasty. *Clin Orthop Relat Res* 1987; 220: 86-98.

34. Herndon JH. Trapeziometacarpal arthroplasty. *Clin Orthop Relat Res* 1987; 220: 99-105.

35. Poppen NK, Niebauer JJ. 'Tie-in' trapezium prosthesis: long-term results. *J Hand Surg* 1978; 3A(5): 446-9.

36. Eaton RG. Replacement of the trapezium for arthritis of the basal articulations: a new technique with stabilization by tenodesis. *J Bone Joint Surg* 1979; 61A(1): 76-82.

37. Sotereanos DG, Taras J, Urbaniak JR. Niebauer trapeziometacarpal arthroplast: a long-term follow-up. *J Hand Surg* 1993; 18A: 560-4.

38. Rajan S, Nylander G, Fransson SG. The Niebauer-Cutter prosthesis in excision arthroplasty of the trapezium. *Hand* 1982; 14(3): 295-303.

39. Ferlic DC, Greer AB, Clayton ML. Degenerative arthritis of the carpometacarpal joint of the thumb: a clinical follow-up of 11 Niebauer prostheses. *J Hand Surg* 1977; 2A(3): 212-5.

40. Crawford GP. Ligament augmentation with replacement arthroplasty of the carpometacarpal joint. *Hand* 1980; 12(1): 91-4.

41. Perez-Ubeda M-J, Garcia-Lopez A, Martinez MF. Results of the cemented SR trapeziometacarpal osteoarthritis. *J Hand Surg* 2003; 28A(6): 917-25.

42. Merritt K, Rodrigo JJ. Immune response to synthetic materials. Sensitization of patients receiving orthopaedic implants. *Clin Orthop Relat Res* 1996; 326: 71-9.

43. Minami A, Iwasaki N, Kutsumi K, Suenaga N, Yasuda K. A long-term follow-up of silicone-rubber interposition arthroplasty for osteoarthritis of the thumb carpometacarpal joint. *Hand Surgery* 2005; 10(1): 77-82.

44. Cooney WP, Linscheid RL, Askew LJ. Total arthroplasty of the thumb metacarpal joint. *Clin Orthop Relat Res* 1987; 220: 35-45.

45. Wachtl SW, Sennwald GR. Non-cemented replacement of the trapeziometacarpal joint. *J Bone Joint Surg* 1996; 78B: 787-92.

46. Badia A, Sambandam SN. Total joint arthroplasty in the treatment of advanced stages of thumb carpometacarpal joint osteoarthritis. *J Hand Surg* 2006; 31A(10): 1605-14.

47. Parker W, Moran SL, Hormel KB, Rizzo M, Beckenbaugh RD. Non-rheumatoid metacarpal joint arthritis. Unconstrained pyrolytic carbon implants: indications, technique and outcomes. *Hand Clinics* 2006; 22: 183-93.

48. Lundborg G, Branemark P, Carlsson I. Metacarpalphalangeal joint arthroplasty based on the osseointegration concept. *J Hand Surg* 1993; 18B: 693-703.

49. Cook S, *et al.* Long-term follow-up of pyrolytic carbon metacarpophalangeal implants. *J Bone Joint Surg* 1999; 81A(5): 635-48.

50. Rettig LA, Luca L, Murphy MS. Silicone implant arthroplasty in patients with idiopathic osteoarthritis of the metacarpophalangeal joint. *J Hand Surg* 2005; 30A: 667-72.

51. Harris D, Dias JJ. Five-year results of a new total replacement prosthesis for the finger metacarpo-phalangeal joints. *J Hand Surg* 2003; 28B(5): 432-8.

52. Goldfarb CA, Stern PJ. Metacarpophalangeal joint arthroplasty in rheumatoid arthritis. A long-term assessment. *J Bone Joint Surg* 2003; 85A (10): 1869-78.

53. Wilson RL, Carlblom ER. The rheumatoid metacarpophalangeal joint. *Hand Clinics* 1989; 5(2): 223-37.

54. Kirschenbaum D, *et al.* Arthroplasty of the metacarpophalangeal joints with the use of silicone rubber implants in patients who have rheumatoid arthritis. *J Bone Joint Surg* 1993; 75A(1): 3-12.

55. Bieber EJ, Weiland AJ, Volenec Dowling S. Silicone rubber implant arthroplasty of the metacarpophalangeal joints for rheumatoid arthritis. *J Bone Joint Surg* 1986; 68A(2): 206-9.

56. Schmidt K, *et al.* Ten-year follow-up of silicone arthroplasty of the metacarpalphalangeal joints in rheumatoid hands. *Scand J Plastic Recon Hand Surg* 1999; 33(4): 433-8.

57. Bass RL, Stern PJ, Nairus JG. High implant fracture incidence with Sutter silicone metacarpophalangeal joint arthroplasty. *J Hand Surg* 1996; 1A(5): 813-8.

58. Beevers DJ, Seedham BB. Metacarpophalangeal joint prosthesis: a review of clinical results of past and current designs. *J Hand Surg* 1995; 20(2): 125-36.

59. Moller K, *et al.* Avanta versus Swanson silicone implants in the MCP joint - a prospective randomized comparison of 30 patients followed for 2 years. *J Hand Surg* 2005; 30A(1): 8-13.

60. Pellegrini VD, Burton RI. Osteoarthritis of the proximal interphalangeal joint of the hand: arthroplasty or fusion. *J Hand Surg* 1990; 15A(2): 195-208.

61. Swanson AB, Mauoin MD, Gajjar NV, de Groot Swanson G. Flexible implant arthroplasty in the proximal interphalangeal joint of the hand. *J Hand Surg* 1985; 10A: 796-805.

62. Takigawa S, Meletiou S, Sauerbier M, Cooney WP. Long-term assessment of Swanson implant arthroplasty in the proximal interphalangeal joint of the hand. *J Hand Surg* 2004; 29A: 785-95.

63. Johnstone BR. Proximal interphalangeal joint surface replacement arthroplasty. *Hand Surgery* 2001; 6(1): 1-11.

64. Belsky MR, Feldon P, Millender LH, Nalebuff EA, Phillips C. Hand involvement in psoriatic arthritis. *J Hand Surg* 1982; 7A(2): 203-7.

65. Iselin F, Conti E. Long-term results of interphalangeal joint resection arthroplasties with a silicone implant. *J Hand Surg* 1995; 20A: S95-97.

66. Tuttle HG, Stern PJ. Pyrolytic carbon proximal interphalangeal joint resurfacing arthroplasty. *J Hand Surg* 2006; 31A: 930-9.

67. Pettersson K, Wagnsjo P, Hulin E. Replacement of proximal interphalangeal joints with new ceramic arthroplasty: a prospective series of 20 proximal interphalangeal joint replacements. *Scand J Plastic Recon Surg Hand* 2006; 40: 291-6.

68. Linscheid RL, Murray PM, Vidal M-A, Beckenbaugh RD. Development of a surface replacement arthroplasty for proximal interphalangeal joints. *J Hand Surg* 1997; 22A: 286-98.

69. Bravo CJ, Rizzo M, Hormel KB, Beckenbaugh RD. Pyrolytic carbon proximal interphalangeal joint arthroplasty: results with a minimum two-year follow-up. *J Hand Surg* 2007; 32A: 1-11.

70. Herren DB, Simmen BR. Palmar approach in flexible implant arthroplasty of the proximal interphalangeal joint. *Clin Orthop Relat Res* 2000; 371: 131-5.

71. Wilder FV, Barrett JP, Farina EJ. Joint-specific osteoarthritis of the hand. *Osteoarthritis and Cartilage* 2006; 4(9): 953-7.

72. Rehart S, Kerschbaumer F. Endoprosthesis of the hand. *Orthopade* 2003; 32(9): 779-83.

73. Brown LG. Distal interphalangeal joint flexible arthroplasty. *J Hand Surg* 1989; 14A(4): 653-6.

74. Snow JW, Boyes JG, Greider JL. Implant arthroplasty of the distal interphalangeal joint of the finger for osteoarthritis. *Plast Reconstr Surg* 1977; 60(4): 558-60.

75. Zimmerman NB, Suhey PV, Clark GL, Wilgis EF. Silicone interpositional arthroplasty of the distal interphalangeal joint. *J Hand Surg* 1989; 14(5): 882-7.

76. Schwartz DA, Peimer CA. Distal interphalangeal joint arthroplasty in a musician. *J Hand Therapy* 1998; 11(1): 49-52.

77. Oxman AD, Cook DJ, Guyatt. User's guides to the medical literature: VI How to use an overview. *JAMA* 1994; 272: 1367-75.

78. Kubik NJ, Lubahn JD. Intra-rater and inter-rater reliability of the Eaton classification of basal joint arthritis. *J Hand Surg*; 27A: 882-8.

79. Moskowitz RW. Osteoarthritis cartilage histopathology: grading and staging. *Osteoarthritis and Cartilage* 2006; 14: 1-2.

80. Haffajee D. Endoprosthetic replacement of the trapezium for arthrosis in the carpometacarpal joint of the thumb. *J Hand Surg* 1977; 2A(2); 141-8.

81. Kvarnes L, Reikeras O. Osteoarthritis of the carpometacarpal joint of the thumb. An analysis of operative procedures. *J Hand Surg* 1985; 10B(1): 117-20.

82. van Cappelle HGJ, Deutman R, van Horn JR. Use of Swanson silicone trapezium implant for treatment of primary osteoarthritis. *J Bone Joint Surg* 2001; 83A(7): 999-1004.

83. Bezwada HP, Sauer ST, Hankins ST, Webber JB. Long-term results of trapeziometacarpal silicone arthroplasty. *J Hand Surg* 2002; 27A: 409-17.

84. Tagil M, Kopylov P. Swanson versus APL arthroplasty in the treatment of osteoarthritis of the trapeziometacarpal joint: a prospective and randomized study in 26 patients. *J Hand Surg* 2002; 27B(5): 452-6.

85. Lovell ME, Nuttall D, Trail IA, Stilwell J, Stanely JK. A patient-reported comparison of trapeziectomy with Swanson silastic implant or sling ligament reconstruction. *J Hand Surg* 1999; 24B(4): 453-5.

86. MacDermid JC, Roth JH, Rampersaud R, Main GI. Trapezial arthroplasty with silicone rubber implantation for advanced osteoarthritis of the trapeziometacarpal joint of the thumb. *Can J Surg* 2003; 46(2): 103-10.

87. Swanson AB, *et al*. Carpal bone titanium implant arthroplasty. *Clin Orthop Relat Res* 1997; 342: 46-58.

88. Naidu SH, Kulkarni N, Saunders M. Titanium basal joint arthroplasty: a finite element analysis and clinical study. *J Hand Surg* 2006; 31A(5): 760-5.

89. Alnot JY, Saint Laurent Y. Total trapeziometacarpal arthroplasty. Report on seventeen cases of degenerative arthritis of the trapeziometacarpal joint. *Ann Chir Main* 1985; 4(1): 11-21.

90. Boeckstyns ME, Sinding A, Elholm KT, Rechnagel K. Replacement of the trapeziometacarpal joint with a cemented (Caffiniere) prosthesis. *J Hand Surg* 1989; 14A: 83-9.

91. Sondergaard L, Konradsen L, Rechnagel K. Long-term follow-up of the cemented Caffiniere prosthesis for trapeziometacarpal arthroplasty. *J Hand Surg* 1991; 16B: 428-30.

92. Nicholas RM, Calderwood JW. de la Caffiniere arthroplasty for basal joint osteoarthritis. *J Bone Joint Surg* 1992; 74B(2): 309-11.

93. Chakrabarti AJ, Robinson AHN, Gallagher P. de la Caffiniere thumb carpometacarpal replacements. *J Hand Surg* 1997; 22B(6): 695-8.

94. Burton RI, Campolattaro RM, Ronchetti PJ. Volar plate arthroplasty of the proximal interphalangeal joint: a preliminary report. *J Hand Surg* 2002; 27A: 1065-72.

Chapter 18

Monitoring of microvascular free tissue transfers

Iain S Whitaker BA (Hons) MA MB BChir MRCS 1
Specialist Registrar, Plastic Surgery
David W Oliver BSc MB ChB FRCS FRCS (Plast.) 2
Consultant Plastic Surgeon

1 THE WELSH CENTRE FOR BURNS AND PLASTIC SURGERY
MORRISTON HOSPITAL, SWANSEA, UK
2 ROYAL DEVON AND EXETER HOSPITAL, EXETER, UK

Introduction

Accurate assessment of the perfusion of free tissue transfers has always been a challenge for surgeons undertaking microvascular reconstructive procedures. In many cases, the complexities of flap microcirculation are difficult to assess, despite all the subjective and objective examination techniques available today [1]. This is further compounded when the free tissue transfer is not visible for monitoring, for example in a buried, vascularised bone graft during head and neck reconstruction [2]. Reliable postoperative monitoring of free tissue transfers is mandatory in order to detect vascular occlusion at an early enough stage to allow re-exploration and ultimately improve the chances of flap salvage.

Routine monitoring of free flaps is usually undertaken by nursing staff on the ward. Junior medical staff often have little experience of such monitoring. The ideal method of monitoring flap viability should satisfy the criteria proposed by Creech and Miller [3]:

* Simple and harmless to the patient and free flap.
* Rapid, repeatable, reliable, recordable and responsive.
* Accurate and inexpensive.
* Objective and applicable to all kinds of flaps.
* User friendly.

This chapter reviews the options currently available to monitor free tissue transfers postoperatively, and to present the levels of evidence (where appropriate) to substantiate their use.

Methodology

Sources for this chapter include a comprehensive literature search using the PubMed and EMBASE databases along with relevant textbooks, Selected Readings in Plastic Surgery, and personal experiences of microsurgery.

Established techniques

Clinical tests

Of the techniques currently available to monitor free flaps postoperatively, clinical assessment is the most commonly used [4, 5] **(III/C)**.

Clinical assessment consists of the following:

* Skin colour of the flap/colour of muscle.
* Skin/soft tissue turgor.
* Surface temperature.
* Capillary refill time.
* Bleeding time following pinprick.

Clinical tests are cheap, non-invasive and repeatable, but have certain limitations. There is a need for experienced interpretation. Perception of colour is markedly affected by ambient lighting [6] and transferred skin colour may also be different from that of the recipient site. Subjective assessment of surface temperature is often unreliable [7]. Even more importantly, clinical changes may be subtle initially and by the time they are clinically apparent, salvage of the flap may be impossible because of irreversible tissue damage. It has been demonstrated that capillary bleeding on pinprick, in terms of colour (bright red vs cyanotic), and speed (brisk vs slow) is a particularly reliable indication of microvascular status, and some authors still believe clinical observation to be the gold standard [8] **(IV/C)**.

Adjunctive techniques

Chemical techniques

Several chemical techniques for monitoring of free flaps have been used historically.

Fluorescein

Sodium fluorescein (resorcinol phthalein sodium, $C_{20}H_{10}Na_2O_5$) is a hygroscopic orange red powder readily soluble in water and assumes an intense yellow green visible by the naked eye when viewed under a Wood's lamp in a darkened room. It is an organic dye which is injected intravenously to monitor skin perfusion. In the 1940s, Dingwall and Lord used it to test the circulation in tubed pedicles [9], and Conway et al validated this using tubed pedicles in a single animal study [10]. In a study of 285 pedicled flaps, the fluorescein injection technique predicted flap survival within a distance of three to five millimeters (McCraw et al 1977 [11]).

The fluorescein test involves injecting sodium fluorescein intravenously at 15mg/kg for one minute. The dye diffuses across the capillary wall to the extracellular fluid compartment within 10-15 minutes but does not penetrate cells. The distribution is then observed. The result can even be photographed with a blue filter to allow a record to be kept. The technique is relatively straightforward and inexpensive but is cumbersome to perform and allergic reactions can occur [12]. It is also prone to subjective error in the interpretation of marginal fluorescence [13], and is only suitable for the monitoring of cutaneous free tissue transfers.

These limitations led to the search for a technique which would improve the precision and accuracy of assessing skin flap viability via repeated assessments of skin fluorescence postoperatively. Silverman et al in 1980 reported the use of a fiberoptic dermofluorometer for assessment of skin fluorescence in animal models [14]. It was subsequently demonstrated that skin fluorometry could also be used for repeated assessment of skin fluorescence postoperatively to allow accurate prediction of skin viability in random pattern skin flaps, island skin flaps and skin free flaps in the rabbit, as well as myocutaneous flaps in the pig. The safety of intravenous fluorescein was investigated by Morykwas in 1991 and he made several recommendations for clinical use [12]. Graham et al [15] found this technique useful for monitoring finger replantation **(IIb/B)**. More recently, Issing, in 1996, concluded that fluorescein staining with computer aided digital morphometry (CADM) represented a more precise predictor of flap survival when compared with pH and temperature monitoring in an animal model [16] **(IIa/B)**.

Indocyanine green

Because of the severity of the potential side effects of fluorescein and its unfavourable pharmacokinetic properties, another fluorescent dye, indocyanine green, with far better pharmacokinetic properties, has been investigated for clinical use. Initial results were promising (Eren et al 1995)[17]. This dye has diverse uses including monitoring heart function [18] and guiding sentinel lymph node biopsies. Little work has been done with indocyanine green and flap monitoring, and further research is needed before it becomes a practical tool.

Tissue pH

Monitoring of tissue pH levels has been used in the postoperative assessment of free tissue transfers. Impairment of tissue blood flow causes an increase in anaerobic metabolic products and an accumulation of acid metabolites. The resulting increased concentration of hydrogen ions causes a pH drop in the affected tissues. Subcutaneously and intramuscularly-placed pH probes have been described. Raskin et al [19, 20], in an experiment using a continuous tissue pH monitoring system, showed that selective occlusion of the vessels supplying lower abdominal island flaps in Sprague-Dawley rats resulted in predictable tissue pH changes **(IIb/B)**. This technique could be applied to muscle flaps where colour is difficult to observe.

Radioactive isotopes

Radioactive isotopes have been studied as a means of directly measuring tissue perfusion. The basis of the radioactive tracer techniques is centred upon the Fick dilutional principle. The ideal tracer should be metabolically inert and diffuse between blood and tissue with no significant impairment (Kety, 1951 [21]). Many different isotopes have been used for assessing tissue clearance such as Kry^{85}, Xe^{133}, Na^{22} and $Tech^{99}m$.

Technitium99m

Technitium 99m sestamibi scintigraphy was studied by Aygit [22] in 1999 as a non-invasive option for monitoring free muscle flap viability, but the results were initially unconvincing. The major disadvantages were that measurements with this technique could only be repeated once per day at most, due to residual background radioactivity and, like other radioactive techniques, it suffers from the costly problems of radioactive waste decontamination and the unavoidable radiation dose to the patient. Continuous monitoring and early intervention for flap salvage failure is not practical.

Xenon

Tsuchida [23], in 1990, described blood flow monitoring in 89 patients with deltopectoral flaps using direct injection of $50\mu Ci$ xenon 133 into the flap. He distinguished between surviving and non-surviving flaps by the radioactive clearance rate **(III/C)**.

Sodium

Harrison et al [24] described sodium 22 isotope clearance as a useful technique for monitoring myocutaneous free flaps **(III/C)**.

Instrumental monitoring methods

Several instrumental methods for the monitoring of free tissue transfers have been described.

Hydrogen gas clearance

The technique of hydrogen gas clearance measurement (Auckland [25] 1964) is based on the same principle as radioactive tracer clearance. It allows quantitative measurement of tissue blood flow in ml/g/min using an implantable probe in animal models. Glogovac [26] found this technique useful clinically in a small number of patients following finger replantation **(IIb/B)**. The advantage of implantable probes is that they can be used for monitoring both superficial and buried flaps. Repeated and quantitative measurements of tissue blood flow are possible in different tissue areas at the same time, and the complete monitoring system is available commercially for a relatively low price.

Skin temperature probes

Surface temperature recording is one of the oldest and simplest method of monitoring free flaps. Its usefulness, however, remains poorly documented, and its problems are little understood. Skin temperature can be easily and continually monitored using simple, inexpensive equipment [27] and therefore, much experience has been gained since the 1970s. The blood flow to the skin is related to blood pressure and microcirculation but not in a consistent fashion [28]. It can also be influenced by many factors including core temperature, ambient air temperature, humidity, light and vasomotor responses. Regional variations in the human skin surface temperature of 8°C were described as early as 1931 [29]. There are generally two types of temperature monitors available: infrared thermometry for evaluation of skin flaps and thermoelectric thermometers as described by Jones [7]. May et al developed a removable thermocouple probe implanted adjacent to the blood vessel of interest, with promising early results [30]. In a series of 18 free flaps, two venous thromboses were diagnosed early by this technique.

Most measurements today, however, are made with cutaneous thermocouples. They are made of two different metals producing a small voltage that varies with slight changes in skin temperature. Kaufman's study [31] of muscle flaps suggested that temperature monitoring was not a reliable indicator of flap perfusion, unless all environmental influences were monitored and kept absolutely constant, leaving perfusion as the only variable. Similarly, Issing [16] found temperature measurements in his experiments on pedicled skin flaps difficult to evaluate objectively due to fluctuations in room temperature, convection and individual variations in body temperature. Those flaps that had a more pronounced temperature loss were often more likely to remain viable. By way of

explanation, lowering tissue temperature by 10°C reduces metabolic demand by 50%, hence demand for blood flow is similarly reduced. These results supported the observations of DesPrez and Kiehn (1962) who achieved better survival of pedicled flaps under conditions of hypothermia. When properly applied and interpreted, large studies have shown the sensitivity of surface-temperature recording to be 98%, and its predictive value to be 75%, making it a simple, inexpensive, and reliable technique of free-flap monitoring [32] **(IIb/B)**.

Tissue oxygen tension

Tissue oxygen tension is increasingly recognised as a sensitive and reliable index of tissue perfusion, and preliminary studies suggest that it may be of value in the assessment of free-flap viability. Tissue oxygen tension can be monitored by implantable or surface probes. A pulse oximeter measures the percentage of oxygen saturation of haemoglobin using two separate wavelengths of light (660nm and 940nm) to distinguish between oxygenated and deoxygenated haemoglobin by light absorption differences. Mahoney and Lista in 1980 [33] described an implantable and disposable tissue oxygen tension monitor. Their initial experience with the technique suggested that a value of less than 20mmHg suggested vascular compromise and the need for careful evaluation of the flap. This technique is simple in its application, disposable and easily placed in the soft tissue of any flap. The sensor also provides digital data that are easy to interpret. However, the technique is invasive and further clinical work is needed to assess reliability of results. Hirigoyen et al [34] described the use of an implantable microcatheter oxygen sensor in a rabbit model. This sensor was sensitive, rapidly responsive and easily interpreted by non-specialist staff **(IIb/B)**.

Near-infrared spectroscopy

Near-infrared spectroscopy (NIRS) was introduced in the 1970s by Jöbsis, and clinician friendly systems were developed in the mid to late 1990s. Near infrared spectroscopy measures the percentage of oxygen saturation in haemoglobin and in the tissues, which correlates with tissue oxygenation. This is determined by both the oxygen delivered to the tissues and oxygen consumed [35]. Thorniley et al [36], in 1998, showed that NIRS was able to detect and distinguish between microcirculatory changes occurring as a result of arterial, venous or total vascular occlusion in a pig flap model. Scheufler et al [37], using a human pedicled TRAM flap model, found that postoperative changes in NIRS values corresponded to clinical observations and blood flow in the superior epigastric artery measured by colour-coded duplex ultrasonography **(IIb/B)**. More recently, in 2005, Li advocated the use of NIRS for flap monitoring after trialling the technique on seven head and neck reconstruction patients [38]. Further experience is needed before NIRS can be advocated for routine clinical flap monitoring, and more groups should be reporting on NIRS as a monitoring technique in the coming years [35].

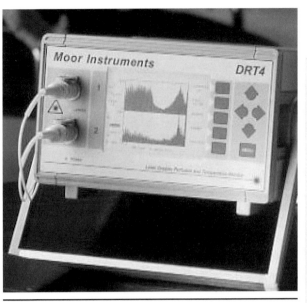

Figure 1. Laser Doppler flow meter monitoring system.

Erlangen microlightguide spectrophotometer

In 1996, Wolff [39] used a non-invasive Erlangen microlightguide spectrophotometer (EMPHO) to measure blood flow and oxygen supply in free flaps in rats and humans **(IIb/B)**. This technique allowed non-invasive examination of the entire flap surface and permitted a statement on the regional circulation and oxygen supply of individual flap areas. In addition, intra-oral flaps could be easily examined. Unfortunately this technique cannot be applied to deep flaps and continuous measurement over several days cannot be made with the EMPHO. Further clinical evaluation EMPHO is required.

Laser Doppler flowmeter (Figure 1)

A well known technique used for adjunctive monitoring of free tissue transfers postoperatively is the laser Doppler flowmeter (LDF), based on the Doppler shifting of laser light. This device allows qualitative blood flow measurements and is commercially available. After a preliminary report on the usefulness of the LDF as a free-flap monitor in 1982, it has become a widely accepted monitoring technique in the US. Laser Doppler flap monitoring can give warning of flap failures many hours before clinical signs are apparent [40]. Signs of a healthy flap

are a pulsatile LD blood flow waveform (on 'FAST' display mode), due to the cardiac cycle and a stable or steadily increasing trend. Fluctuations in LD blood flow are also good signs and are due to vasomotor and physiological responses. Signs of a failing flap include lack of pulsatility, a falling trend and lack of fluctuations. Alarm levels should be set relative to baseline flow rather than for 'normal' values, as even in the same tissues there are a wide range of values [41]. Further guidance on the interpretation of laser Doppler recordings are published elsewhere [42]. LDF is non-invasive and safe, can be used for buried and cutaneous free tissue transfers, provides continuous recording and can be used to assess anastomotic patency both intra- and postoperatively. It is strongly supported by many individuals and although the equipment is relatively expensive, it is perceived as being cost-effective [43, 44] **(IIb/B)**.

Photoplethysmography

Photoplethysmography utilises a green-light-emitting diode to transmit light into a tissue. Reflected light from haemoglobin in dermal capillary red blood cells is received by a photo detector and is analysed as light intensity along a frequency spectrum. This method of analysis facilitates the removal of 'noise' above (stray light and alternating current) and below (room vibrations and respiratory motion) the peak signal (1 to 2Hz) and results in a means by which to distinguish between perfused and non-perfused tissues. It has been shown that spectral analysis of photoplethysmograms from radial forearm free-flap patients provides an accurate and rapid means for determining pedicle vessel patency [45] (IIb/B).

Photoplethysmography may provide a clinically useful tool for postoperative perfusion monitoring of free flaps in the future.

Microdialysis

The metabolic activity of free flaps has been monitored using microdialysis as described by Udesen et al [46]. Microdialysis is a micro-sampling technique that allows a temporal study of the biochemistry in specific organs or tissues. A double-lumen microdialysis catheter or probe, with a dialysis membrane at the end, is introduced into the specific tissue. Perfusion fluid is slowly pumped through the catheter and equilibrates across the membrane with surrounding extracellular concentrations of low-molecular-weight substances. The dialysate is collected in microvials and analysed. Glucose, glycerol, and lactate concentrations were measured in the flaps and compared with those in a reference catheter that was placed subcutaneously. In the study by Udesen, during flap ischaemia, the concentration of glucose was reduced, while the lactate and glycerol levels increased. The differences between the flaps and controls were highly statistically significant. Udesen concluded that microdialysis could reliably detect ischaemia in free flaps at an early stage, making early surgical intervention possible (IIa/B).

Radiological techniques

A small group of experimental radiological techniques have been described in the literature to monitor free tissue transfers using magnetic resonance imaging. Magnetic resonance imaging [47] and nuclear magnetic resonance spectroscopy have been shown to be experimentally useful for examining microsurgical flaps; however, these techniques are too complicated and impractical for clinical use at present (IIb/B).

Implantable venous Doppler

A promising technique commercially available in the US is the Cook-Swartz implantable venous Doppler probe (Figure 2), first described by Swartz in 1994 [48]. This system consists of an implantable probe with a 20 MHz ultrasonic probe in a suturable cuff (an 8 x 5mm^2 thin silicone sheet), which provides direct vessel monitoring of microvascular anastomoses. The probe can be placed around the venous or arterial anastomoses, or both. The absence of the monitor's audible signal alerts the medical staff that a potential problem with perfusion may exist, thus providing the opportunity for early intervention. When vessel monitoring is completed, the probe may be removed by applying minimal traction, leaving only the cuff *in situ*. Several studies have shown this technique to be of use in monitoring free tissue transfers, particularly when the flap is buried [49-51] (IIb/B).

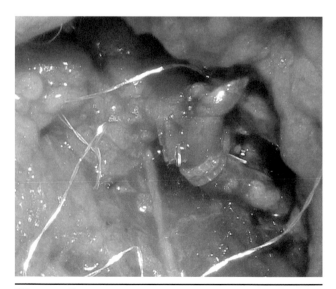

Figure 2. Cook-Swartz venous Doppler probe *in situ.*

Orthogonal polarization spectral imaging

Orthogonal polarization spectral (OPS) imaging represents a major innovation over conventional intravital microscopy, because of its portability and elimination of the need for special preparations. Light from a source is converted to a wavelength of 550 nanometers, the isobestic point for haemoglobin. Haemoglobin becomes the contrast agent allowing for optimal imaging of the microcirculation. The light passes through the first polarizer and is directed towards the tissue by a set of lenses. As the light hits the tissue, it is reflected back through the lenses. Most of the light reflecting off the tissue and returning through the lenses will remain polarized. Ten percent or less of the light will penetrate deeply into the tissue and go through multiple scattering events becoming depolarized. The depolarized light is reflected back through the lenses to a second polarizer or analyser. The analyser, orthogonal (90°) to the first polarizer, eliminates the reflected polarized light and allows the depolarized light to pass through to the CCD (charged couple device) videocamera. The depolarized light forms an image of the microcirculation on the CCD, which can be captured through single frames or on videotape. The image produced is as if the light source is actually placed behind the desired target or transilluminated. Given the success of validation studies on mouse skin flaps, investigators have suggested the technique be used to monitor flaps in humans [52-54].

Conclusions

There is a wide variation in the postoperative monitoring of free tissue transfers in the UK [2, 4, 5]. A huge number of techniques to monitor flaps in the postoperative period have been explored, and it is salient that most surgeons still rely on their own clinical observation. However, with the routine monitoring of free flaps on the ward often being undertaken by junior nurses and inexperienced junior doctors, it is increasingly clear that the development of an adjunctive reliable method of free-flap monitoring would be beneficial in detecting early flap failure (especially in buried free tissue transfers), to expedite successful salvage of such cases.

Over time, flap salvage rates decline significantly and the ideal time to detect a flap with inflow or outflow compromise is before the patient leaves the operating theatre. Implantable probes such as the Cook-Swartz Doppler system offer this exciting opportunity. As the specialty of plastic surgery expands, it is increasingly likely for the surgeon to consider free tissue transfer outside the plastic surgery unit. This will only be possible if reliable adjunctive monitoring techniques are available. Unfortunately, we can no longer assume our medical and nursing staff will always be able to develop the expertise to monitor our flaps effectively. The most reliable methods of postoperative monitoring available at present are clinical tests with adjunctive techniques such as the laser Doppler flow meter **(IIb/B)** or the implantable Cook-Swartz venous Doppler probe **(IIb/B)**. One would be more inclined to use adjunctive techniques in those flaps traditionally considered to be slightly higher risk or where vein grafts have been required [55]. Core temperature, urine output, oxygen saturations, blood pressure and pulse rate should all be closely monitored and charted in the days following the procedure. Close involvement of the anaesthetic staff in the postoperative period is often beneficial. Some of the other adjunctive techniques we describe, although not in routine use at present, may be logistically feasible to allow postoperative care to be optimised in the future.

Chapter 18

Recommendations	Evidence level

- There is a wide variation in practice in the UK. — III/C
- Clinical tests are the most commonly used monitoring technique. — III/C
- Laser Doppler and implantable venous Doppler probes should be considered as adjunctive monitoring methods especially in buried free tissue transfers. — IIb/B
- Newer techniques under evaluation including NIRS, microdialysis, photoplethysmography and orthogonal polarization spectral imaging may be logistically feasible to allow postoperative care to be optimised in the future. — IIb/B

References

1. Whitaker IS, Karoo ROS, Oliver DW, Ganchi PA, Gulati V, Malata CM. Master Class in Plastic Surgery: current techniques in the post-operative monitoring of microvascular free-tissue transfers. *Eur J Plast Surg* 2005; 27(7): 315-21.

2. Whitaker IS, Gulati V, Ross GL, Menon A, Ong TK. Variations in the postoperative management of free tissue transfers to the head and neck in the United Kingdom. *Br J Oral Maxillofac Surg* 2007; 45(1): 16-8.

3. Creech B, Miller S. Evaluation of circulation in skin flaps. In: *Skin Flaps*. Grabb WC, Myers MB, Eds. Boston: Little Brown; 1975.

4. Jallali N, Ridha H, Butler PE. Postoperative monitoring of free flaps in UK plastic surgery units. *Microsurgery* 2005; 25(6): 469-72.

5. Whitaker IS, Oliver DW, Ganchi PA. Postoperative monitoring of microvascular tissue transfers: current practice in the United Kingdom and Ireland. *Plast Reconstr Surg* 2003; 111(6): 2118-9.

6. Edwards EA, Duntley SQ. The pigments and colour of human living skin. *American Journal of Anatomy* 1939; 65(1): 1-33.

7. Jones BM. Monitors for the cutaneous microcirculation. *Plast Reconstr Surg* 1984; 73(5): 843-50.

8. Dagum AB, Dowd AJ. Simple monitoring technique for muscle flaps. *Microsurgery* 1995; 16(11): 728-9.

9. Dingwall JA, Lord JW. The fluorescein test in the management of tubed (pedicle) flaps. *Bulletin Johns Hopkins Hospital* 1943; 73: 129.

10. Conway H, Stark RB, Doktor JP. Vascularisation of tubed pedicles. *Plast Reconstr Surg* 1949; 4: 133-8.

11. McCraw JB, Myers B, Shanklin KD. The value of fluorescein in predicting the viability of arterialized flaps. *Plast Reconstr Surg* 1977; 60(5): 710-9.

12. Morykwas MJ, Hills H, Argenta LC. The safety of intravenous fluorescein administration. *Ann Plast Surg* 1991; 26(6): 551-3.

13. Kreidstein ML, Levine RH, Knowlton RJ, Pang CY. Serial fluorometric assessments of skin perfusion in isolated perfused human skin flaps. *Br J Plast Surg* 1995; 48(5): 288-93.

14. Silverman DG, LaRossa DD, Barlow CH, Bering TG, Popky LM, Smith TC. Quantification of tissue fluorescein delivery and prediction of flap viability with the fiberoptic dermofluorometer. *Plast Reconstr Surg* 1980; 66(4): 545-53.

15. Graham BH, Gordon L, Alpert BS, Walton R, Buncke HJ, Leitner DW. Serial quantitative skin surface fluorescence: a new method for postoperative monitoring of vascular perfusion in revascularized digits. *J Hand Surg (Am)* 1985; 10(2): 226-30.

16. Issing WJ, Naumann C. Evaluation of pedicled skin flap viability by pH, temperature and fluorescein: an experimental study. *J Craniomaxillofac Surg* 1996; 24(5): 305-9.

17. Eren S, Rubben A, Krein R, Larkin G, Hettich R. Assessment of microcirculation of an axial skin flap using indocyanine green fluorescence angiography. *Plast Reconstr Surg* 1995; 96(7): 1636-49.

18. Utoh J, Kunitomo R, Sakaguchi H, Hagiwara S, Uemura S, Uemura K, *et al.* Indocyanine green (JCG) clearance as a monitor to evaluate right heart function. *Kyobu Geka* 2000; 53(3): 212-4.

19. Raskin DJ, Erk Y, Spira M, Melissinos EG. Tissue pH monitoring in microsurgery: a preliminary evaluation of continuous tissue pH monitoring as an indicator of perfusion disturbances in microvascular free flaps. *Ann Plast Surg* 1983; 11(4): 331-9.

20. Raskin DJ, Nathan R, Erk Y, Spira M. Critical comparison of transcutaneous PO_2 and tissue pH as indices of perfusion. *Microsurgery* 1983; 4(1): 29-33.

21. Kety SS. The theory and application of the exchange of inert gas at the lungs and tissues. *Pharmacological Review* 1951; 3: 1-41.

22. Aygit AC, Sarikaya A. Technetium 99m sestamibi scintigraphy for noninvasive assessment of muscle flap viability. *Ann Plast Surg* 1999; 43(3): 338-40.

23. Tsuchida Y. Age-related changes in skin blood flow at four anatomic sites of the body in males studied by xenon-133. *Plast Reconstr Surg* 1990; 85(4): 556-61.

24. Harrison DH, Girling M, Mott G. Experience in monitoring the circulation in free-flap transfers. *Plast Reconstr Surg* 1981; 68(4): 543-55.

25. Aukland K, Bower BF, Berliner RW. Measurement of local blood flow with hydrogen gas. *Cir Res* 1964; 14: 164-87.

26. Glogovac SV, Bitz DM, Whiteside LA. Hydrogen washout technique in monitoring vascular status after replantation surgery. *J Hand Surg (Am)* 1982; 7(6): 601-5.

27. Sloan GM, Reinissch JF. Flap physiology and the prediction of flap viability. *Hand Clinics* 1985; 1(4): 609-19.

28. Tsuchida Y. Rate of skin blood flow in various regions of the body. *Plast Reconstr Surg* 1979; 64: 505.

29. Eddy HC, Taylor HP. Experiences with the Dermatherm in relation to peripheral vascular disease. *American Heart Journal* 1931; 6: 683.

30. May JW Jr, Lukash FN, Gallico GG 3rd, Stirrat CR. Removable thermocouple probe microvascular patency monitor - an experimental and clinical study. *Plast Reconstr Surg* 1983; 72: 366.

31. Kaufman T, Granick MS, Hurwitz DJ, Klain M. Is experimental muscle flap temperature a reliable indicator of its viability? *Ann Plast Surg* 1987; 19(1): 34-41.

32. Khouri RK, Shaw WW. Monitoring of free flaps with surface-temperature recordings: is it reliable? *Plast Reconstr Surg* 1992; 89(3): 495-9.

33. Mahoney JL, Lista FR. Variations in flap blood flow and tissue PO_2: a new technique for monitoring flap viability. *Ann Plast Surg* 1988; 20(1): 43-7.

34. Hirigoyen MB, Blackwell KE, Zhang WX, Silver L, Weinberg H, Urken ML. Continuous tissue oxygen tension measurement as a monitor of free-flap viability. *Plast Reconstr Surg* 1997; 99(3): 763-73.

35. Erdmann D, Klitzman B. Investigation of TRAM flap oxygenation and perfusion ny near-infrared reflection spectroscopy and color-coded duplex sonography. *Plast Reconstr Surg* 2004; 113(1): 153-4.

36. Thorniley MS, Sinclair JS, Barnett NJ, Shurey CB, Green CJ. The use of near-infrared spectroscopy for assessing flap viability during reconstructive surgery. *Br J Plast Surg* 1998; 51(3): 218-26.

37. Scheufler O, Exner K, Andresen R. Investigation of TRAM flap oxygenation and perfusion by near-infrared reflection spectroscopy and color-coded duplex sonography. *Plast Reconstr Surg* 2004; 113(1): 141-52.

38. Li Y, Ding HS, Huang L, Tian FH, Cai ZG. Application of near-infrared spectroscopy to postoperative monitoring of flap in plastic surgery. *Guang Pu Xue Yu Guang Pu Fen Xi* 2005; 25(3): 377-80.

39. Wolff KD, Marks C, Uekermann B, Specht M, Frank KH. Monitoring of flaps by measurement of intracapillary haemoglobin oxygenation with EMPHO II: experimental and clinical study. *Br J Oral Maxillofac Surg* 1996; 34(6): 524-29.

40. Jones BM, Mayou BJ. The laser Doppler flowmeter for microvascular monitoring: a preliminary report. *Br J Plast Surg* 1982; 35: 147-9.

41. Hellner D, Schmeize R. Laser Doppler monitoring of free microvascular flaps in maxillofacial surgery. *J Cranio-Maxillo-Facial Surg* 1993; 21: 25-9.

42. Svensson H, Holmberg J, Svedman P. Interpreting laser Doppler recordings from free flaps. *Scand J Plast Reconstr Hand Surgery* 1992; 27: 81-7.

43. Yuen JC, Feng Z. Monitoring free flaps using the laser Doppler flowmeter: five-year experience. *Plast Reconstr Surg* 2000; 105(1): 55-61.

44. Yuen JC, Feng Z. Reduced cost of extremity free flap monitoring. *Ann Plast Surg* 1998; 41(1): 36-40.

45. Stack BC Jr, Futran ND, Shohet MJ, Scharf JE. Spectral analysis of photoplethysmograms from radial forearm free flaps. *Laryngoscope* 1998; 108(9): 1329-33.

46. Udesen A, Lontoft E, Kristensen SR. Monitoring of free TRAM flaps with microdialysis. *J Reconstr Microsurg* 2000; 16(2): 101-6.

47. Elias DL, Nelson RC, Herbst MD, Zubowicz VN. Magnetic resonance imaging for detection of arterial and venous occlusion in canine muscle flaps and bowel segments. *Ann Surg* 1987; 206(5): 624-7.

48. Swartz WM, Izquierdo R, Miller MJ. Implantable venous Doppler microvascular monitoring: laboratory investigation and clinical results. *Plast Reconstr Surg* 1994; 93(1): 152-63.

49. Oliver DW, Whitaker IS, Giele H, Critchley P, Cassell O. The Cook-Swartz venous Doppler probe for the post-operative monitoring of free tissue transfers in the United Kingdom: a preliminary report. *Br J Plast Surg* 2005; 58(3): 366-70.

50. Pryor SG, Moore EJ, Kasperbauer JL. Implantable Doppler flow system: experience with 24 microvascular free-flap operations. *Otolaryngol Head Neck Surg* 2006; 135(5): 714-8.

51. Kind GM, Buntic RF, Buncke GM, Cooper TM, Siko PP, Buncke HJ, Jr. The effect of an implantable Doppler probe on the salvage of microvascular tissue transplants. *Plast Reconstr Surg* 1998; 101(5): 1268-73.

52. Olivier WA, Hazen A, Levine JP, Soltanian H, Chung S, Gurtner GC. Reliable assessment of skin flap viability using orthogonal polarization imaging. *Plast Reconstr Surg* 2003; 112(2): 547-55.

53. Erdmann D, Sweis R, Wong MS, Eyler CE, Olbrich KC, Levin LS, *et al*. Current perspectives of orthogonal polarization spectral imaging in plastic surgery. *Chirurg* 2002; 73(8): 827-32.

54. Langer S, Biberthaler P, Harris AG, Steinau HU, Messmer K. *In vivo* monitoring of microvessels in skin flaps: introduction of a novel technique. *Microsurgery* 2001; 21(7): 317-24.

55. Kroll SS, Schusterman MA, Reece GP, Miller MJ, Evans GR, Robb GL, *et al*. Choice of flap and incidence of free flap success. *Plast Reconstr Surg* 1996; 98(3): 459-63.

Chapter 18

Chapter 19

Use of the anterolateral thigh flap for intra-oral reconstruction

Emma Hormbrey BSc MB BS FRCS (Plast.)

Fellow in Head and Neck Surgery

Oliver Cassell MB ChB FRCS (Plast.) MS

Consultant Plastic and Reconstructive Surgeon

THE JOHN RADCLIFFE HOSPITAL, OXFORD, UK

Introduction

Oral cavity reconstruction after removal of locally advanced tumours is particularly challenging. Anatomical restoration must accurately reproduce the complex original structures; this enables effective and fast rehabilitation of mastication, swallowing and phonation. The requirements for intra-oral reconstruction are many and varied. Small flaps may be needed to allow mobility or replace thin defects. Larger flaps are required post-glossectomy or for the reconstruction of through and through defects. More than one flap may be required for reconstruction of more composite defects with associated bone loss.

Tumour resection is performed in conjunction with a neck dissection; therefore, a long flap pedicle may be required, depending on donor vessel availability. Furthermore, the defects themselves may extend down to include neck skin when extensive nodal masses are removed.

A wide variety of options are available for reconstruction of the oral cavity. Classically, a radial forearm free flap has been the mainstay for small intra-oral defects or subtotal tongue resection and the rectus abdominis free flap where bulk is required. These techniques have high success rates, can repair almost any soft tissue oral defect that might be encountered, and are still in common use today [1-3] **(IV/C)**. However, the anterolateral thigh flap can be modified to reconstruct the full range of intra-oral defects.

The anterolateral thigh flap was first described by Song and co-workers in 1984 [4]. It has become a key flap for many reconstructive surgeons in head and neck surgery over the last 10-15 years in Japan, Taiwan and the West [5-9] **(IV/B)**. Here we review its application with respect to intra-oral reconstruction.

Methodology

A Medline search was undertaken using the terms 'anterolateral thigh flap', 'ALT', 'complications', 'oral cavity' and 'reconstruction' for all publications listed. This was further supplemented by a datastar search by the Cochrane review team in Oxford using the mesh terms: anterolateral, antero, lateral, flap, intra-oral, intra, oral, oropharynx, pharynx, tongue, mandible, face, head, and neck with matches retrieved between 1983 and 2006. No clinical paper was identified to offer higher than grade III/B evidence for reconstruction of intra-oral defects. We review the evidence regarding the anatomy of the flap, its planning, marking, the technique of flap harvest, closure, alternative options, pedicle availability, flap size and versatility as it relates to intra-oral reconstruction.

Flap anatomy (Figure 1)

Arterial supply

The anterolateral thigh flap is but one component supplied by the lateral circumflex system, a branch of the profunda femoris artery.

The profunda femoris artery, as classically described in *Gray's Anatomy*, is a large branch arising laterally from the femoral artery about 3.5cm distal to the inguinal ligament. It then spirals posterior to the femoral artery and vein passing between pectineus and adductor longus.

It gives off the lateral circumflex femoral artery near its root. This artery runs laterally between the divisions of the femoral nerve, posterior to sartorius and rectus femoris, dividing into ascending, transverse and descending branches.

The ascending branch ascends along the intertrochanteric line under the tensor fascia lata. Lateral to the hip joint it anastomoses with the superior gluteal, deep circumflex femoral and the medial circumflex femoral arteries.

The transverse branch, the smallest, passes laterally anterior to vastus intermedius and pierces vastus lateralis to wind around the femur anastomosing with the medial circumflex, inferior gluteal and first perforating arteries, as the cruciate anatomosis, just distal to the greater trochanter.

The descending branch runs in the intermuscular septum between rectus femoris and vastus lateralis. It supplies rectus femoris with a branch which enters the muscle in its proximal third approximately 10cm below the inguinal ligament. It continues its descent in close relation with the nerve to vastus lateralis. Branches supply vastus lateralis and then the vessel extends as a long ramus within the muscle to anastomose with the lateral superior genicular branch of the popliteal artery.

The anterolateral thigh flap is a cutaneous flap based on perforators from the descending branch of the lateral circumflex femoral artery.

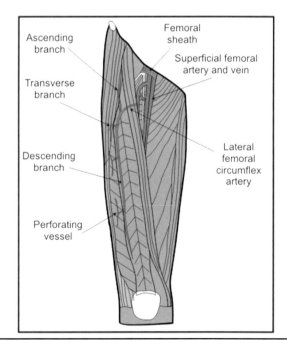

Figure 1. Anterolateral thigh flap anatomy. *Reproduced with the kind permission of Dr. Rudy Buntic, MD (microsurgeon.org).*

Table 1. Perforator classification [12].

Type	Perforator source from lateral circumflex femoral /direction across vastus lateralis	Percentage (n=37)
I	Musculocutaneous: descending branch/vertical	57 (21/37)
II	Musculocutaneous: transverse branch/horizontal	27 (10/37)
III	Septocutaneous: descending branch/vertical	11 (4/37)
IV	Septocutaneous: transverse branch/horizontal	5 (2/37)

The perforators supply thigh skin directly via septocutaneous vessels running in the intermuscular space, or more commonly, indirectly through branches to the vastus lateralis muscle as musculocutaneous perforators [5]. These perforators travel through the vastus lateralis muscle piercing the deep fascia and terminate in the anterolateral thigh skin after giving off numerous branches to the muscle from the side and posteriorly.

In the largest series to date, reported by Wei et al [5] after performing 672 cases, musculocutaneous perforators occurred in 87% of flaps, with only 13% of skin branches travelling in the septum [5, 10]. However, Yu et al found after a total of 72 flaps that no perforator could be identified in 6% of cases and the flap could not be raised [6, 11].

Not only is there variation in perforator anatomy but also in the main arterial vessel. This flap is classically described arising from the descending branch but in a significant number of cases, 32% in one study, the perforator arises from the transverse branch [12]. Furthermore, Kimata et al found that the vessel originated from the descending branch of the lateral circumflex artery in 84%, from the lateral circumflex femoral artery directly in 13%, from the profunda femoris artery in 1.4% and directly from the femoral artery in 1.4% [13].

Due to the variation in anatomy, different perforator classifications have been suggested. Shieh et al [12] created a four-part classification based on their experience in 37 flaps raised (Table 1), adding to the perceived complexity.

Depending on the flap vessel and perforator, the pedicle length varies between 8-15cm, with a vessel diameter of larger than 2mm, as evidenced from anatomical dissections of 42 unembalmed cadavers [14] and multiple clinical papers [4, 5, 6, 11] **(IV/C)**.

The variable route of vessels has also generated confusing 'perforator' flap terminology which Professor Wei attempted to clarify in 2005. He states that the term perforator should only be applied to flap harvest requiring intramuscular dissection of the supplying vessel: "If a skin only flap is harvested on a vessel which is of adequate calibre and divided before piercing the fascia it should be called a cutaneous anterolateral thigh cutaneous vessel flap. If the skin vessel is septocutanous, traversing between the rectus femoris and vastus lateralis muscles, it should be referred to as a cutaneous anterolateral thigh septocutaneous vessel flap. If the skin vessel pierces the vastus lateralis muscle and an intramuscular dissection is performed taking this vessel with the flap it should be called a cutaneous anterolateral thigh myocutaneous perforator flap" [15]. Furthermore, if only skin is harvested the flap should be prefixed cutaneous; if more than skin is harvested on the same vessel it should be prefixed as compound; if components based on alternative branches are included the flap should be described as combined.

The branches of the lateral circumflex femoral artery supply multiple components that can be harvested based on this system. There are many variations of combined flaps available with an anterolateral thigh flap incorporating anteromedial skin, vacularised lateral femoral cutaneous nerve, fascia lata, vastus lateralis, rectus femoris, tensor fascia lata, and iliac crest [16-20]. These components may be based on separate branches facilitating flap insetting to the complex three-dimensional defects created by resections in the oral cavity.

Venous anatomy

Little is written specifically addressing the venous drainage of this flap but in general one or two venae commitantes are mentioned running with the main arterial vessel and from personal experience are of a smaller calibre than the artery until the main root of the pedicle is dissected.

Nerves

For sensory innervated anterolateral thigh flaps, branches of the lateral cutaneous nerve of the thigh that emerge from below the inguinal ligament can be harvested [21]. This nerve divides into two or three branches: the largest branch (1.5-2.0mm in diameter) proceeds downward along the anterior aspect of the thigh and innervates the inferiolateral thigh. The smaller branches (0.5-1.0mm in diameter) innervate the midlateral aspect of the thigh and are included for tongue reconstruction [19].

Fascia

The classic flap is raised in a plane beneath the fascia lata, thereby retaining the fascia with the flap. However, no fascia is taken in a pure suprafascial cutaneous flap but a small cuff may be taken where the perforator pierces the fascia. The other extreme is to incorporate fascial extensions for reconstructive use such as to recreate oral continence [17, 22, 23] or for protection of the great vessels (personal experience) when intra-oral surgery is combined with radical neck dissections and vessel exposure.

Planning

Patient assessment

A general assessment of the patient is essential prior to surgery both in terms of their general health and suitability to undergo free flap surgery. Appraisal of the donor sites will influence the site of flap harvest.

Relevant considerations include:

- Body mass index (BMI). Yu *et al* [6] found in their study of the Western characteristics of the anterolateral thigh flap that patient BMI correlated with flap thickness. This will impact on skin laxity and hence donor-site closure and cosmesis. The BMI will also influence the bulk of the flap and the potential need for flap thinning **(IV/B)**.
- Previous trauma or surgery may preclude the use of this flap.
- Pre-existent peripheral vascular disease may influence its use. A vascular history and assessment of the peripheral pulses, especially the popliteal, will give a guide. The anterolateral thigh flap has been raised in patients with known peripheral vascular disease as the profundus system appears to be spared and forms part of the collateral network allowing distal perfusion. However, partial necrosis of the foot and calf after flap harvest has been documented. Therefore, pre-operative angiography with planning for potential venous bypass grafting has been recommended in patients without a palpable popliteal pulse, as the descending branch of the lateral circumflex artery may prove to be a critical collateral on flap pedicle microclamping [24] **(IV/C)**.

Others have also associated increased complications of marginal necrosis and flap dehiscence in patients with both peripheral vascular disease and diabetes [25] **(IV/C)**.

Surface marking

The description seems largely standard: the patient is placed in a supine position and a line is drawn between the anterior superior iliac spine to the superolateral border of the patella. This line represents the muscular septum between the rectus femoris and the vastus lateralis muscles.

The cutaneous vessels can be mapped pre-operatively by a portable hand-held pencil Doppler probe, centred over the midpoint of this line. Lida *et al*

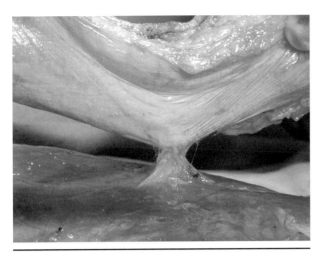

Figure 2. Intramuscular perforator ascending the elevated flap with the fascia lata.

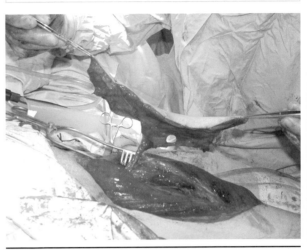

Figure 3. A raised ALT flap and island on its pedicle.

found after assessing 17 anterolateral thigh flap patients that pre-operative colour Doppler flowmetry provides 100% concordance with intra-operative perforator location in comparison to only 40% with acoustic Doppler [26, 27] **(Ib/A)**. The majority of the skin perforators are located within a circle with a 3cm radius centred on this midpoint. Xu *et al* [28] located at least one perforator in the inferolateral quadrant of this circle in 80% of cases **(III/B)** (although further perforators throughout the anterolateral thigh flap have been documented [6]). The flap is centred over the location of these vessels, and its long axis is designed parallel to that of the thigh.

Operation

Two key steps are involved in elevating the anterolateral thigh flap. The first is to locate the cutaneous perforators at the subfascial level where they exit the muscle or septum to enter the fascia. The second is to follow these perforators from the subfascial level to their origin from the main pedicle (Figures 2 and 3).

The technique of dissection appears standard and begins at the medial border of the flap, which should be located over the rectus femoris muscle, as recommended by Wei *et al* [29] **(IV/C)**. A long 15cm incision is made [6] and extended through the fascia lata. The flap is raised laterally for a short distance until the intermuscular septum between the rectus

femoris and vastus lateralis is reached. At this stage a septocutaneous vessel may be seen and the descending branch of the lateral femoral circumflex artery is then identified in the groove between the rectus femoris and vastus lateralis, facilitating further dissection. However, septocutaneous vessels are only encountered in 10-18% of cases. Therefore, in the majority of cases flap harvest requires careful dissection laterally through the septum to identify a suitable intramuscular perforator.

Once the musculocutaneous perforator is found the main pedicle is then defined. The lateral limit of the flap is then incised. The course of the perforator from the skin to the main pedicle is then exposed by careful division of the muscle overlying it. The small muscular branches are ligated. If the perforator is large, skeletonisation is acceptable, but if small, Wei [5] advises that a 'muscle cuff' should be included with the perforator. This is a painstaking dissection unnecessary in alternative flaps, such as the radial forearm and rectus abdominis.

In the majority of cases, as discussed previously, the main pedicle is the descending branch of the lateral circumflex femoral artery. The vessel is dissected proximally and divided according to pedicle length requirements whilst preserving the motor branch to vastus lateralis, which is closely related to it [29].

In general, the pedicle to rectus femoris is preserved to avoid the potential risk of muscle necrosis; however, Kimata documented 17 cases wherein the branch was sacrificed and found that donor-site dysfunction, i.e. fatigue on walking, climbing stairs and manual muscle tests, correlated with the extent of intramuscular dissection of the vastus lateralis not directly with ligation of the rectus blood supply [30]. Unfortunately, it is not clear in the text whether these situations are mutually exclusive and preservation if possible seems prudent.

Thus the most significant problem documented with this flap has been the technical demands of raising it. This is because of variability in the perforator anatomy and the necessity of a relatively difficult intramuscular perforator dissection with concomitant risk to the pedicle.

Perforators may arise from different branches of the lateral circumflex femoral artery. Mourougayan recommended microclamping the pedicles in turn and if flap viability was threatened anastomosing both to separate recipient vessels [31].

The variability in vessel location in comparison with other flaps with more reliable anatomy naturally generates insecurity in the occasional user. Such problems may discourage many from its use.

Closure

In their series of 672 flaps, Wei et al describe repair of the muscle dissection and fascial repair if the fascial harvest is less than 2-3cm. They describe that flaps of 6-9cm in width can be closed directly over drains [5] (IV/C). Chen et al found that large donor defects greater than 8-10cm in width will require skin grafting [32] (IV/C). Hallock has shown that pre-expansion allows primary donor defect closure; this is not possible in ablative cancer cases due to the time delay required for expansion [33].

Donor-site advantages

As there is no special positioning on the operating table, a simultaneous two-team approach reduces operative time and allows the reconstructive surgeon to start harvesting the flap [8] (IV/C) as the tumour resection is being carried out. Furthermore, as a large flap can be raised and the donor site directly closed,

the flap dimensions can be tailored after the recipient vessel identification and tumour removal has taken place. This is important as the time for flap harvest can vary considerably depending on whether harvest is easy or requires a difficult and time-consuming intramuscular dissection.

The anterolateral thigh flap causes minor donor-site sequelae in the majority of cases. These range from mild contour defects (22%), sensory disturbance in the thigh (50%), cold intolerance if skin grafts are required (13%), but no significant impairment in range of motion and muscle strength of the donor leg [9, 34] (II/B). This is especially important in elderly patients with significant comorbidity, common in many head and neck cancer patients, who often have chronic obstructive pulmonary disease and minimal pulmonary reserve due to smoking.

The ability to achieve early mobilisation and hence a quick recovery decreases postoperative complications and shortens hospital stay benefiting both the patient and hospital.

Donor-site disadvantages

Seroma is a common donor-site complication occurring in up to 13%, despite large bore drain use [35]. However, it does not have a major impact on rehabilitation (IV/C).

Either handling or harvest of the lateral cutaneous nerve of the thigh to innervate an intra-oral reconstruction may cause some patients to experience numbness within its distribution (IV/C).

Donor-site dysfunction has been found to correlate with the degree of damage to the vastus lateralis muscle as a result of tissue harvest. The most incapacitating procedure, however, appears to be the use of skin grafts. Kimata et al found that three out of five patients grafted had limited range of motion in the hip and knee compared with primary closure [30] (III/B).

The donor-site scars associated with skin grafts in reconstructing massive intra-oral defects may preclude its use on aesthetic grounds, particularly in female patients (IV/C).

Pedicle length

The pedicle of this flap is long, up to 15cm [36], and of large calibre, making it particularly useful for intra-oral and combined midfacial reconstruction when recipient vessels are at a distance in the neck or their availability is compromised by radical neck dissections [8] **(IV/C)**.

Furthermore, the continuation of the descending branch of the lateral circumflex femoral artery is of sufficient calibre that it can be used for anastomosis of a second flap in chimeric fashion, e.g. the fibula flap in oromandibular reconstruction.

Flap size

The size range of flap that can be raised is wide whilst still allowing direct closure. This is particularly applicable to head and neck cancer patients who have increased skin laxity due to weight loss. Anatomical studies have shown that the total area which can be harvested can extend to 12 x 30cm [28] and successful clinical cases of up to 18 x 25cm have been documented [37]. Hence, both the small intra-oral floor of the mouth or partial tongue defects are accommodated, as well as the more extensive tongue and tonsillar reconstructions **(IV/C)**.

Flap thickness

Thigh skin itself is thicker than forearm skin and is not normally put through as great a range of movement as the forearm. However, as yet there has not been any documented disadvantage relating to this in terms of intra-oral pliability to set a precedent for flap choice.

The anterolateral thigh flap is often of thin to moderate thickness in this group of patients, due to associated problems of oral intake and weight loss, making it pliable and easily adaptable to the structural peculiarities resulting from lip, buccal, retromolar trigone, palatal, and tongue defects [17, 18, 25] **(IV/C)**.

The anterolateral thigh flap was first made popular in Asia where the general population is thinner compared with Western patients [6]. The flap (skin and subcutaneous tissue) is on average 7mm thick in Asian patients, which compares favourably with the radial forearm (2mm) and inferior epigastric territory (13mm) [38]. However, it is almost double this thickness in the Western population, correlating with the BMI of the patient, and is significantly thicker in women compared with men [6]. This bulk may make it unsuitable for certain areas, such as the alveolus or floor of the mouth where a thin flap is required **(IV/C)**. When too thick, the flap can be modified by raising it suprafascially [39] or by direct thinning **(IV/C)**.

Primary thinning has been successful to a thickness of 3-5mm, with careful preservation of a small rim of fat at the level of the perforator vessels [25, 29, 38, 40] **(III/B)**. Kimura *et al* determined that the safe radius of a thin anterolateral thigh flap with a thickness of 3-4mm was approximately 9cm from the point where the perforator met the skin. This was based on the retrospective review of 31 thinned flaps as the skin blood supply beyond this limit was unreliable and resulted in marginal necrosis [22, 41] **(III/B)**. Longer flaps have been raised by preserving subcutaneous fat in a 3-4cm area around the perforator along with the subdermal fat and its associated venous network to ensure venous drainage [23] **(IV/C)**. This concept is supported by recent cadaveric CT angiography studies demonstrating that vascular communications between the fascial, adipose and dermal layers of the flap were maximised within a 5cm radius of the perforator entry within the flap [42] **(III/B)**. However, clinical success has not been universal and others advocate thinning as a secondary procedure. This decision is based on both clinical experience [43] and anatomical cadaveric injection dye studies demonstrating damage to the fascial plexus and oblique vessels supplying the subdermal plexus [44] **(III/B)**.

Alternative thinning techniques of 'lipectomy' are evolving. In this technique fat globules are painstakingly removed while preserving the vascular network (personal communication). This may offer added security in the future. Therefore, although one-stage flap thinning is possible, it is time-consuming, requires meticulous dissection and may jeopardise flap survival in inexperienced hands.

On the contrary, a thicker flap is more desirable for subtotal or total glossectomy defects for which a rectus abdominis flap is commonly used [45] **(IV/C)**. Harvesting an anterolateral thigh flap with part of the vastus lateralis muscle provides a suitable alternative.

Flap versatility

Different insetting techniques can be applied to the standard flap or various combined flaps can be raised based on the lateral circumflex axis creating a larger armamentarium for the reconstructive surgeon.

In large full-thickness cheek defects, the flap skin paddle can be tailored to recreate both surfaces by either folding the flap with the intervening folded portion being de-epithelialised, or by splitting the flap into two skin paddles based on separate cutaneous perforators [46] **(IV/C)**.

For the reconstruction of extensive composite oromandibular defects involving large lip, cheek, and intra-oral resection, double flaps are usually required [8]. Ao describes use of the free fibular flap for mandibular reconstruction combined with the anterolateral thigh flap to reconstruct the alveolus, floor of mouth and tongue defects in six cases. They utilised the long pedicle and continuation of the descending branch as flow through for the fibular anastomosis since recipient vessels were absent in the vicinity due to previous radiotherapy or surgery [47] **(IV/C)**.

Jeng et al have addressed the difficult problem of massive intra-oral, mandibular and lip resection by combining a fibula flap for the mandible and an anterolateral thigh flap for the associated cheek and lip defects. A long sheet of fascia lata was harvested from the thigh donor site and tunnelled subcutaneously to recreate the oral sphincter [17] and restore oral continence. Alternatively, the flap has been harvested by Vildirim et al with 5cm fascial extensions in continuity at the superior and inferior margins. These strips were then split longitudinally into two and are used to recreate sphincter function suturing one to the other and the orbicularis via a tunnel through the orbicularis muscle in the upper lip and anchoring the second to the zygoma for static support [18].

Where intra-oral defects have a significant volume deficit, folded de-epithelialised segments or part of the vastus lateralis muscle have been used to fill in dead space in the neck, the floor of the mouth or the cheek, to give a good contour to the recipient site and avoid a long-term sunken appearance, improving cosmesis [25]. This is especially true of the dead space left by extirpation of the masseter muscle, buccal fat pad and the parotid gland with extensive oral and midface resections. Similarly, total glossectomy defects require significant bulk to restore height and volume to the reconstructed tongue and an anterolateral thigh flap may be used in preference to a rectus abdominis musculocutaneous flap for its donor-site benefits **(IV/C)**.

Flap innervation

Sensory innervation with neurorrhaphy to a transected lingual nerve has been recommended for large tongue defects when direct neurotisation will be less effective. The anterolateral thigh flap may be innervated by harvesting branches of the lateral cutaneous nerve of the thigh, a more straightforward procedure than harvesting an innervated rectus abdominis with its multiple intercostal branches. Yu et al [6] compared 13 innervated with 16 non-innervated flaps for hemiglossectomy reconstructions and found better touch, pin prick, temperature and two-point discrimination pressure sensory recovery in the innervated group, with the greatest recovery in the innervated anterolateral thigh group (8), compared with the innervated rectus abdominis group (5) **(III/B)**. However, numbers were small and none achieved protective sensation.

Although rarely used, motor re-innervation with vastus lateralis muscle is possible in complex defects involving the upper lateral face where facial dynamics need to be reconstructed [48].

Conclusions

Providing a reconstruction with the ideal aesthetic, functional, and donor-site outcomes places increasing demands on modern-day practice. The anterolateral thigh flap is versatile and useful for a variety of intra-oral reconstructive problems.

Advances in perforator flaps have provided familiarity with the technique required for safe dissection with success rates of over 96% in experienced hands making this a reliable flap once raised [5].

The anterolateral thigh flap can be harvested with a skin paddle as large as that of abdominal perforator flaps and avoids the issue of abdominal donor-site complications when musculocutaneous flaps are raised. The flap can be harvested as thin as the radial forearm flap but its main advantage is the reduced donor-site morbidity. The anterolateral thigh flap can therefore be used in most intra-oral reconstructions where previously the radial forearm or rectus abdominis flap has been the preferred option.

Patient positioning allows a two-team approach with harvest of the flap able to proceed simultaneously with the tumour resection, and therefore has clear advantages over scapular, parascapular and latissimus dorsi flaps. The anterolateral thigh flap, therefore, provides a versatile option for all intra-oral defects.

Recommendations	Evidence level
◆ Pre-operative colour Doppler flowmetry accurately maps perforator location.	Ib/A
◆ Careful flap elevation minimises functional donor-site morbidity and facilitates early postoperative ambulation.	II/B
◆ Vascular communications between fascial, adipose and dermal layers of the ALT flap are maximal within 5cm of the point at which the perforator enters the flap.	III/C
◆ Large intra-oral reconstructions can be undertaken using multiple skin paddles or by combining the ALT flap with other flaps as a chimeric free tissue transfer.	IV/C
◆ The ALT flap can be innervated by coaption of its sensory nerve to the lateral cutaneous nerve of the thigh.	III/B

References

1. Zhang B, Yamada A. Donor site choice of free flaps in head and neck reconstruction after tumor surgery. *Zhongguo Xiu Fu Chong Jian Wai Ke Za Zhi* 2005; 19(10): 777-9.

2. Andry G, Hamoir M, Leemans CR. The evolving role of surgery in the management of head and neck tumors. *Curr Opin Oncol* 2005; 17(3): 241-8.

3. Jeng SF, Kuo YR, Wei FC, Su CY, Chien CY. Reconstruction of concomitant lip and cheek through-and-through defects with combined free flap and an advancement flap from the remaining lip. *Plast Reconstr Surg* 2004; 113(2): 491-8.

4. Song YG, Chen GZ, Song YL. The free thigh flap: a new free flap concept based on the septocutaneous artery. *Plast Reconstr Surg* 1984; 37: 149-59.

5. Wei FC, Jain V, Celik N, Chen HC, Chuang DC, Lin CH. Have we found an ideal soft-tissue flap? An experience with 672 anterolateral thigh flaps. *Plast Reconstr Surg* 2002; 109(7): 2219-26; discussion 2227-30.

6. Yu P. Characteristics of the anterolateral thigh flap in a western population and its application in head and neck reconstruction. *Head and Neck* 2004; 26(9): 759-69.

7. Kuo Y-R, Jeng S-F, Kuo M-H, Liu Y-T, Lai P-W. Versatility of the free anterolateral thigh flap for reconstruction of soft tissue defects: review of 140 cases. *Ann Plast Surg* 2002; 48(2): 161-6.

8. Koshima I, Hosoda S, Inagawa K, Urushibara K, Moriguchi T. Free combined anterolateral thigh flap and vascularised fibula for wide through-and-through oromandibular defects. *J Reconstr Microsurg* 1998; 14(8): 529-34.

9. Huang CH, Chen HC, Huang YL, Mardini S, Feng GM. Comparison of the radial forearm flap and the thinned anterolateral thigh cutaneous flap for reconstruction of tongue defects and evaluation of donor-site morbiditiy. *Plast Reconstr Surg* 2004; 114(7): 1704-10.

10. Yildirim S, Avci G, Akoez T. Soft-tissue reconstruction using a free anterolateral thigh flap: experience with 28 patients. *Ann Plast Surg* 2003; 51(1): 37-44.

11. Kimata Y, Uchiyama K, Sakubara M, Ebihara S, Nakatsuka T, Harii K. Anterolateral thigh flap for reconstruction of head and neck defects. *Jpn J Plast Reconstr Surg* 2001; 44(2): 127-45.

12. Shieh SJ, Chiu HY, Yu JC, Pan SC, Tsai ST, Shen CL. Free anterolateral thigh flap for reconstruction of head and neck defects following cancer ablation. *Plast Recontr Surg* 2000; 105(7): 2349-57.

13. Kimata Y, Uchiyama K, Ebihara S, Nakatsuka T, Harii K. Anatomic variations and technical problems of the anterolateral thigh flap: a report of 74 cases. *Plast Reconstr Surg* 1998; 102(5): 1517-23.

14. Shimizu T, Fisher DR, Carmichael SW, Bite U. An anatomic comparison of septocutaneous free flaps from the thigh region. *Ann Plast Surg* 1997; 38(6): 604-10.

Table 1. Nahabedian classification of muscle-sparing TRAM flaps.

Muscle-sparing technique	Definition (rectus abdominis)
MS-0	Full width, partial length.
MS-1	Preservation of lateral segment
MS-2	Preservation of lateral and medial segments
DIEP (MS-3)	Preservation of entire muscle

Further complicating any meaningful comparison between the various flaps is the variety of methods used across studies to assess donor-site morbidity. Methods of assessment have variously included: rates of postoperative abdominal wall asymmetry/bulge/fascial laxity/hernia; the ability to perform sit-ups/curl-ups; physiotherapist assessment; structured interviews; specific activities of daily living (ADL)/symptom questionnaires; generic health questionnaires (e.g. SF-36); isokinetic dynamometry; postoperative morphine requirements; length of hospital stay; and CT and MRI assessment. This, of course, generates a further question: which of these outcome measurements are clinically meaningful?

A final problem relates to statistical analysis. Put simply, many studies are underpowered to detect statistically significant differences between the study groups [12]. This is particularly the case where the outcome measurement of interest is expressed as a rate or percentage, e.g. hernia formation. It is, therefore, prudent to examine trends within results as well as the hard statistics.

Methodology

To compare TRAM and DIEP flaps a Medline search was performed to identify relevant studies using the search terms, 'transverse rectus abdominis myocutaneous', 'transverse rectus abdominis musculocutaneous', 'TRAM', 'deep inferior epigastric artery perforator', 'DIEP', 'DIEaP', 'breast reconstruction'. Studies reporting on outcomes from TRAM and/or DIEP flap breast reconstruction were then reviewed. An evidence level and grade were assigned where an appropriate conclusion could be reached.

Aesthetic results and patient satisfaction

The aesthetic results of TRAM or DIEP flap breast reconstructions are generally good to excellent as rated by patients, surgeons or independent observers [13-22] **(IIb/B)**. Moreover, these results persist over time with 94% of patients maintaining an acceptable aesthetic result at five-year follow-up [16]. Several studies have failed to find any statistically significant differences between free and pedicled TRAM flap reconstructions in terms of patient satisfaction [20, 23-25] **(IIb/B)**. Similarly, free TRAM and DIEP flaps have comparable levels of patient satisfaction [21, 22] **(IIb/B)**.

While patient satisfaction is similar, no study has been undertaken to directly compare the aesthetic results of free TRAM and DIEP flap breast reconstructions. However, there are comparative studies that report higher satisfaction with breast shape [26], symmetry [14] and overall aesthetic result [14] among free TRAM flap patients compared with pedicled TRAM patients. By contrast, other studies report that pedicled TRAM flaps produce superior aesthetic results [16].

In a retrospective study of 237 free or pedicled TRAM flap reconstructions, Kroll *et al* [27] analysed numerous potential factors affecting aesthetic outcome. Nine independent judges rated the aesthetic result using postoperative photographs. Bilateral reconstructions were found to be aesthetically superior to unilateral reconstructions and immediate reconstructions were superior to delayed reconstructions. Mean aesthetic results were also higher for the free TRAM flap versus the pedicled TRAM flap group, but when tested by multiple regression analysis, this trend was not statistically significant **(III/B)**.

In addition to the aesthetic quality of the neo-breast, it is also worth considering the aesthetic impact of TRAM and DIEP flap surgery upon the abdomen. In a review of 150 pedicled TRAM flap patients 5-7 years after surgery, Mizgala *et al* [24] found self-reported improvement in the aesthetic appearance of the abdomen as a result of surgery in 72.4% of respondents. In addition, the aesthetic appearance of the abdomen was rated more highly than matched controls. Similarly, in a smaller study, Dulin *et al* [28] reported a mean improvement from 5.1 to 6.8 (on a scale of 1-10) in the aesthetic appearance of the abdomen following pedicled TRAM flap surgery. Similarly, Schaverien *et al* [22] reported very high rates of satisfaction with the results of surgery on the abdomen following both free MS-0 TRAM and DIEP flaps. By contrast, Blondeel *et al* compared free MS-0 TRAM flaps with DIEP flaps and approximately one third of patients in each group reported an improvement in appearance, while 47% and 25% of patients, respectively, reported deterioration in aesthetic appearance of the abdomen (non-significant) [21].

Contour abnormalities and hernia

Contour abnormalities include defects variously described as fascial laxity, upper and lower abdominal bulge and epigastric fullness. Some authors would also include within this group abdominal asymmetry, on the premise that the underlying pathology is the same. Contour abnormalities and hernia following abdominal flap surgery are likely to represent a continuum commencing with abdominal wall laxity and attenuation manifest as an abdominal bulge, through to a true fascial defect and resultant hernia formation. In an attempt to reduce these complications, there has been a trend away from pedicled TRAM flaps towards muscle-sparing techniques.

With regard specifically to hernia formation, many large series report very low or no incidences with all varieties of TRAM flap and the DIEP flap [8, 9, 29-33]. Although some authors advocate the routine use of mesh [34, 35], none of the cited series did so routinely, suggesting that this is not a prerequisite for low rates of hernia formation even when using pedicled TRAM flaps **(III/B)**.

Close attention to the method of fascial closure is important in preventing postoperative contour abnormalities, including hernia formation. Kroll *et al* [36] reviewed 130 pedicled TRAM flap patients each of whom had undergone one of three different methods of abdominal wall closure. Patients who had a two-layer fascial closure had a significantly lower rate of abdominal wall bulge when compared with single-layer fascial closure groups (8% vs 33-40%).

The role of muscle sparing per se in preventing contour abnormalities is harder to elucidate. Studies directly comparing incidences of contour abnormality and hernia between free and pedicled TRAM flaps have recorded mixed results but have mostly found no significant differences [2, 30, 32, 36]. Similarly, comparative studies of free TRAM and DIEP flaps have found mixed results [37-39]. Most of these studies, however, are limited by their small sample size.

In a series of studies, Nahabedian has comprehensively evaluated the relationship between muscle sparing flaps and abdominal wall contour abnormalities [8, 9, 29, 30]. These studies have coincided with an evolution in the authors' practice away from pedicled and free MS-0 TRAM flaps toward MS-2 TRAM and DIEP flaps. The earliest of these studies demonstrated significantly higher rates of contour deformity associated with pedicled TRAM flaps when compared with free TRAM flaps (22% vs 6%); an excess of upper abdominal abnormalities in the former group accounted for a large part of this disparity **(III/B)**. Similarly, bilateral TRAM flaps resulted in a higher incidence of contour abnormalities when compared with unilateral TRAM flaps (27% vs 7%) **(III/B)**. These findings remained significant after controlling for confounding factors using multiple regression analysis. Interestingly, it was only in the case of bilateral reconstructions that muscle-sparing TRAM flaps (MS-1 + MS-2) demonstrated a significant advantage over non-muscle-sparing (MS-0) TRAM flaps in terms of reducing contour abnormalities. In subsequent studies, MS-2 TRAM flaps were compared directly with DIEP flaps. These studies found no significant differences in the rates of contour abnormalities between the groups, although there was a trend towards reduced contour abnormalities in the DIEP flap group, particularly for bilateral reconstruction (unilateral reconstructions, 4.6% vs 1.5%, respectively; bilateral reconstructions, 21% vs 4.5%, respectively). Similarly, Bajaj et al [10] found a non-significant trend for increased postoperative bulge in MS-2 TRAM flaps when compared with DIEP flaps (7% vs 4%).

Postoperative pain and recovery

Kroll et al demonstrated that postoperative morphine requirements **(IIb/B)** and length of hospital stay were significantly lower amongst DIEP flap patients when compared with free MS-0 TRAM flap patients, although the reduction in length of stay was less than one full day [40] **(III/B)**. Other authors have failed to find any significant increase in length of hospital stay following MS-0 TRAM flap compared with DIEP flap reconstructions [22].

Reporting on the prevalence of long-term pain, Mizgala et al [24] found varying degrees of abdominal pain and discomfort in 28% of patients at 5-7 years following pedicled TRAM flap reconstruction. Amongst matched unoperated controls, the rate was 15.2%, although this difference was not statistically significant. Similarly, back pain was more frequent amongst patients than controls (46% versus 24%), but again, this was not statistically significant. In contrast Lejour and Dome found no excess of back pain amongst pedicled TRAM flap patients on long-term follow-up [23].

Several studies have directly compared free TRAM with DIEP flaps. Futter et al [38] found that long-term abdominal pain was a more frequent complaint amongst a cohort of muscle-sparing (not specified) free TRAM flap patients than in DIEP flap patients (22% versus 6%, respectively). Blondeel et al [21] similarly found higher rates of chronic abdominal pain amongst MS-0 free TRAM flap patients when compared with DIEP flap patients (47% versus 25%).

None of the above differences were, however, statistically significant. By contrast, in a direct comparison of free MS-0 TRAM flaps with DIEP flap groups at least six months post-surgery, Schaverien et al [22] found that both groups only 'rarely' suffered from abdominal pain

In a further study directly comparing DIEP flaps with MS-2 TRAM flaps (203 flaps), there were no significant differences in postoperative abdominal or back pain reported between the two groups [10]. In both groups the vast majority of patients (80% and 72%, respectively) reported abdominal pain dissipating completely within a few days to a few weeks following their operation.

Vascular complications

A perceived benefit of free TRAM flaps when compared with pedicled TRAM flaps is their superior vascularity. This has been confirmed by in vivo haemodynamic studies demonstrating the superior cutaneous blood flow in the free TRAM flap as opposed to the pedicled TRAM flap [41, 42]. A number of studies have demonstrated significantly higher rates of fat necrosis in pedicled TRAM than in free TRAM flaps [3, 43] **(III/B)**. Kroll et al [44] assessed fat necrosis using mammography and clinical examination, and found significantly higher rates of fat necrosis in pedicled TRAM flaps as opposed to free TRAM flaps (26.9% vs 8.2%; 13.4% vs 2%, respectively). A number of authors have also reported higher rates of partial flap necrosis in pedicled TRAM compared with free TRAM flaps (13-33% versus 0%) [3, 4, 45] **(III/B)**.

One of the primary concerns with regard to DIEP flaps is the reliability of their blood supply when compared with traditional MS-0 TRAM flaps. An increased incidence of partial flap loss and fat necrosis has been reported by experienced microsurgeons during their early experience with the DIEP flap [6]. In a series of unselected patients, Kroll reported very high rates of fat necrosis (62.5%) and partial flap loss (37.5%) [6]. Subsequently, DIEP flaps were only performed in individuals with a perforator with a palpable pulse and a vein of at least 1mm diameter. In addition, at least 30% of the flap

Table 2. Vascular complication rates with DIEP and TRAM flaps.

First author and reference	Year	Flap	No. of flaps	Major/total flap necrosis (%)	Partial flap necrosis (%)	Fat necrosis (%)	Venous congestion (%)	Return to theatre (%)
Patterson [47]	1995	Pedicled TRAM	729	0	5	11	NR	NR
Blondeel [37]	1999	DIEP	100	2	7	6	NR	6
Kroll [6]	2000	MS-0 free TRAM	279	1.1	2.2	12.9	NR	NR
		DIEP (unselected)	8	0	37.5	62.5	NR	NR
		DIEP (selected)	23	0	8.7	17.4	NR	NR
Nahabedian [8]	2002	(MS-0, 1 + 2) free TRAM	143	3.5	0	9.8	1.4	11
		DIEP	20	5	0	10	0	15
Gill [33]	2004	DIEP	758	0.5	2.5	12.9	3.8	5.9
Nahabedian [9]	2005	MS-2 free TRAM	113	1.8	0/1.8	7.1	2.7	NR
		DIEP	110	2.7	0/2.7	6.4	4.5	NR
Bajaj [10]	2006	MS-2 free TRAM	155	0	0.6	5.8	NR	6.4
		DIEP	48	4.2	2.1	8.3	NR	8.4
Garvey [49]	2006	Pedicled TRAM	94	8.5	NR	58.5	2.1	NR
		DIEP	96	3.1	NR	17.7	3.1	NR
Tran [7]	2007	DIEP	100	1	0	12	15 (11 intra-operative 4 post-op)	4
Chen [48]	2007	MS-1 + 2	159	0.6	2	20	NR	NR
		DIEP	41	0	0	5	NR	NR

NR = not recorded

(presumably zone IV) was routinely discarded. Application of these criteria reduced fat necrosis and partial flap loss rates in line with MS-0 TRAM flaps. Venous congestion is also cited more frequently amongst DIEP flaps [7, 46]. In one prospective series of 100 DIEP flap breast reconstructions, venous congestion was recorded in 15 cases necessitating venous bypass surgery in five of those cases [7].

Despite concerns about precarious vascularity, recently published series of experience with the DIEP flap report vascular complication rates comparable with free and pedicled TRAM flap series (Table 2) [6-10, 33, 37, 47-49] **(III/B)**. It should be recognised, however, that these are results from established centres of excellence often with vast experience with the DIEP flap. Whether similarly low complication rates are the norm elsewhere remains to be seen.

Abdominal strength

Numerous studies have sought to objectively quantify the impact of abdominal flaps on trunk strength using isometric dynamometry. Three prospective studies found mean flexion strength deficits of between 7-23% (non-significant) following unilateral pedicled TRAM flap surgeries [2, 28, 50]. Each of these studies was small ($n <= 17$), and their findings failed to reach statistical significance. Following bilateral pedicled TRAM flaps, Dulin et al [28] demonstrated a mean decrease in flexion strength to 60% of pre-operative levels one year after surgery (p<0.01) **(IIa/B)**. Alderman et al prospectively assessed three groups totalling 183 patients for two years following: a) a free TRAM; b) a pedicled TRAM or c) a breast implant/expander. At two years post-surgery, TRAM flap patients (free and pedicled) had significantly decreased peak flexion torque compared with the implant expander group **(IIa/B)**. Greatest decreases in peak flexion torque (12-19%) were noted amongst the bilateral TRAM flap reconstruction patients **(IIa/B)**. There were no significant differences in strength recorded between the free and pedicled TRAM flaps groups, consistent with the findings of previous studies [31, 50, 51] **(IIa/B)**.

Two studies have retrospectively compared abdominal strength following free TRAM [38] and DIEP [21] flaps with a healthy control group. Both studies reported similar results, with a consistent trend for lower abdominal wall strength (multiple variables measured) amongst free TRAM patients when compared with both DIEP flap patients and healthy controls **(IIb/B)**. This trend attained statistical significance on some, but not all, variables measured. In the same study, Blondeel et al prospectively followed the DIEP flap group and found no significant differences between pre and postoperative values of abdominal strength [21] **(IIa/B)**.

Bonde et al [52] used isokinetic dynamometry to retrospectively compare abdominal wall strength between two groups following either free MS-2 TRAM flaps or DIEP flaps. Both groups were almost identical in terms of demographics and follow-up period (mean two years) and were operated upon by the same surgical team over a one-year period. They found a trend towards higher abdominal strength (corrected for body weight) in the DIEP group, although this only reached statistical significance for eccentric (muscle lengthening under tension, e.g. lifting) muscle strength **(IIb/B)**. The statistical power of the study was limited by the relatively small sample size (DIEP group n=17; MS-2 group n=15)

Sit-ups or curl-ups are a simple and popular means for assessing abdominal wall strength and function. Sit-up or curl-up performance is significantly decreased after free TRAM [2, 53] or pedicled TRAM flap surgery [2, 24], although this is offset by muscle-sparing techniques [8, 9, 54] **(IIb/B)**. In a review of 268 TRAM flap breast reconstructions, Kroll et al [54] found significant differences in sit-up performance between free versus pedicled reconstructions (58.3% versus 38.2%) and unilateral versus bilateral reconstructions (61.7% versus 35.6%) **(III/B)**. The vast majority of patients undergoing DIEP flap surgery retain their pre-operative ability to perform curl-ups or sit-ups [9, 21] **(IIa/B)**.

In a direct comparison of MS-2 TRAM flap reconstructions and DIEP flap reconstructions, Nahabedian found very high rates of postoperative sit-up performance amongst unilateral reconstructions (97% versus 100%, respectively; not significant) and bilateral reconstructions (83% versus 95%; not significant) [9] **(IIb/B)**.

Despite the popularity of both sit-ups and isometric dynamometry in assessing abdominal wall strength and function, some surgeons question their validity as outcome measures of donor-site morbidity arguing that neither accurately reflects what is truly important: the ability of an individual to return to their pre-operative functional status in the absence of any significant symptoms attributable to their procedure.

Postoperative morphological changes within the abdominal wall

A number of studies have used radiological investigations to assess changes in the abdominal wall following TRAM or DIEP flap surgery. These can be helpful in determining the efficacy of muscle-sparing techniques and assessing compensatory changes within the abdominal wall following surgery.

Both ultrasound and MRI studies have confirmed attenuation of the remaining caudal rectus abdominis muscle after resection of a full width segment as part of a free (MS-0) TRAM flap procedure [32, 55] **(IIa/B)**. In addition, medial migration and thinning of the oblique muscles have been observed after both free and pedicled TRAM flap reconstruction [53]. By contrast, following DIEP flap surgery, normal abdominal wall anatomic proportions are maintained, and less than

20% of patients show significant (>5%) muscle atrophy or fatty infiltration **(IIa/B)**. Furthermore, using electromyographic assessments, Bottero et al [56] demonstrated the capacity of the rectus abdominis muscle to functionally recover following DIEP flap surgery. At nine weeks post-surgery, muscle activity (linear correlation with strength) was 50% of the contralateral muscle, rising to 70% by 15 months post-surgery **(IIa/B)**.

The selective preservation of a strip of the rectus abdominis muscle as part of a pedicled TRAM flap is a practice that has been called into question [23, 36]. Lejour and Dome performed CT scans on four patients who had previously undergone such a procedure and could find no evidence of any remaining muscle in three. Galli et al reported that preservation of a lateral strip of muscle results in denervation of that strip of muscle in 60% of cases (tested intra-operatively), although ultrasound examination at six months post-surgery suggested that only 40% of patients had any significant attenuation in this strip of muscle [57]. There are no radiological studies that we are aware of that have reported on the appearance of the anterior abdominal wall following muscle-sparing MS-2 free TRAM flaps.

Activities of daily living (ADLs) and health-related quality of life (HRQL)

Lejour and Dome [23] assessed ADLs in 57 patients following pedicled TRAM flap surgery. Patients reported that their sit-up and sporting activity was for the most part unchanged, and that they had less back pain. Despite their questionnaire responses, however, a physical therapist assessment of the abdomen demonstrated decreased function of the abdomen which was more prevalent and of a greater degree in the case of bilateral reconstructions.

Kind et al [50] prospectively investigated 25 patients undergoing various forms of TRAM flap breast reconstruction. Activities of daily living were assessed using a Human Activity Profile questionnaire pre-operatively and at six weeks, three months, six months and one year post-surgery. At one year postoperatively, mean scores were 102+/-4% and 103+/-3% of pre-operative levels in pedicled and free

TRAM flap groups, respectively. There were no significant changes in score at any recorded point.

Mizgala et al [24] reviewed 150 patients 5-7 years after muscle-sparing pedicled TRAM flaps. Patient questionnaires revealed that the ability to exercise, perform housework, render child care, perform jobs and lift objects was unchanged in the majority of patients (72.0%-94.4%). A high proportion of patients did, however, report reduced abdominal strength and increased difficulty getting up from a prone position (45.5% and 42.7%, respectively). Lower scores were also consistently noted amongst the bipedicled/bilateral TRAM flap group compared with the unilateral group. With regard to participation in specific sports, walking, swimming and jogging were unaffected in most cases but around one quarter of those participating in aerobics and tennis noted impaired performance. Similarly, other studies have failed to demonstrate a change in patients' ability to participate in sport following free or pedicled TRAM flap surgery [22].

Retrospective comparative studies of free (MS-0, 1 + 2) TRAM and DIEP flap patients have failed to demonstrate any significant difference in ADL performance between the groups [21, 22, 38]. Two of these studies did, however, report that difficulty with housework, sport or hobbies was more prevalent amongst TRAM flap patients (11-26%) than DIEP flap patients (0-4%) (not significant) [21, 38]. In a direct comparison of 89 patients who had undergone either a MS-2 TRAM flap or a DIEP flap, there were no statistically significant differences in ADL performance between the groups, nor were there any consistent trends favouring either group [10].

A number of studies have used the validated SF-36 questionnaire to record changes in health-related quality of life associated with breast reconstruction [14, 22, 38, 58]. In a comparative study of free and pedicled TRAM flaps, no significant differences were found, but both groups did score significantly less than the reference population on some parameters [14]. By contrast, a prospective controlled study by Veiga et al [58] followed a cohort of mastectomised patients and found statistically significant progressive improvements in seven of eight SF-36 domain scores following pedicled TRAM flap reconstruction. Two studies have directly compared postoperative SF-36 scores between free TRAM (MS-0) [22], (MS 1+2) [38] and DIEP flap breast reconstruction groups at a minimum of six months post-surgery. Neither study demonstrated any significant difference in scores between the two groups on the three physically orientated domains of the questionnaire: physical functioning (PF), role-physical (RP) and bodily pain (BP). Futter et al [38] did, however, find a trend toward higher SF-36 scores amongst DIEP flap patients compared with the (MS 1+2) TRAM flap patients.

Conclusions

Breast reconstruction with all varieties of TRAM flaps and DIEP flaps results in high levels of patient satisfaction and good to excellent aesthetic breast results. These findings are independent of the method of breast reconstruction selected **(IIa/B)**. Furthermore, the majority of patients report an improvement in the aesthetic appearance of their abdomen, again independent of the method of breast reconstruction **(IIa/B)**.

There are no significant differences in rates of abdominal wall hernia between the various forms of TRAM and DIEP flap, nor is mesh placement routinely required to prevent hernia **(IIa/B)**. Upper abdominal contour abnormalities are more frequent with pedicled TRAM flap reconstructions than with free TRAM and DIEP flap reconstructions **(IIb/B)**. Bilateral free TRAM flap reconstructions lead to higher incidences of contour abnormalities than unilateral reconstructions **(IIb/B)**. Muscle-sparing flaps may lead to reduced contour abnormalities particularly in the case of bilateral reconstructions compared with non-muscle sparing flaps **(IV/C)**.

DIEP flaps appear to lead to reduced pain in the immediate postoperative period when compared with MS-0 TRAM flaps **(IIb/B)**. There is no conclusive evidence at present that muscle-sparing techniques (MS-2 or DIEP) offer any benefit in terms of reduced incidence of long-term abdominal or back pain.

Pedicled TRAM flaps have significantly higher rates of fat necrosis and partial flap necrosis than free TRAM flaps **(III/B)**. Free TRAM flaps (all varieties) and DIEP flaps have comparable rates of vascular complications **(III/B)**.

Both pedicled and free TRAM flap breast reconstructions result in a quantitative decrease in abdominal wall strength as measured by isokinetic dynamometry **(IIa/B)**. This decrease in strength is most marked following bilateral TRAM flap reconstructions, as is impaired ability to perform sit-ups/curl-ups **(IIb/B)**. Decreased sit-up/curl-up performance with TRAM flap reconstructions is offset by muscle-sparing techniques **(IIb/B)**. There is no significant difference between MS-2 TRAM and DIEP flaps in ability to perform sit-ups postoperatively **(IIb/B)**. DIEP flap patients retain/regain their pre-operative ability to perform sit-ups/curl-ups and their abdominal strength as measured by isokinetic dynamometry **(IIb/B)**. Consistent with this finding, EMG and radiological studies have demonstrated functional recovery of the rectus abdominis muscle following DIEP flap harvest **(IIa/B)**.

The impact of donor-site morbidity upon ADLs and HRQL following any variety of TRAM or DIEP flap is for the most part minimal and/or well compensated **(IIb/B)**. An exception to this is bilateral pedicled TRAM flaps that lead to a subjective reduction in abdominal strength and function **(III/C)**. In spite of the superiority of DIEP flaps in preserving quantitative abdominal strength there is no conclusive evidence that DIEP flaps offer benefits over TRAM flaps with regard to maintaining ADLs and HRQL **(IIb/B)**.

Recommendations	Evidence level
◆ TRAM and DIEP flaps produce comparable aesthetic breast reconstructions and comparable patient satisfaction.	IIa/B
◆ Pedicled TRAM flaps result in a higher rate of postoperative abdominal contour deformities than do free TRAM or DIEP flaps.	IIb/B
◆ In large series there are no significant differences in the rates of vascular complications associated with DIEP and free TRAM flaps.	IIb/B
◆ DIEP flaps are associated with reduced pain in the immediate postoperative period when compared with free MS-0 TRAM flaps.	III/B
◆ Pedicled TRAM flaps have higher rates of fat necrosis and partial flap loss than do free TRAM flaps.	IIa/B
◆ Free and pedicled TRAM flaps lead to a quantitative decrease in abdominal wall strength. This is most marked with bilateral reconstructions.	IIb/B
◆ Sit-up/curl-up ability is reduced following free or pedicled TRAM flap surgery, although this is offset by increasing degrees of muscle sparing.	IIb/B
◆ Despite the superiority of DIEP flaps in preserving abdominal wall strength, there is no conclusive evidence that this translates to better maintenance of ADLs and HRQL.	IIb/B
◆ The impact of donor-site morbidity upon ADLs and HRQL following any variety of TRAM or DIEP flap is for the most part minimal and/or well compensated.	IIb/B

Chapter 20

References

1. Hartrampf CR, Scheflan M, Black PW. Breast reconstruction with a transverse abdominal island flap. *Plast Reconstr Surg* 1982; 69(2): 216-25.

2. Edsander-Nord A, Jurell G, Wickman M. Donor-site morbidity after pedicled or free TRAM flap surgery: a prospective and objective study. *Plast Reconstr Surg* 1998; 102(5): 1508-16.

3. Baldwin BJ, Schusterman MA, Miller MJ, Kroll SS, Wang BG. Bilateral breast reconstruction: conventional versus free TRAM. *Plast Reconstr Surg* 1994; 93(7): 1410-6; discussion 1417.

4. Gherardini G, Arnander C, Gylbert L, Wickman M. Pedicled compared with free transverse rectus abdominis myocutaneous flaps in breast reconstruction. *Scand J Plast Reconstr Surg Hand Surg* 1994; 28(1): 69-73.

5. Allen RJ, Treece P. Deep inferior epigastric perforator flap for breast reconstruction. *Ann Plast Surg* 1994; 32(1): 32-8.

6. Kroll SS. Fat necrosis in free transverse rectus abdominis myocutaneous and deep inferior epigastric perforator flaps. *Plast Reconstr Surg* 2000; 106(3): 576-83.

7. Tran NV, Buchel EW, Convery PA. Microvascular complications of DIEP flaps. *Plast Reconstr Surg* 2007; 119(5): 1397-405; discussion 1406.

8. Nahabedian MY, Momen B, Galdino G, Manson PN. Breast reconstruction with the free TRAM or DIEP flap: patient selection, choice of flap, and outcome. *Plast Reconstr Surg* 2002; 110(2): 466-75; discussion 476.

9. Nahabedian MY, Tsangaris T, Momen B. Breast reconstruction with the DIEP flap or the muscle-sparing (MS-2) free TRAM flap: is there a difference? *Plast Reconstr Surg* 2005; 115(2): 436-44; discussion 445.

10. Bajaj AK, Chevray PM, Chang DW. Comparison of donor-site complications and functional outcomes in free muscle-sparing TRAM flap and free DIEP flap breast reconstruction. *Plast Reconstr Surg* 2006; 117(3): 737-46; discussion 747-50.

11. Lindsey JT. Integrating the DIEP and muscle-sparing (MS-2) free TRAM techniques optimizes surgical outcomes: presentation of an algorithm for microsurgical breast reconstruction based on perforator anatomy. *Plast Reconstr Surg* 2007; 119(1): 18-27.

12. Chung KC, Kalliainen LK, Spilson SV, Walters MR, Kim HM. The prevalence of negative studies with inadequate statistical power: an analysis of the plastic surgery literature. *Plast Reconstr Surg* 2002; 109(1): 1-6; discussion 7-8.

13. Moscona RA, Holander L, Or D, Fodor L. Patient satisfaction and aesthetic results after pedicled transverse rectus abdominis muscle flap for breast reconstruction. *Ann Surg Oncol* 2006; 13(12): 1739-46.

14. Edsander-Nord A, Brandberg Y, Wickman M. Quality of life, patients' satisfaction, and aesthetic outcome after pedicled or free TRAM flap breast surgery. *Plast Reconstr Surg* 2001; 107(5): 1142-53; discussion 1154.

15. Veiga DF, Neto MS, Garcia EB, *et al*. Evaluations of the aesthetic results and patient satisfaction with the late pedicled TRAM flap breast reconstruction. *Ann Plast Surg* 2002; 48(5): 515-20.

16. Clough KB, O'Donoghue JM, Fitoussi AD, Vlastos G, Falcou MC. Prospective evaluation of late cosmetic results following breast reconstruction: II. Tram flap reconstruction. *Plast Reconstr Surg* 2001; 107(7): 1710-6.

17. Hamdi M, Weiler-Mithoff EM, Webster MH. Deep inferior epigastric perforator flap in breast reconstruction: experience with the first 50 flaps. *Plast Reconstr Surg* 1999; 103(1): 86-95.

18. Bruner S, Frerichs O, Schirmer S, Cervelli A, Fansa H. [Patients' satisfaction and social reintegration after breast reconstruction with the DIEP/TRAM flap]. *Handchir Mikrochir Plast Chir* 2006; 38(6): 417-25.

19. Banic A, Boeckx W, Greulich M, *et al*. Late results of breast reconstruction with free TRAM flaps: a prospective multicentric study. *Plast Reconstr Surg* 1995; 95(7): 1195-204; discussion 1205.

20. Serletti JM, Moran SL. Free versus the pedicled TRAM flap: a cost comparison and outcome analysis. *Plast Reconstr Surg* 1997; 100(6): 1418-24; discussion 1425.

21. Blondeel N, Vanderstraeten GG, Monstrey SJ, *et al*. The donor site morbidity of free DIEP flaps and free TRAM flaps for breast reconstruction. *Br J Plast Surg* 1997; 50(5): 322-30.

22. Schaverien MV, Perks AG, McCulley SJ. Comparison of outcomes and donor-site morbidity in unilateral free TRAM versus DIEP flap breast reconstruction. *J Plast Reconstr Aesthet Surg* 2007; 60: 1219-24.

23. Lejour M, Dome M. Abdominal wall function after rectus abdominis transfer. *Plast Reconstr Surg* 1991; 87(6): 1054-68.

24. Mizgala CL, Hartrampf CR, Jr., Bennett GK. Assessment of the abdominal wall after pedicled TRAM flap surgery: 5- to 7-year follow-up of 150 consecutive patients. *Plast Reconstr Surg* 1994; 93(5): 988-1002; discussion 1003-4.

25. Ducic I, Spear SL, Cuoco F, Hannan C. Safety and risk factors for breast reconstruction with pedicled transverse rectus abdominis musculocutaneous flaps: a 10-year analysis. *Ann Plast Surg* 2005; 55(6): 559-64.

26. Shaikh-Naidu N, Preminger BA, Rogers K, Messina P, Gayle LB. Determinants of aesthetic satisfaction following TRAM and implant breast reconstruction. *Ann Plast Surg* 2004; 52(5): 465-70; discussion 470.

27. Kroll SS, Coffey JA, Jr., Winn RJ, Schusterman MA. A comparison of factors affecting aesthetic outcomes of TRAM flap breast reconstructions. *Plast Reconstr Surg* 1995; 96(4): 860-4.

28. Dulin WA, Avila RA, Verheyden CN, Grossman L. Evaluation of abdominal wall strength after TRAM flap surgery. *Plast Reconstr Surg* 2004; 113(6): 1662-5; discussion 1666-7.

29. Nahabedian MY, Dooley W, Singh N, Manson PN. Contour abnormalities of the abdomen after breast reconstruction with abdominal flaps: the role of muscle preservation. *Plast Reconstr Surg* 2002; 109(1): 91-101.

30. Nahabedian MY, Manson PN. Contour abnormalities of the abdomen after transverse rectus abdominis muscle flap breast reconstruction: a multifactorial analysis. *Plast Reconstr Surg* 2002; 109(1): 81-7; discussion 88-90.

31. Nahabedian MY, Momen B. Lower abdominal bulge after deep inferior epigastric perforator flap (DIEP) breast reconstruction. *Ann Plast Surg* 2005; 54(2): 124-9.

32. Suominen S, Asko-Seljavaara S, von Smitten K, Ahovuo J, Sainio P, Alaranta H. Sequelae in the abdominal wall after pedicled or free TRAM flap surgery. *Ann Plast Surg* 1996; 36(6): 629-36.

33. Gill PS, Hunt JP, Guerra AB, *et al*. A 10-year retrospective review of 758 DIEP flaps for breast reconstruction. *Plast Reconstr Surg* 2004; 113(4): 1153-60.

34. Zienowicz RJ, May JW, Jr. Hernia prevention and aesthetic contouring of the abdomen following TRAM flap breast reconstruction by the use of polypropylene mesh. *Plast Reconstr Surg* 1995; 96(6): 1346-50.

35. Moscona RA, Ramon Y, Toledano H, Barzilay G. Use of synthetic mesh for the entire abdominal wall after TRAM flap transfer. *Plast Reconstr Surg* 1998; 101(3): 706-10; discussion 711-02.

36. Kroll SS, Marchi M. Comparison of strategies for preventing abdominal-wall weakness after TRAM flap breast reconstruction. *Plast Reconstr Surg* 1992; 89(6): 1045-51; discussion 1052.

37. Blondeel PN, One hundred free DIEP flap breast reconstructions: a personal experience. *Br J Plast Surg* 1999; 52(2): 104-11.

38. Futter CM, Webster MH, Hagen S, Mitchell SL. A retrospective comparison of abdominal muscle strength following breast reconstruction with a free TRAM or DIEP flap. *Br J Plast Surg* 2000; 53(7): 578-83.

39. Arnez ZM, Khan U, Pogorelec D, Planinsek F. Rational selection of flaps from the abdomen in breast reconstruction to reduce donor site morbidity. *Br J Plast Surg* 1999; 52(5): 351-4.

40. Kroll SS, Sharma S, Koutz C, *et al*. Postoperative morphine requirements of free TRAM and DIEP flaps. *Plast Reconstr Surg* 2001; 107(2): 338-41.

41. Tuominen HP, Asko-Seljavaara S, Svartling NE. Cutaneous blood flow in the free TRAM flap. *Br J Plast Surg* 1993; 46(8): 665-9.

42. Tuominen HP, Asko-Seljavaara S, Svartling NE, Harma MA. Cutaneous blood flow in the TRAM flap. *Br J Plast Surg* 1992; 45(4): 261-9.

43. Elliott LF, Eskenazi L, Beegle PH, Jr., Podres PE, Drazan L. Immediate TRAM flap breast reconstruction: 128 consecutive cases. *Plast Reconstr Surg* 1993; 92(2): 217-27.

44. Kroll SS, Gherardini G, Martin JE, *et al*. Fat necrosis in free and pedicled TRAM flaps. *Plast Reconstr Surg* 1998; 102(5): 1502-7.

45. Schusterman MA, Kroll SS, Weldon ME. Immediate breast reconstruction: why the free TRAM over the conventional TRAM flap? *Plast Reconstr Surg* 1992; 90(2): 255-61; discussion 262.

Chapter 20

46. Blondeel PN, Arnstein M, Verstraete K, *et al.* Venous congestion and blood flow in free transverse rectus abdominis myocutaneous and deep inferior epigastric perforator flaps. *Plast Reconstr Surg* 2000; 106(6): 1295-9.

47. Watterson PA, Bostwick J, 3rd, Hester TR, Jr., Bried JT, Taylor GI. TRAM flap anatomy correlated with a 10-year clinical experience with 556 patients. *Plast Reconstr Surg* 1995; 95(7): 1185-94.

48. Chen CM, Halvorson EG, Disa JJ, *et al.* Immediate postoperative complications in DIEP versus free/muscle-sparing TRAM flaps. *Plast Reconstr Surg* 2007; 120: 1477-82.

49. Garvey PB, Buchel EW, Pockaj BA, *et al.* DIEP and pedicled TRAM flaps: a comparison of outcomes. *Plast Reconstr Surg* 2006; 117(6): 1711-9; discussion 1720.

50. Kind GM, Rademaker AW, Mustoe TA. Abdominal-wall recovery following TRAM flap: a functional outcome study. *Plast Reconstr Surg* 1997; 99(2): 417-28.

51. Alderman AK, Kuzon WM, Jr., Wilkins EG. A two-year prospective analysis of trunk function in TRAM breast reconstructions. *Plast Reconstr Surg* 2006; 117(7): 2131-38.

52. Bonde CT, Lund H, Fridberg M, Danneskiold-Samsoe B, Elberg JJ. Abdominal strength after breast reconstruction using a free abdominal flap. *J Plast Reconstr Aesthet Surg* 2007; 60(5): 519-23.

53. Blondeel N, Boeckx WD, Vanderstraeten GG, *et al.* The fate of the oblique abdominal muscles after free TRAM flap surgery. *Br J Plast Surg* 1997; 50(5): 315-21.

54. Kroll SS, Schusterman MA, Reece GP, Miller MJ, Robb G, Evans G. Abdominal wall strength, bulging, and hernia after TRAM flap breast reconstruction. *Plast Reconstr Surg* 1995; 96(3): 616-9.

55. Suominen S, Asko-Seljavaara S, Kinnunen J, Sainio P, Alaranta H. Abdominal wall competence after free transverse rectus abdominis musculocutaneous flap harvest: a prospective study. *Ann Plast Surg* 1997; 39(3): 229-34.

56. Bottero L, Lefaucheur JP, Fadhul S, Raulo Y, Collins ED, Lantieri L. Electromyographic assessment of rectus abdominis muscle function after deep inferior epigastric perforator flap surgery. *Plast Reconstr Surg* 2004; 113(1): 156-61.

57. Galli A, Adami M, Berrino P, Leone S, Santi P. Long-term evaluation of the abdominal wall competence after total and selective harvesting of the rectus abdominis muscle. *Ann Plast Surg* 1992; 28(5): 409-13.

58. Veiga DF, Sabino Neto M, Ferreira LM, *et al.* Quality of life outcomes after pedicled TRAM flap delayed breast reconstruction. *Br J Plast Surg* 2004; 57(3): 252-7.

Chapter 20

A comparison of TRAM and DIEP
flaps for breast reconstruction

Chapter 21

Immediate versus delayed breast reconstruction

Tom WL Chapman BSc MB ChB MRCS 1
Specialist Registrar, Plastic and Reconstructive Surgery
Robert J Morris FRCS (Plast.) 2
Consultant Plastic Surgeon

1 FRENCHAY HOSPITAL, BRISTOL, UK
2 DERRIFORD HOSPITAL, PLYMOUTH, UK

Introduction

As reconstructive techniques have evolved over the past 20 years, so ever greater emphasis has been placed upon the preservation of breast aesthetics, quality of life and body image after extirpative surgery for breast cancer. Not only is there now a myriad of techniques available for breast reconstruction, but patients have a choice as to the timing of the reconstructive surgery itself. Traditional delayed reconstruction is no longer mandatory and a proportion of patients can now be offered immediate reconstruction, i.e. at the same time as tumour resection. Controversy remains as to which patients are potentially better served by immediate reconstruction, but in an era of increasing patient expectations and autonomy we need to understand the possible benefits and disadvantages of immediate versus delayed reconstruction. Where possible, such understanding should be evidence-based rather than anecdotal. In this chapter we aim to outline the practical, psychological, economical, oncological and surgical considerations that mediate in the decision making process.

Methodology

A Medline search was used to gather evidence using the search words 'immediate breast reconstruction', 'delayed breast reconstruction' and 'immediate and/or delayed breast reconstruction'.

Oncological considerations

One of the initial concerns with immediate reconstruction was that early local recurrence may be masked and difficult to detect, or adjuvant therapy delayed by surgical complications, both potentially adversely affecting overall survival. There is now good evidence to show that immediate reconstruction does not delay the onset of radiotherapy [1, 2] and survival is no different in patients treated by immediate reconstruction compared with those treated by mastectomy alone and delayed reconstruction [1] **(IIb/B)**. Local recurrence is similarly no more frequent after immediate reconstruction and this is true for either implant or autologous reconstruction techniques [3]. Immediate reconstruction appears to be safe even for high-risk patients with advanced (T3 or node positive) stages of breast carcinoma [4] and possibly also for those with ductal carcinoma *in situ* [5]. When local recurrence occurs, an immediate reconstruction does not appear to delay its detection. In addition, recurrence is often a marker of systemic metastatic disease so survival rates are unlikely to be influenced by earlier detection [6]. While much of this evidence is retrospective, the overwhelming evidence is that immediate reconstruction is an oncologically safe alternative to mastectomy with or without delayed reconstruction.

Practical considerations

Inherent with immediate reconstruction is the increased operating time required and the difficulties in co-ordinating two surgical teams and theatre space at relatively short notice. The emergence of oncoplastic surgery through 'cross-fertilisation' between specialties, however, may obviate the need for both general breast and reconstructive plastic surgeons in the future. As the proportion of patients undergoing immediate reconstruction rises, some of the practical issues associated with ad hoc arrangement of long procedures will no doubt be overcome by greater centralisation.

Surgical considerations

Reconstruction of the breast involves replacement of breast skin, and restoration of shape and volume. Skin-sparing mastectomy with immediate reconstruction potentially delivers the best cosmetic results due to maximal preservation of good quality breast skin and the inframammary fold. Delayed reconstruction necessitates the replacement of a larger amount of skin and is compromised by inferior quality skin flaps. Greater overall volume loss also means balancing surgery on the contralateral breast is more likely to be required. The end result of delayed reconstruction may, therefore, not be as cosmetically pleasing or at least the achievement of good cosmesis more challenging. There is little objective evidence, however, to suggest that the overall aesthetic result is superior in immediate compared with delayed reconstruction.

It has been postulated that surgical complications correlate with operative time. There is some evidence to demonstrate that wound complications are at least doubled in immediate reconstruction patients [2] **(III/B)**.

Wound healing may be significantly delayed after immediate, compared with delayed, free TRAM flaps [7] **(III/B)**. However, there is little evidence to suggest a significantly higher rate of partial or total flap loss in immediate versus delayed groups when free autologous reconstruction is used [8] **(III/B)**. As surgical and anaesthetic teams become more experienced in immediate reconstruction, complication rates may fall and approach those of delayed reconstruction. At present, however, patients should probably be made aware in the pre-operative discussion of a possible increased risk of short-term complications with immediate compared with delayed reconstructive breast surgery. Patients with significant comorbidities, such as severe cardiovascular disease, morbid obesity or pulmonary disease, may be better treated by delayed reconstruction.

The significant advantage to delayed reconstruction is that any detrimental effects of radiotherapy or chemotherapy upon the reconstruction can be avoided. In particular, postoperative radiotherapy may cause fibrosis, scarring and contracture in the irradiated field (which includes the reconstructed breast), leading ultimately to a disappointing aesthetic result. Such effects, however, are difficult to predict and depend partly upon the choice of reconstructive technique.

It is thought that the long-term results of implant-based reconstructions are generally poor after radiotherapy as a result of skin and capsular contracture, although much of the evidence is limited to older and retrospective studies. Placement of prostheses should be subpectoral to minimise contracture, extrusion and infection, and to minimise the risks of locally recurrent disease being masked. Expandable implants are unlikely to be successful as expansion after radiotherapy is limited by fibrosis and thinning of the overlying dermis. Expandable implants should, therefore, be avoided if postoperative radiotherapy is anticipated, but remain a good option in prophylactic skin-sparing mastectomy. Implant only reconstructions are inappropriate if there is a significant skin deficiency after tumour resection. Contralateral surgery is also likely to be required in the form of mastopexy, reduction or augmentation, but where bilateral reconstruction is undertaken, symmetry is more readily achieved using implants compared with autologous techniques. However, a higher rate of revisional procedures are required with implants, although reported rates of 30-50% implant extrusion are probably an exaggeration when applied to modern implants in well selected cases. In a recent large cohort from Scandinavia, only 7% of patients with subpectoral permanent implants required removal and later salvage reconstruction, with an overall complication rate of 13% [8]. The majority of these patients had undergone radiotherapy which had not been predicted pre-operatively. With careful selection of those patients unlikely to need radiotherapy, implant-based reconstruction may provide good results, particularly in smaller volume, minimally ptotic breasts, and the majority of such patients are satisfied with the aesthetic outcome of this relatively simple procedure [8].

Autologous tissue reconstructions are generally more durable, natural appearing and can better tolerate radiotherapy, but are not immune to the problems of scarring and contracture within the irradiated field. Rates of fat necrosis with volume loss requiring further surgery have been quoted around 6% [9] to 28% [10] in immediate free TRAM reconstruction, requiring further flaps to correct distorted contour. Significant differences of fat necrosis, fibrosis and contracture have also been reported in irradiated compared with non-irradiated DIEP flaps [11]. For this reason, some authors have advocated abandoning immediate reconstruction even with autologous tissue in those patients with poor prognoses or who are likely to need radiotherapy. The complicating factor is that it is not always possible to predict which patients will require postoperative radiotherapy as this is guided by the definitive histology and resection margin status. Consequently, 'delayed-immediate' breast reconstruction has been advocated with mastectomy and tissue expander reconstruction followed, at a second stage, by autologous reconstruction [12] (III/B). There is no evidence, however, of an advantage in aesthetic, practical or psychological terms for patients undergoing delayed-immediate reconstruction.

Immediate nipple reconstruction is feasible but requires well vascularised autologous tissue. However, small flaps used to reconstruct the nipple may be compromised by adjuvant radiotherapy. In addition, the exact nipple location can be difficult to assess. There is little evidence for a significant advantage to immediate nipple reconstruction and therefore at present it is rarely performed. Areolar reconstruction is normally in the form of tattooing which is best performed two or three months after nipple reconstruction.

Ultimately, it is impossible to predict pre-operatively the final result of any procedure and patients need to be aware that postoperative radiotherapy, if needed, may compromise the aesthetic outcome whatever the reconstructive technique. It should be remembered, however, that a compromised aesthetic result for a surgeon, knowing what can be achieved in optimum circumstances, can still be a good result from the perspective of the patient. Immediate reconstruction should not be avoided simply to satisfy the aesthetic pride of the surgeon, and there is evidence that most patients are equally satisfied with their autologous reconstruction whether they have had radiotherapy or not [13] (III/B). These issues, therefore, highlight the importance of pre-operative decision making in a multi-disciplinary setting involving the patient, breast surgeon, reconstructive surgeon, oncologist, radiologist and pathologist for a consensus decision upon the appropriate and most practical surgical plan.

Economical considerations

Cost efficiency has become an important consideration in health care provision. It has been suggested that the cost of immediate reconstruction, with one operation, one anaesthetic and one recovery period, is less than mastectomy and later reconstruction. There is now good evidence for this to be true, certainly for autologous reconstruction techniques [14, 15] (III/B). When the costs of the initial mastectomy are removed from the equation, there is little difference in cost between an immediate and delayed free tissue transfer [16]. It should be remembered, however, that procedure tariffs rarely accurately reflect the real costs of providing care. In the UK National Health Service, hospital Trusts are remunerated for each separate procedure undertaken, based on its complexity. Combined procedures are assumed to be more cost-effective and the remuneration is based upon the most complex part of the overall procedure only. There may, therefore, be little economic advantage to immediate reconstruction as NHS hospital Trusts are remunerated for the reconstruction but not the mastectomy. In addition, actual costs to the Trust can be spread into different financial years if delayed reconstruction follows some months after the initial mastectomy. Practical problems, such as cancellation of other procedures at short notice to accommodate an immediate reconstruction or under-use of ring-fenced lists, may incur further penalties and costs. Such matters are rarely considered in economic comparisons between immediate and delayed reconstruction.

Psychological considerations

There is no doubt that the emotional problems associated with mastectomy are significant; these include mood disturbance, a negative body image with loss of feminine identity, and anxieties concerning the recurrence and spread of cancer. Immediate reconstruction of the breast may help counteract some of these emotional problems while patients waiting for delayed reconstruction have to live with the physical and psychological problems of a mastectomy. However, emotional and psychological issues are difficult to objectively measure, and the majority of studies have been non-randomised. Certainly, women undergoing immediate reconstruction appear to have less distress in recalling surgery, are less repulsed by their naked appearance and have more freedom to dress compared with those women who do not have reconstruction or in whom reconstruction has been delayed [17, 18]. There may, however, be a selection bias in that patients who want and demand immediate reconstruction are a self-selected and well motivated group. Breast reconstruction, also, is not a panacea for the emotional consequences of mastectomy and women still feel conscious of altered body image one year postoperatively, regardless of whether they have had a reconstruction or not [19]. It should not, therefore, be assumed that reconstruction is psychologically beneficial to all patients. Most women, if given the choice of immediate breast reconstruction, choose this over delayed reconstruction [20], and clearly patient

preference is integral to satisfaction and psychological well-being.

However, patients with newly diagnosed cancer undergoing major surgery, need extra support compared with those undergoing late reconstructions, and a proportion of women seeking immediate reconstruction show a relatively higher incidence of psychosocial impairment and functional disability [21] **(III/B)**. Pre-operative psychosocial distress may have important implications for clinical decision making and surgical outcome in those seeking immediate reconstruction. In addition, the decision making time is reduced and anxieties concerning cancer and basic survival may cloud patients' ability to 'take in' information regarding their reconstruction. For this reason, most surgeons would advocate at least two pre-operative discussions prior to immediate reconstruction which may, in some circumstances, cause practical difficulty. Younger patients (35-44 years of age) are more likely to choose immediate or at least early delayed breast reconstruction, compared with those over 55 years who are significantly less likely to want any type of reconstruction [22]. Younger patients are more likely to have increased sensitivity concerning body image and, although this patient group may benefit more from immediate reconstruction, they may also be more difficult to satisfy when it comes to the aesthetic result. Some might argue that patient satisfaction is more likely in patients who have first undergone mastectomy as their expectations are lower or more realistic. In other words, coping with the exchange of an apparently normal breast for a reconstructed breast is more challenging than coping with exchange of a mastectomy scar for a reconstructed breast. One large prospective study found that the greater the time lapse between mastectomy and reconstruction, the greater the patients' satisfaction overall with the reconstruction [23].

Ultimately a judgment must be reached based on the personality of the patient, their mood, anxiety, body image, coping strategies, psychosocial support and expectations. Some patients are likely to benefit emotionally and psychologically from immediate reconstruction, but not all, and distinguishing those patients who will benefit may prove difficult.

Conclusions

Immediate breast reconstruction is a safe and acceptable procedure after mastectomy for cancer with no evidence of untoward oncological sequelae. The appropriate timing of breast reconstruction, however, remains controversial. The practical problems in performing immediate reconstruction, and difficulty in predicting the effects of postoperative radiotherapy, need to be weighed against psychological and economical considerations. Implant-based techniques are simple but good cosmesis is difficult to achieve.

Autologous techniques are more robust, natural appearing and likely to withstand radiotherapy, but are longer procedures and not without complications. Time must be given to discuss each option and the likely advantages and disadvantages for individual patients in an appropriate multi-disciplinary environment. Whatever the choice and outcome, patients are likely to be satisfied provided they are adequately informed, a good rapport has been developed and appropriate peri-operative emotional and practical support has been given.

Chapter 21

Recommendations	Evidence level
◆ Immediate breast reconstruction is oncologically safe and does not affect timing of adjuvant therapy with patient survival rates comparable with delayed reconstruction.	IIb/B
◆ Wound complications appear higher in immediate reconstruction compared with delayed reconstruction, although rates of partial and total flap failure using autologous techniques are similar in each setting.	III/B
◆ Implant-based immediate reconstruction is not favoured in the UK when postoperative radiotherapy is likely to be required, as the effects of subsequent capsular contracture have been aesthetically disappointing.	III/B
◆ Effects of radiotherapy on an autologous reconstruction are difficult to predict. Revisional surgery may be required, but most patients are satisfied with the result.	III/B
◆ Immediate reconstruction would appear to be more cost-efficient than mastectomy and delayed reconstruction.	III/B
◆ There may be a psychological benefit to immediate over delayed reconstruction, especially in younger patients and those with an enhanced perception of body image.	III/B

References

1. Gouy S, Rouzier R, Missana MC, Atallah D, Youssef O, Barreau-Pouhaer L. Immediate reconstruction after neo-adjuvant therapy: effect on adjuvant treatment starting and survival. *Ann Surg Oncol* 2005; 12(2): 161-6.

2. Mortenson MM, Scheider PD, Khatri VP, Stevenson TR, Whetzel TP, Sommerhaug EJ, Goodnigh JE Jr, Bold RJ. Immediate breast reconstruction after mastectomy increases wound complications; however, initiation of adjuvant therapy is not delayed. *Arch Surg* 2004; 139(9): 988-91.

3. Murphy RX Jr, Wahhab S, Rovito PF, Harper G, Kimmel SR. Impact of immediate reconstruction on local recurrence of breast cancer after mastectomy. *Ann Plast Surg* 2003; 50(4): 333-8.

4. Downes KJ, Glatt BS, Kanchwala SK, Mick R, Fraker DL, Fox KR, Solin LJ, Bucky LP, Czernieki BJ. Skin-sparing mastectomy and immediate reconstruction is an acceptable treatment option for patients with high-risk breast carcinoma. *Cancer* 2005; 103(5): 906-13.

5. Speigel AJ, Butler CE. Recurrence following treatment of ductal carcinoma *in situ* with skin-sparing mastectomy and

immediate breast reconstruction. *Plast Reconstr Surg* 2003; 111(2): 706-11.

6. Langstein HN, Cheng MH, Singletary SE, Robb GL, Hoy E, Smith TL, Kroll SS. Breast cancer recurrence after immediate reconstruction: patterns and significance. *Plast Reconstr Surg* 2003; 111(2): 712-22.

7. DeBono R, Thompson A, Stevenson JH. Immediate versus delayed free TRAM breast reconstruction: an analysis of peri-operative factors and complications. *Br J Plast Surg* 2002; 55(2): 111-6.

8. Lagergren J, Jurell G, Sandealin K, Rylander R, Wickman M. Technical aspects of immediate breast reconstruction with implants: five-year follow-up. *Scan J Plast Recon Surg Hand Surg* 2005; 35(3): 147-52.

9. Foster RD, Hansen SL, Esserman LJ, Hwang ES, Ewing C, Lane K, Anthony JP. Safety of immediate transverse rectus abdominis myocutaneous breast reconstruction for patients with locally advanced disease. *Arch Surg* 2005; 140(2): 196-200.

10. Tran NV, Chang DW, Gupta A, Kroll SS, Robb GL. Comparison of immediate and delayed free TRAM flap breast reconstruction in patients receiving postmastectomy radiation therapy. *Plast Reconstr Surg* 2001; 108(1): 78-82.

11. Rogers NE, Allen RJ. Radiation effects on breast reconstruction with the deep inferior epigastric perforator flap. *Plast Reconstr Surg* 2002; 109(6): 1919-24.

12. Kronowitz SJ, Hunt KK, Kuerer HM, Babiera G, McNeese MD, Buchholz TA, Strom EA, Robb GL. Delayed-immediate breast reconstruction. *Plast Reconstr Surg* 2004; 113(6): 1617-28.

13. Salhab M, Al Sarakbi W, Joseph A, Sheards S, Travers J, Mokbel K. Skin-sparing mastectomy and immediate breast reconstruction: patient satisfaction and clinical outcome. *Int J Clin Oncol* 2006; 11(1): 51-4.

14. Neyt MJ, Blondeel PN, Morrison CM, Albrecht JA. Comparing the cost of delayed and immediate autologous breast reconstruction in Belgium. *Br J Plast Surg* 2005; 58(4): 493-7.

15. Elkowitz A, Colen S, Slavin S, Seibert J, Weinstein M, Shaw W. Various methods of breast reconstruction after mastectomy: an economic comparison. *Plast Reconstr Surg* 1993; 92(1): 77-83.

16. Cheng MH, Lin JY, Ulusal BG, Wei FC. Comparisons of resource costs and success rates between immediate and delayed breast reconstruction using DIEP or SIEA flaps under a well controlled clinical trial. *Plast Reconstr Surg* 2006; 117(7): 2139-42.

17. Dean C, Chetty U, Forrest APM. Effects of immediate breast reconstruction on psychosocial morbidity after mastectomy. *Lancet* 1983; 1: 459-62.

18. Steven LA, McGrath MH, Druss RG, Kirster SJ, Gump FE, Forde KA. The psychological impact of immediate breast reconstruction for women with early breast cancer. *Plast Reconstr Surg* 1984; 73: 619-28.

19. Harcourt DM, Rumsey NJ, Ambler NR, Cawthorn SJ, Reid CD, Maddox PR, Kenealy JM, Rainsbury RM, Umpleby HC. The psychological effect of mastectomy with or without breast reconstruction: a prospective, multicenter study. *Plast Reconstr Surg* 2003; 111(3): 1060-8.

20. Ananian P, Houvenaeghel G, Protiere C, Rounanet P, Arnaud S, Moatti JP, Tallet A, Braud AC, Julian-Reynier C. Determinants of patients' choice of reconstruction with mastectomy for breast cancer. *Ann Surg Oncol* 2004: 11(8): 762-71.

21. Roth RS, Lowery JC, Davis J, Wilkins EG. Quality of life and affective distress in women seeking immediate versus delayed breast reconstruction after mastectomy for breast cancer. *Plast Reconstr Surg* 2005; 116(4): 993-1002.

22. Alderman AK, McMahon L Jr, Wilkins EG. The national utilization of immediate and early delayed breast reconstruction and the effect of sociodemographic factors. *Plast Reconstr Surg* 2003; 111(2): 695-703.

23. Psychological impact of treatments for breast cancer. Rolland JH. In: *Surgery of the Breast: Principles and Art.* Spear SL, Little JW, Lippman ME, Wood WC, Eds. Philadelphia, Pennsylvania: Lipincott-Raven, 1998: 295-313.

Chapter 21

Chapter 22

Strategies for minimising palpable implant rippling in the augmented breast

Jonny Hobman MB BS MRCS MRCS (Glas)
Registrar, Plastic Surgery
David T Sharpe OBE MA FRCS
Consultant Plastic Surgeon

BRADFORD ROYAL INFIRMARY, BRADFORD, UK

Introduction

The tremendous advance in breast augmentation first described by Cronin and Gerow in 1964 [1] heralded the development of modern methods of breast enlargement and has enabled millions of women to benefit worldwide.

As is well known, the use of silicone, saline, and gel-filled prostheses has not been without problems. Now that concerns regarding the potential toxicity of silicone have largely been allayed, the debate centred upon the reliability and efficacy of these devices has turned more towards the local complications associated with the technique [2]. Questions have been raised regarding the incidence of capsular contracture, the life expectancy of breast implants, and the problems of rippling and wrinkling of the prosthesis which are palpable to both patient and surgeon, and the subject of this chapter.

Interestingly, in Cronin and Gerow's first paper there was the first description of "a palpable rolling or curling of the upper edge of the prosthesis" that was attributed to inadequacy of the implant pocket dissection.

Methodology

An internet search was performed using PubMed. Search terms used were 'breast implant', 'breast implant operations', 'breast ripple' and 'breast implant complication'. Papers found using these search terms were then analysed for further relevant publications.

Diagnosis and assessment

As will be discussed, certain physical characteristics in patients predispose to implant palpability. These factors cannot be controlled, but can be ameliorated by careful pre-operative patient counselling and appropriate selection of both implant and plane of insertion.

In certain patients implant palpability is inevitable. If this is explained pre-operatively then it may dissuade the patient from breast augmentation, or at least make the symptom less troublesome when it does occur. It is not uncommon for a surgeon to be able to feel the implant edge, but for this not to be reported as a problem by the patient.

The problem of palpability and rippling has been more keenly felt in North America as a result of David Kessler's moratorium [3] on silicone gel-filled implants in 1991, which has only just been rescinded. In the absence of silicone gel, saline-filled implants have been used. Because of the lack of cohesiveness of the saline filler, rippling and creasing of the implants has been much more apparent and has stimulated attempts to try and resolve the problem, some of which are described in this chapter.

Young [4] describes two rating scales for skin wrinkling and implant palpability:

Skin wrinkling scale:

* Grade I. No visible wrinkling in any position.
* Grade II. Minimal wrinkling that is not visible in a swimsuit or low-cut clothes (minimal problem for patient).
* Grade III. Wrinkling readily visible in nude (standing or lying down) and in swimsuit or low-cut clothes (major problem for patient).

Implant palpability scale:

* Grade I. No palpability; neither surgeon nor patient can feel the implant.
* Grade II. The surgeon can feel the implant; however, the patient and her partner do not (not a problem for the patient).
* Grade III. The implant is easily felt by the surgeon, patient, and partner (major problem for the patient).

Aetiology of palpable implant rippling

The aetiology of any complication in breast implant surgery can be broken down into three main groups, namely: patient factors, surgical technique and implant-related.

Patient factors

Over time breasts become ptotic due to the effects of gravity and aging. The effect of thinning of the breast tissue overlying the implant, due to pressure from the implant, can result in the shell becoming more palpable. It has been estimated that approximately 25% of the breast tissue overlying the implant can be lost in ten years and this is accelerated when larger implants are used. Patients therefore need to be warned of this effect, particularly where there is low pre-operative breast volume, and advised that excessively large implants will result in a more rapid deterioration in their aesthetic appearance.

This is analogous to the effects of breastfeeding. When the breasts are engorged with milk they can - subsequent to the cessation of breastfeeding - become saggy and thin. In the same way, tissue expansion of the breast can adversely affect the thickness of the breast tissue envelope by causing fat atrophy.

Surgical technique

If a patient is considered appropriate for augmentation mammaplasty, the most critical decision facing the surgeon is the surgical plane in which the implant will be placed.

Based upon personal experience and published studies, Spear [5] recommends subpectoral placement of implants in thin, small-breasted women, especially if saline-filled implants are used, to avoid implant palpability, visibility and rippling. Subglandular placement is reserved for those women with adequate breast tissue and subcutaneous fat **(III/B)**.

He identified the ptotic breast with thin, attenuated skin as a particular problem, since subpectoral placement runs the risk of double-bubble deformity, whilst subglandular placement runs the risk of palpability and visibility. For this last group of patients he recommends that mastopexy be performed as an adjunctive procedure, particularly if saline-filled implants are to be used **(IV/C)**.

The combination of mastopexy and implant augmentation, although initially providing excellent results, can result in long-term patient dissatisfaction not only with the scars necessitated by the mastopexy but also with the change of position of the implant, bottoming out of the breast and the scar rising up onto the breast mound. Sensitive and detailed counselling needs to be given to women undergoing mastopexy as to the level of their self-consciousness resulting from visible scarring.

In 1993, Mladick [6] published a retrospective analysis of 2,863 breast augmentations using saline implants in 1,327 patients. Initially, his practice was to place under-filled implants in the submammary plane. Because of the complications encountered with this method, the technique evolved to using over-filled implants subpectorally. Wrinkles were reported by 22/666 (3.3%) patients with subpectoral implants. Mladick attributed this difference to the increased soft tissue cover provided by the pectoralis major muscle **(III/B)**.

In the author's experience, an incidence of wrinkling of 3.3% is low, particularly with saline implants, and the problem is hugely more apparent as time progresses. Unfortunately, many of the papers published on rippling and wrinkling do not clearly establish the plane in which the implant is inserted, nor do they distinguish between saline and silicone implants, and the period of follow-up is often very short or vague. Consequently, it is quite difficult to get accurate figures of the incidence of rippling and wrinkling.

Retrospective studies, particularly when carried out by the operating surgeon, are very unlikely to be unduly critical. Indeed, in the commercial world it is very rare that the surgeon will point out to a patient attending for follow-up many years following surgery, the imperfections of their surgical result. This criticism is not easily invited and if a patient is happy then it is often best left undiscussed.

In reply to a letter regarding one of his own papers, Dr Tebbetts [7] states what he feels to be the main reasons for re-operation in patients with edge palpability or visibility secondary to tissue thinning. These are:

- Using excessively large implants.
- Placing implants below inadequate breast tissue (submammary placement in thin patients).
- Dividing medial origins of pectoralis.
- Thin subcutaneous tissue cover or placing any implant at all in very thin patients.

In particular, he describes how large implants with inadequate soft tissue cover predispose a patient to traction rippling (caused by the implant pulling on a capsule attached to thin overlying soft tissue). Palpable breast implants are more common following implant exchange, especially with extensive capsulotomy.

A plane deep to pectoralis major muscle fascia and superficial to the muscle may overcome problems seen with both conventional planes for implant placement. Graf [8] states that subglandular implant placement has higher rates of capsular contracture and implant palpability than subpectoral placement, whereas subpectoral placement is prone to distortion when the overlying muscle contracts. Placing the implant deep to the pectoral fascia obviates both these problems. In their study, McGhan FM 410™ cohesive silicone gel implants were used. Although the duration of follow-up is not reported, none of their 263 patients complained of noticeable implant edges **(III/B)**. It is felt that this technique would require an excessive amount of skill to maintain the integrity of the fascia at the lower pole of dissection.

Implant factors

The contour of the anterior implant wall depends upon the degree of implant fill, the visco-elastic property of the filler, and the elasticity of the shell wall [9].

Implant fill volume

All breast implants need to be adequately filled regardless of the properties of the shell and filler materials used. With pure silicone-filler implants there is no scope to alter the degree of fill but with saline-filled implants this is not so. Overfill is a fill volume in a saline implant which exceeds the manufacturer's recommended fill range. Underfill can mean using a fill volume below the manufacturer's fill range [10].

At the absolute limit for overfilling, a deformity called edge scalloping is likely to develop as the shell deforms into indentations and protrusions along the implant periphery. If an implant is overfilled, it will be firm, mimicking capsular contracture.

If implants are underfilled, there is a greater likelihood of implant creases and folds which are easily palpable. These creases also predispose to implant failure, especially with a saline filler. When the patient is upright, the implant filler migrates inferiorly leaving a relatively underfilled upper pole and overfilled lower pole. Vertical tension on the implant exceeds horizontal tension and therefore vertical ripples develop. The more viscous the filler, the less likely this is to occur.

Tebbetts describes a tilt test to achieve optimal fill [10]. It assesses the amount of fill required to prevent upper pole collapse when the implant is placed upright. Before implantation, the implant is supported in both the surgeon's hands. If the implant is adequately filled, there will be no upper pole collapse or creases. An implant has to pass the tilt test before insertion and this, allied with careful pocket selection (never placing a subglandular implant in a patient with less than 2cm pinch thickness superior to the breast parenchyma), has largely eliminated visible rippling or wrinkling **(III/B)**.

Filler material

In 2002, McGhan [11] published results from their own research, having examined complications in a heterogeneous group of patients from 1995. No information is available regarding the plane of implant placement or the surface characteristics. One study (A95) looked at 901 patients undergoing primary breast augmentation, whilst another included 237 patients undergoing breast reconstruction (R95). At five years post-surgery, in the primary augmentation group, 14% of patients complained of implant wrinkling and 12% of implant palpability or visibility. In the reconstruction group, at five years post-surgery, 25% of patients complained of implant wrinkling and 27% of implant palpability or visibility. Patients were re-operated upon in 4% of the primary augmentation patients for both wrinkling and implant palpability/visibility, and 3% of the reconstruction group by the fifth postoperative year.

Cohesive gel filler

The problems encountered with traction wrinkles in saline-filled and conventional silicone-filled breast implants provoked the development of cohesive gel-filled implants. Because the filler is less susceptible to inferior migration under the influence of gravity, traction wrinkling should not be seen. Early clinical studies support this theoretical advantage. Disadvantages of this filler are that it is firmer than conventional silicone and more expensive, although this is probably due to marketing rather than raw material costs.

Also, in a submammary pocket, the cohesive gel implant moves as a more solid structure rather like a saucer, and can, under certain circumstances, have a very artificial appearance not dissimilar to gross capsular contracture **(IV/C)**.

Cohesive gel-filled implants are manufactured by several companies including Silimed, Mentor and McGhan. Brown [12] reports on his experience with the first 118 patients in whom he implanted McGhan 410 cohesive gel implants (117 bilateral and one unilateral). The indications for using these implants specifically included patients considered to be at high risk of postoperative rippling. Both subglandular and submuscular pockets were used for the primary augmentation. Interestingly he reported no cases of implant rippling **(III/B)**.

In a larger series published by Heden et al [13], 823 patients with McGhan style 410 anatomical cohesive gel implants were examined. Fourteen patients (1.7%) complained of irregularities of the upper pole. This was usually associated with capsular contracture and subglandular placement. In two cases this buckling was visible (0.2%). They attributed this buckling to inadequate superior pocket dissection at the original implant insertion, exacerbated by capsular contracture **(III/B)**. It is not possible to be clear on the time for which these patients were followed up. The remarkable absence of implant palpability may reflect a relatively short follow-up period.

Hodgkinson [14] has reported on two cases of palpable upper pole deformity in breasts augmented using McGhan style 410 implants. The patients presented within six months of augmentation with palpable upper pole breast masses. At operation he found that the fibrous tissue capsule around the implants had contracted, causing corrugations which imprinted on the cohesive gel and resulted in buckling of the superior pole and a palpable superior mass. To avoid this complication in future, he recommended submuscular placement of the superior aspect of the implant **(IV/C)**.

Newer cohesive implants with a softer gel, such as the Mentor Contour Profile® gel implant, have been used where revisional surgery is required to correct visible wrinkling [15]. The outcome following long-term follow-up remains to be seen.

Other filler materials

In one study of Trilucent™ implants [16] before their compulsory withdrawal from sale, a postal survey found that 13.7% of patients complained of implant rippling. The authors defined rippling as shell surface irregularities with or without skin wrinkling.

It is interesting to note that the bulletin published by the makers of Trilucent implants within the first few years of their sale made no reference to rippling when discussing complications, although this was apparent to many of those practitioners who used them.

Implant shell factors

Polyurethane-coated implants were found to produce lower capsular contracture rates than smooth-surfaced implants when they were first introduced. There were, however, concerns that the breakdown products of polyurethane could be toxic and that late delamination of the coating produced capsular contracture. Collis and Sharpe [17] noted that the incidence of capsular contracture reached 25% as the polyurethane detached itself from its surface. This is possibly because the underlying surface no longer presented a textured interface, and the underlying shell was smoother. The difference in capsular contracture between smooth and textured implants was originally reported in 1989 [18]. Textured-surface silicone implants, or rather textured-silicone-surface implants were becoming popular by the mid-80s and the associated reduction in the incidence of capsular contracture was becoming apparent.

Different methods are used by different manufacturers to produce the irregular surface.

Mentor achieves their Siltex® surface by negative contact imprinting off a texturing foam. Biocell™ surfaces are produced by McGhan using a lost salt technique. Textured implants have a thicker shell when compared with smooth-walled breast implants and are therefore stiffer, predisposing to palpability and visibility of wrinkles in an implant [4]. When textured implants are placed in the subglandular plane they are especially prone to producing palpable folds in the implant shell, especially if placed in association with a capsulectomy or parenchymal atrophy [19].

Handel et al [20] found a correlation between surface texture and wrinkles. Wrinkling appeared more frequently in patients with Biocell (10.0%) and polyurethane-covered implants (4.7%) than Siltex (2.2%) and smooth (0.4%) **(III/B)**.

This is supported by Young [4] who assessed 154 patients with 308 implants for primary breast augmentation using round McGhan or Mentor saline implants in the submuscular position. When looking at surface coating he found that overall, 13% of the smooth and 44% of the textured breasts had implant ripples palpable by the surgeon. This was a problem for the patient with 3% of the smooth implants and 29% of the textured implants. Another aspect of textured implants is that if tissue re-growth occurs into the texturing then, particularly in saline-filled implants, traction wrinkling occurs when the patient is upright **(III/B)**.

Buckling and kinking of the implants and palpable folds in the inframammary position appear to have a direct relationship to the thickness of the implant shell. This can be seen *in vitro* when comparing different types of implants. Thinner-shelled implants, when judged by micrometre thickness, have a softer palpable feel and this is born out in practice when they are used in the submammary position.

Strategy for treating palpable implant rippling

Non-operative treatment

A palpable implant may be detected by the examining surgeon or by the patient. When it is the

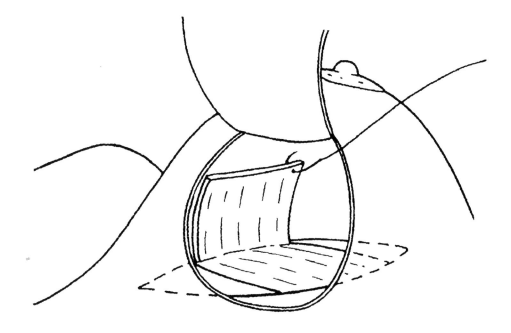

Figure 1. Pectoralis major trapdoor flap being transposed through the capsulotomy and sutured to the inside medial implant capsule. *Reproduced with permission from Lippincott Williams & Wilkins, © 2001* [19].

patient who detects the implant she may simply require reassurance as to what she is feeling and then no further action need be taken. If the patient has recently lost weight, it is often the case that a small amount of weight gain corrects the problem without recourse to surgical intervention. In patients who smoke, it is worth recommending that they try to stop smoking, not only because of the obvious health benefits, but also because it can cause a subtle enough gain in weight and therefore the soft breast tissue envelope to mask the palpable implant.

In addition, a database compiled by Collis and Sharpe shows that smoking is associated with a two-fold increase in the incidence of capsular contracture [21] **(III/B)**.

Operative treatment

Other surgical techniques for correcting established, symptomatic, implant rippling have been described. The principle of treatment is autologous soft tissue interposition between the implant and skin.

If it is not felt sensible to move the implant from a subglandular to subpectoral plane, then various options are available. These involve recruiting local tissues or using tissue grafts from a remote location.

A small segmental medially-based pectoralis major 'trapdoor' flap has been described by Collis *et al* [19]. After removal of the implant, a medial capsulotomy is used to provide access to the pectoralis major muscle. A medially-based flap is then raised from lateral to medial, approximately 8cm in length and two ribs wide. Intercostal pedicles are preserved. This flap is then sutured to the inside of the anterior capsule wall and the implant replaced. This muscle flap was used in five patients over a three-year period. No complications were found. The pre-operative contour deformity had been corrected when patients were seen postoperatively, but the exact duration of follow-up is not stated **(III/B)** (Figure 1).

To treat one patient who presented with palpable subglandular implant wrinkling at the medial border and atrophic overlying skin, but was otherwise happy with the implant position, rather than reinserting an

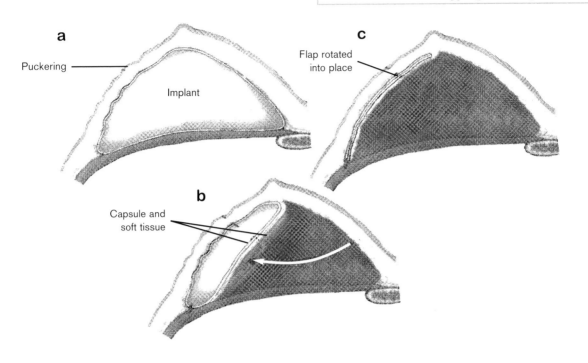

a Puckering — Implant

c Flap rotated into place

b Capsule and soft tissue

Figure 2. a) **A schematic view of the rippling skin over the implant (pre-operatively). b) The flap of capsular scar tissue with the lining of adipose and soft tissues is elevated from thicker areas, is hinged on its base, and is sutured in place. c) Final stage before insertion of the implant.** *Reproduced with permission from Lippincott Williams & Wilkins, © 2002* [23].

implant subpectorally, Gargano *et al* [22] elected to reinsert the implant in the original subglandular plane. Overlying soft tissue augmentation was achieved by releasing the capsule laterally and superolaterally to allow rotation of a flap of the capsule to lie deep to the thinned skin. When seen in the sixth postoperative week, the patient reported resolution of her symptoms. No follow-up is available after this time **(III/B)**.

Massiha [23] describes a technique similar in principle to that of Gargano *et al.* The implant is removed from its capsule. The capsule is then dissected off the chest wall and breast anteriorly and sutured onto itself. Massiha claims good results but there is no comment on follow-up **(III/B)** (Figure 2).

In the same paper, Massiha also describes using fat injections in one patient to correct severe widespread ripples. This is highly controversial. Bircoll [24] first described breast augmentation using fat harvested following suction lipectomy. Numerous problems have been described in the relatively small

number of patients in whom this has been performed, including sepsis [25]. Perhaps the most serious of these are discrete areas of firmness within the breast and calcifications seen on mammography, both of which could mimic the appearance of carcinoma of the breast [26]. To retain perspective it should be noted that breast masses and calcification are both common following routinely performed breast reduction surgery. These legitimate concerns may explain the paucity of reports supporting Massiha's practice.

Dr Emanuel Delay [27] suggests that fat injection may be associated with fewer risks when carried out using refined techniques of multiple tissue passes and small pieces of fat cells. Incidents of calcification and fat loss may be much reduced, and opinion may change in the next few years.

McGregor [28] corrected the problem of palpable implant rippling in two patients using a fascia lata patch applied within or outside the area of the capsule where the problem exists. In a personal communication from Mr. McGregor [29], he reveals that follow-up of these two

Chapter 22

patients has been at least two years. The most severe case has seen the rippling improved but the problem has not been completely corrected. Both patients are happy with the results achieved. Mr McGregor goes on to explain that further patients have declined to have fascia lata patches to correct palpable implant ripples due to concerns about the donor site (although the donor sites of the two patients in his original series have not caused problems) **(III/B)**.

Conclusions

In conclusion, the best strategy for minimising palpable implant rippling, is to be realistic in the selection of appropriate patients for breast augmentation. Care must be taken in the thin patient with ptotic breasts. Planning for the operation must include consideration of the anatomical plane of implant insertion and the type of filler material used to best avoid a palpable implant. The subpectoral plane and cohesive fillers are least likely to result in a palpable implant. Descriptions of techniques to correct this problem are not plentiful in the literature and, therefore, no single technique can be prescribed. With time, and the popularity of breast augmentation using silicone prostheses, thinning of the overlying breast tissue will result in the deformity rivalling capsular contracture as the most intractable barrier to the optimal aesthetic result.

Recommendations	Evidence level
◆ Patients at high risk of experiencing palpable breast implants such as those with very small amounts of breast tissue (<2cm at the upper pole), revision augmentation with capsulectomy, and following reconstruction, must be identified and appropriately counselled.	III/B
◆ If a previously augmented breast does not require capsulectomy the risk of implant palpability is less.	III/B
◆ If a thin, small-breasted patient requests breast augmentation, the subpectoral plane is less likely to result in a palpable implant.	III/B
◆ Where adequate upper pole breast tissue exists, subglandular augmentation is acceptable. This may need to be performed in conjunction with a mastopexy if the breast is very ptotic.	III/B
◆ Large and, therefore, broad-based implants, are more likely to be palpable. Patients need to be warned of this pre-operatively.	IV/C
◆ Saline-filled implants are more likely to be palpable than silicone gel-filled implants.	III/B
◆ Cohesive gel-filled implants have the lowest incidence of implant palpability (when compared with conventional silicone and saline fillers).	III/B
◆ Textured implants, especially in the subglandular plane, are more likely to be palpable.	III/B
◆ Non-operative treatment of palpable breast implants includes conscious subtle weight gain by the patient, helped, where possible, by the cessation of smoking.	IV/C
◆ Operative strategies for correcting palpable implants include implant exchange (using cohesive gel or using a softer shell) and altering the plane of insertion from subglandular to submuscular.	III/B
◆ With the exception of fat injection, the methods used to correct established implant palpability are all reported to work well, at least in the short term. No long-term follow-up is available.	III/B
◆ The use of fat injection to treat implant palpability cannot presently be recommended because of concerns about confusing artefacts on mammography.	III/B

References

1. Cronin TD, Gerow FJ. Augmentation mammaplasty: a new 'natural feel' prosthesis. Transactions of the 3rd International Congress of Plastic and Reconstructive Surgery, Amsterdam, Excerpta Medica 1964: 41-9.

2. Kulmala I, McLaughlin JK, Pakkanen M, Lassila K, Hölmich LR, Lipworth L, Boice JD, Raitanen J, Luoto R. Local complications after cosmetic breast implant surgery in Finland. *Ann Plast Surg* 2004; 53(5): 413-9.

3. Kessler DA. Statement on silicone gel breast implants, Jan 1992, www.fda.gov/.

4. Young VL Watson ME. Breast implant research. Where have we been, where we are, where we need to go. *Clin Plastic Surg* 2001; 28 (3): 451-82.

5. Spear SL, Elmaraghy M, Hess C. Textured-surface saline-filled silicone breast implants for augmentation mammaplasty. *Plast Reconstr Surg* 2000; 105 (4): 1542-52.

6. Mladick RA. 'No-touch' submuscular saline breast augmentation technique. *Aesthetic Plast Surg* 1993; 17: 183-92.

7. Tebbetts JB. Reply. *Plast Reconstr Surg* 2003; 111: (4) 1565-7.

8. Graf RM, Bernardes A, Rippel R, Araujo LRR, Damasio RCC, Auersvald A. Subfascial breast implant: a new procedure. *Plast Reconstr Surg* 2003; 111(2): 904-8.

9. Nicolle FV. Capsular contracture and ripple deformity of breast implants. *Aesthetic Plast Surg* 1996; 20: 311-4.

10. Tebbetts JB. Patient's acceptance of adequately filled breast implants using the tilt test. *Plast Reconstr Surg* 2000; 106 (1): 139-47.

11. *Making an Informed Decision. Saline-Filled Breast Implant Surgery.* Inamed Corporation, 2002.

12. Brown MH, Shenker R, Silver SA. Cohesive silicone gel breast implants in aesthetic and reconstructive breast surgery. *Plast Reconstr Surg* 2005; 116 (3): 768-79.

13. Hedén P, Jernbeck J, Hober M. Breast augmentation with anatomical cohesive gel implants. The world's largest current experience. *Clin Plast Surg* 2001; 28(3): 531-52.

14. Hodgkinson DJ. Buckled upper pole breast style 410 implant presenting as a manifestation of capsular contraction. *Aesthetic Plast Surg* 1999; 23: 279-81.

15. Fruhstorfer BH, Hodgson ELB, Malata CM. Early experience with an anatomical soft cohesive silicone gel prosthesis in cosmetic and reconstructive breast implant surgery. *Ann Plast Surg* 2004; 53 (6): 536-42.

16. Rizkalla M, Duncan C, Matthews RN. Trilucent™ breast implants: a 3-year series. *Br J Plast Surg* 2001; 54: 125-7.

17. Collis N, Sharpe DT. Silicone gel-filled breast implants integrity: a retrospective review of 478 explanted implants. *Plast Reconstr Surg* 2000; 105: 1979-85.

18. Collis N, Coleman D, Foo ITF, Sharpe DT. Ten-year review of a prospective randomised controlled trial of textured versus smooth subglandular silicone gel breast implants. *Plast Reconstr Surg* 2000; 106: 786-90.

19. Collis N, Platt AJ, Batchelor AG. Pectoralis major 'trapdoor' flap for silicone breast implant medial knuckle deformities. *Plast Reconstr Surg* 2001; 108(7): 2133-5.

20. Handel N, Jensen JA, Black Q, Waisman JR, Silverstein MJ. The fate of breast implants: a critical analysis of complications and outcomes. *Plast Reconstr Surg* 1995; 96(7): 1521-33.

21. Collis N, Sharpe DT. Recurrence of subglandular breast implant capsular contracture: anterior versus total capsulectomy. *Plast Reconstr Surg* 2000; 106: 792-7.

22. Gargano F, Moloney DM, Arnstein PM. Use of a capsular flap to prevent palpable wrinkling of implants. *Br J Plast Surg* 2002; 55(3): 269.

23. Massiha H. Scar tissue flaps for the correction of post-implant breast rippling. *Ann Plast Surg* 2002; 48(5): 505-7.

24. Bircoll M. Cosmetic breast augmentation utilizing autologous fat and liposuction techniques. *Plast Reconstr Surg* 1987; 79(2): 267-71.

25. Valdatta L, Thione A, Buoro M, Tuinder S. A case of life-threatening sepsis after breast augmentation by fat injection. *Aesthetic Plast Surg* 2001; 25: 347-9.

26. Dixon PL. Autologous fat injection and breast augmentation. *Med J Aust* 1988; 148: 537.

27. Sinna R, Delay E, Garson S, Mojallel A. Scientific basis of fat transfer - critical review of the literature. *Ann Chir Plast Esthet* (French) 2006; 51(3): 223-30.

28. McGregor J, Bahia H. A possible new way of managing breast implant rippling using an autogenous fascia lata patch. *Br J Plast Surg* 2004; 57(4): 372-4.

29. McGregor J. Personal communication, 2006.

Strategies for minimising palpable implant
rippling in the augmented breast

Chapter 22

Chapter 23

Gynaecomastia: an algorithmic approach to surgical management (with special emphasis on liposuction)

Charles Malata BSc (HB) MB ChB LRCP MRCS FRCS (Glasg) FRCS (Plast.)
Consultant Plastic and Reconstructive Surgeon
Devor Kumiponjera MB BS AFRCS Ed FCS-ECSA
Clinical Fellow, Plastic Surgery
Catherine Lau MB ChB MRCS
Clinical Fellow, Plastic Surgery

ADDENBROOKE'S UNIVERSITY HOSPITAL
CAMBRIDGE UNIVERSITY HOSPITALS NHS TRUST, CAMBRIDGE, UK

Introduction

Abnormal male breast enlargement is a common benign condition for which treatment is sought if it fails to resolve spontaneously or is too socially embarrasing. Although medical therapies have been described, the gold standard of treatment is surgery. There is a plethora of reported surgical techniques for the correction of gynaecomastia. In contrast there is a paucity of published work on an integrated surgical approach in general and the roles of the different treatment modalities in particular. Common to many plastic surgery conditions the evidence levels for proposed treatments is low.

This chapter outlines the main surgical techniques and presents an algorithmic approach which can assist a surgeon in achieving predictable and safe results. It also provides the evidence for the proposed roles of the different treatment modalities.

Methodology

A PubMed search was used to gather evidence, using the key words 'gynaecomastia', 'classifications', 'open excision' and 'liposuction'. Secondary references were then obtained from these primary sources.

Aetiology

Gynaecomastia, or abnormal breast tissue enlargement in men, is the most common breast pathology among males. At puberty, 30-65% of boys have gynaecomastia [1]. This usually lasts for a few months and in almost 75% of them the breast enlargement subsides within two years. The incidence of clinical gynaecomastia in adult males is 36% and its prevalence gradually increases with age [2] to over 60% in the seventh decade [3].

Table 1. Causes of gynaecomastia. *Adapted from Neuman (1997)* [4] *and Wiesman et al (2004)* [5].

I: Idiopathic

II: Physiological
a.   Neonatal
b.   Pubertal
c.   Aging

III: Pathological
a.   *Congenital disorders*: Klinefelter's, anorchia (vanishing testis syndrome), hermaphroditism, androgen resistance syndromes, enzyme defects of testosterone synthesis (sometimes late onset), increased peripheral tissue aromatase)
b.   *Endocrine causes:* castration, mumps, Cushing's syndrome, congenital adrenal hyperplasia, ACTH deficiency, hyperthyroidism, hypothyroidism, panhypopituitarism, hyperprolactinaemia
c.   *Tumours*: testicular (choriocarcinoma, sertoli, Leydig cell tumours); adrenal (adenoma, carcinoma); pituitary adenoma; breast carcinoma; tumours that secrete HCG (lung, liver, kidney, stomach and lymphopoietic)
d.   *Drugs*: hormones (oestrogens, androgens, gonadotrophins); anti-androgens (cimetidine, spironolactone, digitalis, progesterone, cyproterone, flutamide); stimulators of prolactin (phenothiazines, reserpine, hydroxyzine); drugs of abuse (marijuana, heroin, methadone, amphetamines); anti-TB drugs (isoniazid, ethionamide, thiacetazone)
e.   *Metabolic:* thyrotoxicosis (altered testosterone/oestrone binding); renal failure (acquired testes failure); cirrhosis (increased substrate for peripheral aromatisation); starvation (same as cirrhosis); alcoholism
f.   *Miscellaneous:* HIV, chest wall trauma, cystic fibrosis, physiological stress

Most cases of gynaecomastia are idiopathic (25%) [6]. The known causes of gynaecomastia broadly fall into two categories: physiological or pathological (Table 1). Physiological gynaecomastia occurs in three different age groups: newborn, adolescent and elderly. In the newborn, gynaecomastia is attributed to the influence of transplacental transfer of circulating maternal oestrogen during intra-uterine life. At puberty and in the elderly, however, a relative imbalance between serum oestrogen and androgen levels may be responsible [2]. In the elderly, this results from both declining levels of testosterone and peripheral conversion of testosterone to oestrogen (peripheral aromatisation).

Three basic pathophysiological mechanisms account for the pathological type of gynaecomastia: relative or absolute excess of oestrogens, a decrease of circulating androgens or a defect in androgen receptors. Regardless of the aetiology, the ultimate cause of gynaecomastia is an increase in the effective oestrogen to testosterone ratio, since oestrogens stimulate breast development while androgens inhibit it. Drugs are the most common cause of pathological breast development. Testicular tumours are an important although less common cause. Tumours of the Leydig cells of the testis and those originating in the germinal elements act through the production of HCG (human chorionic gonadotropin). Other tumours such as bronchial carcinoma may also induce gynaecomastia via the same mechanism, whereas adrenal tumours cause excessive production of adrenal androgens which are then converted to oestrogen. In hepatic cirrhosis, liver clearance of adrenal androgens is reduced and therefore more are available for conversion to oestrogen in the periphery.

Classification of gynaecomastia

There are many classifications for gynaecomastia [7-9], the most practical being that proposed by Simon [7] (Table 2), as it takes into consideration not only the size of the breast but also the amount of redundant skin. There is still an overlap between the categories leading to subjectivity and inter-observer variability. The classification by Rohrich where the fatty and glandular tissue is determined by pinch test medially, laterally and beneath the nipple-areola complex and grades III and IV have either mild or severe ptosis, has similar limitations [8]. Therefore, we have simplified the Simon classification into two practical categories namely, small-to-moderate size with no or minimal skin excess (Simon's grades I and IIa), and moderate-to-large size with moderate-to-marked skin excess (grades IIb and III) [10]. In addition, breast consistency must be noted as it influences treatment options. Based on its consistency, gynaecomastia has been subdivided by Fodor into true (predominantly glandular hypertrophy), pseudo (predominantly adipose tissue), and mixed (combination of both) types [9].

Patient evaluation

The commonest presenting complaint is social embarrassment, but in some patients breast pain secondary to enlargement can be problematic (55% in grade I) [11]. Pubertal boys with gynaecomastia in the presence of normal growth do not merit complicated laboratory investigations. In patients with abnormal growth, however, approximately half will have an abnormality responsible for their gynaecomastia [3].

Referring clinicians (commonly paediatricians, endocrinologists or general breast surgeons) need to exclude possible underlying medical causes of gynaecomastia. A detailed medical and drug history with special attention to possible thyroid and liver abnormalities is taken. Testicular examination should also be performed to rule out tumours or atrophy. In addition, a biochemical assessment (prolactin, liver function tests, testosterone, oestrogen, T4/TSH, U/Es) is recommended along with mammography and breast ultrasound with or without fine-needle aspiration/core biopsy if indicated [11]. Most cases of gynaecomastia are bilateral and hence unilateral breast swelling should not be assumed to be gynaecomastia unless breast cancer has been excluded. Clinically the most difficult condition to differentiate from gynaecomastia is adipose hypertrophy without glandular proliferation (pseudo-gynaecomastia). Additional tests (α-FP, ß-hCG, γ-GT, PSA, DHEAs, urinary 17-ketosteroids) may be indicated based on clinical findings and may be necessary in cases of recent or symptomatic gynaecomastia [12]. Extensive work-up is rarely indicated and often does not influence treatment [6].

In the first consultation with the plastic surgeon, a detailed history and clinical examination of the enlarged breasts is necessary in order to evaluate the severity of the gynaecomastia and formulate an appropriate management plan. The salient history includes the patient's age, duration and onset of breast enlargement, symptoms of pain, tenderness, medications, recreational drug use, psychological and social effects and systems review including weight changes and cancer. On inspection, note is made whether the condition is unilateral or bilateral, the

Table 2. Simon's classification of gynaecomastia.

I.	Small visible breast enlargement, no skin excess
II.	Moderate breast enlargement
	a. Without skin redundancy
	b. With skin redundancy
III.	Marked breast enlargement and marked skin redundancy

patient is obese or not obese, and whether there is skin excess, ptosis, or developed inframammary folds. The skin quality is assessed into poor, fair or normal depending on its potential ability to contract postoperatively. On palpation, the presence of glandular (or parenchymal) tissue, its extent, distribution and proportion versus fat is noted. Any tenderness and discrete masses especially firm sub-areolar discs are determined. The consistency of breasts is also determined (soft, moderate, and firm/hard). Then an appropriate management plan is formulated.

Medical management

Most cases of gynaecomastia especially those occurring during adolescence are benign and self-limiting [1-3]. Therefore, pubertal males should be reassured and observed in the first instance. If there is an underlying cause, this should, however, be corrected (or withdrawn). Treatment is sought when gynaecomastia fails to resolve spontaneously or its emotional and/or psychological impact is unbearable. Medical therapies using testosterone (the non-aromatisable androgen dihydrotestosterone), anti-oestrogens (clomiphene and tamoxifen) and danazol (androgen and pituitary gonadotrophin inhibitor) or testolactone (aromatase inhibitor) have limited success and are probably most effective during the active, proliferative phase of gynaecomastia. Irradiation has also been used prophylactically in patients with prostatic cancer treated by anti-androgens [13-15]. In patients with longstanding gynaecomastia (>12 months), the breast glandular tissue should be removed surgically [16] because it will often have progressed to irreversible dense fibrosis and hyalinization [3, 16, 17]. Most patients do not need a trial of drug treatment and are best treated with surgery, which is the mainstay of treatment.

Surgical management

The aim of surgery is restoration of a normal male chest contour while minimising the evidence of surgery and maintaining the viability of the nipple-areola complex. It is indicated in cases of severe gynaecomastia, failed medical therapies or on the patient's request. Post-pubertal gynaecomastia also requires aggressive management in the form of surgery. There are many surgical techniques for treating gynaecomastia varying from open excision and skin reduction to minimally invasive liposuction. Open surgery, primarily through excisional techniques is long established and continues to have a significant role. Over the last two decades conventional liposuction (SAL) and, more recently, ultrasound-assisted liposuction (UAL) have been demonstrated to be effective treatment options. The salient features of the main available surgical modalities are outlined below.

Open techniques (open excision alone /open excision with skin reduction)

Simple open excision of excess breast tissue and overlying skin, as the treatment for gynaecomastia to improve mammary appearance was first described by Paulus Aegineta (625-690 AD) [18]. Although the glandular resection remains the same, many types of incision have been proposed and this subject has been excellently illustrated by Aslan et al [19]. They include circumareolar, peri-areolar, transareolar and circumthelial incisions. Today open excision via an inferior peri-areolar approach as reported by Webster in 1946 remains the standard worldwide [20]. Excisional methods, although effective, leave patients with visible (sometimes large) scars. In patients with skin excess (Simon grades IIb and III), skin reduction may be indicated. The optimal timing and method to undertake skin resection remain controversial. The available skin reduction techniques are peri-areolar, lateral wedge, elliptical, inverted-T and LeJour [10, 21-23]. The concentric peri-areolar technique is the most popular because of the less noticeable scarring [21, 22]. In patients with true ptosis or those aiming for completely flat breasts, skin reduction can be undertaken using the LeJour vertical mammaplasty skin pattern [10]. The open transaxillary approach [24] has not gained popularity. All these scars are noticeable even after 12-18 months (Figure 1). Patients with very large and/or ptotic breasts are suitable candidates for elliptical mastectomy and free nipple grafting [7, 23, 25] (IV/C). This also avoids the telltale features of female-type breast reduction scars. It should, however, be avoided in dark coloured skin because of nipple-areola de-pigmentation.

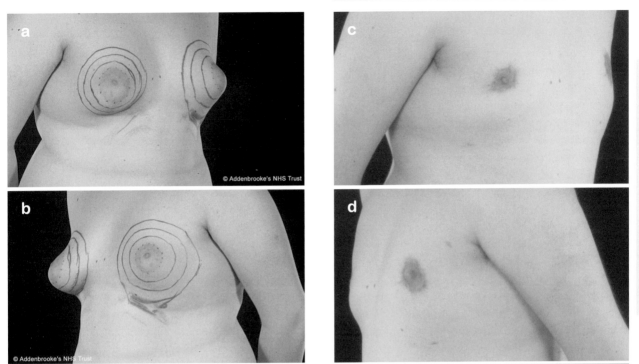

Figure 1. a) and b) A 14-year-old child with idiopathic severe gynaecomastia and moderate skin excess.
c) and d) He was successfully treated with SAL, open excision and concentric skin reduction. Note the
peri-areolar puckered scars one year postoperatively.

Table 3. Complications of open excision techniques for correcting gynaecomastia.

- ◆ Bleeding and haematoma
- ◆ Nipple-areolar or skin necrosis
- ◆ Contour irregularities (spectrum)
  - ● unevenness
  - ● depressed nipple-areola
  - ● large contour deformities
  - ● saucer deformity
  - ● nipple inversion
- ◆ Noticeable and deforming scars especially with skin reduction techniques

Patients with massive gynaecomastia [21, 26] and those with large anabolic steroid-induced hypertrophy of parenchymal breast tissue [27], are best treated by subcutaneous mastectomy and reduction mammaplasty, because of the extensive glandular enlargement well beyond the areola **(IV/C)**. Patients with Klinefelter's syndrome should also be treated by mastectomy because of the increased risk of breast cancer. Rosenberg, however, contends that suction-assisted lipectomy (SAL) with adequate cannulae can adequately treat both early hypertrophy and late fibrous hyalinization of steroid-induced gynaecomastia [28].

In an attempt to reduce unsightly scarring and risk of nipple deformities, less invasive excisional techniques have recently been advocated but have no proven track records. These include endoscopically-assisted techniques [29, 30], the so-called pull-through technique [31] and ultrasound-guided mammatome excision [32]. Open excisional techniques have been associated with high complication rates [32-34] (Table 3), hence the emergence of liposuction as a popular treatment modality. The aim of liposuction is to achieve a smooth, even feel with well-feathered edges.

Suction-assisted lipectomy (SAL)

This conventional liposuction uses a vacuum to aspirate fat through a stab incision via a hollow metal cannula. In gynaecomastia treatment, the liposuction access incisions have been variously sited, on the lateral chest wall (at the level of the nipple), peri-areolar and intra-areolar locations [35-42]. The more distal incisions tend to allow better access to the sub-areolar tissue [43]. Others prefer a separate inframammary fold or anterior axillary fold stab incision [10, 44], because sub-areolar tissue is especially hard to remove (suction) via the peri-areolar margin [45].

The breast tissue is infiltrated with liposuction solution (wet, super wet, tumescent techniques) to minimise complications such as bleeding. The hydro-dissection of the tumescent technique also facilitates suctioning in the tissue-dense areas and allows easier open excision should this become necessary during liposuction. It is commonly accepted that SAL is useful in selected patients with predominantly fatty breasts and well-located nipple-areolar complexes [10]. Teimourian, in 1983, was the first to apply SAL to treat gynaecomastia successfully [35]. This was further supported by Rosenberg who contended that all degrees of enlargement, as well as relative proportions of adipose and parenchymal tissue, could be treated with suction lipectomy [39]. He achieved this by using cannulas of different sizes and different cutting types through the peri-areolar incision to remove the tissue beneath the nipple-areolar complex. Rosenberg has also advocated aggressive suctioning and broad undermining, increasing with the size of gynaecomastia and the presence or absence of excess skin.

SAL alone

Complete removal of the fat and parenchymal tissue of gynaecomastia with SAL alone has been widely reported [10, 32, 37-41, 46, 47]. Special gynaecomastia cannulas are often necessary to achieve adequate correction of the deformity [28, 46-48]. Cross-suctioning for larger breasts, ptotic breasts, excess skin or well defined inframammary folds makes SAL more effective because it enables more consistent skin contraction and redraping with less waviness and irregularity (IV/C). The inframammary crease can be obliterated by sharp dissection [38] or by suction cannulae [48].

SAL combined with open excision

SAL has been used in conjunction with surgical excision since the early 1980s [32, 35, 36, 38]. Teimourian and later, Lewis, were the first to use SAL in moderate to large cases of gynaecomastia with excision of glandular tissue (by extending the incision if necessary) [35, 36]. The SAL was utilised in the periphery to smooth the contour. After vigorous suction, the nodules of parenchymal tissue can be sharply removed by scissors, cautery or knife. Rosenberg, however, contends that the individual nodules can be easily suctioned (and sent for histology) [28]. This, however, is not our experience. In patients with severe large soft gynaecomastia with skin excess and/or ptosis, we combine liposuction with concentric skin reduction as popularised by Botta (1998) [49].

In the senior author's experience, conventional liposuction (SAL) alone is useful for diffuse soft to moderately firm breast enlargement, especially in overweight and obese patients (IV/C). However, a residual sub-areolar nodule is a frequently encountered complication with this technique [10]. The postoperative persistence of these nodules is often uncomfortable to patients leading to requests for further surgery. Additionally, SAL is not suitable for severe cases or in breasts with primarily fibrous tissue and is associated with a high (up to 50%) incidence of intra-operative conversion to open excision [8, 10] (IV/C). It can be effective in soft breasts even if large, but good skin quality is important for later contraction and avoidance of skin resection. Superficial subcutaneous liposuction also helps to increase the degree of skin contraction [46, 48].

The complications of SAL are minimal (Table 4) and SAL alone has high patient satisfaction similar to ultrasound-assisted liposuction (UAL) [50].

Table 4. Reported complications of SAL.

- Haematoma
- Irregularity
- Seroma
- Skin redundancy
- Infection
- Asymmetry
- Residual lump (+/- painful or tender)

Ultrasound-assisted liposuction (UAL)

This technique employs ultrasonic energy transmitted by means of excited piezo-electric crystals located at the terminal ends of suction cannulae to emulsify fat (in tissues infiltrated with a wetting solution), while preserving adjacent nervous, vascular and connective tissue elements [8]. Emulsification is effected through cavitation of fat cells in tumesced fields [8, 51]. After application of the US energy to the tissues, the target area is contoured mechanically by using ordinary SAL cannulae for evacuation and remodelling [51-57].

UAL has been successfully applied to all three degrees of gynaecomastia by a number of workers [8, 10, 52, 53, 55, 56, 58] and is said to have a number of advantages over SAL **(III/B)** (Table 5). It is documented to be more effective over SAL in dense fibrous lipodystrophy areas of the body such as gynaecomastia, buttocks, back, flanks, upper abdomen and as a secondary procedure. It has thus extended the role of lipoplasty in body contouring in these difficult areas [55, 57]. At higher energy settings it removes the denser fibrotic parenchymal tissue that SAL is ineffective at eradicating [6]. It is, therefore, more effective for firmer breasts than SAL [8, 53, 56, 58]. The incidence of intra-operative conversion to open excision is very low (4%; two out of 49 consecutive breasts in the senior author's series) [10, 58]. Four other breasts required skin reduction because they were very large and ptotic with skin excess. The UAL amplitude, however, needs to be high (80-95%) [6, 58]. There is a very low rate of revisional or repeat surgery (three out of 49 breasts, 6% versus 26% for SAL after five years). It has also been suggested that postoperatively, UAL results in less bruising and swelling [50, 58, 59], a smoother breast contour and better skin contraction [55, 58, 60] **(IV/C)**. There was no difference in postoperative ecchymosis, swelling, complication rates and skin contraction in one prospective comparison of UAL and SAL [50].

Similar to SAL, UAL when used alone cannot correct extremely large gynaecomastia or marked skin redundancy (ptosis). It can, however, decrease the need for skin excisional procedures because of the induced skin retraction (although this is not specific to gynaecomastia) [50, 55, 58, 60]. For instance, Kloehn [61]

Table 5. Advantages claimed for UAL versus SAL.

- Selective emulsification of fat (leaving higher density structures undamaged)
- More efficient removal of fat in areas with higher densities of fibroconnective tissues such as male breasts
- Removal of denser fibrotic parenchymal tissue that SAL is inefficient at removing - at higher energy settings
- Better skin retraction in postoperative healing period
- Decreased physical demand

Table 6. Reported potential complications of UAL. *After Gingrass, 1999* [59] *and Rohrich et al, 2000* [67].

◆ Thermal and friction burns	◆ End hits
◆ Seroma (other sites 10 - 20%)	◆ Numbness: temporary
◆ Dysaesthesiae reversible - can be prolonged	◆ Haematoma
◆ Contour irregularities	◆ Asymmetries
◆ Minor surface irregularities	◆ Fibrosis
◆ Skin necrosis	◆ Blood loss
◆ Infection	◆ Scars
◆ Hyperpigmentation	

reported that gynaecomastia cases were easy to treat with UAL, but often required some sub-areolar tissue excision. The latter has not been our experience to date. With UAL, there is less physical effort by the surgeon which is important in fibrous areas such as gynaecomastia [56, 57, 61-63]. The advantages of less bruising and swelling, smoother breast contour and better postoperative skin retraction, are difficult to quantify. UAL has more potential complications than SAL (Table 6) and therefore requires meticulous safety precautions.

Power-assisted liposuction (PAL)

Power-assisted liposuction (PAL) is also a useful treatment modality. It represents another aggressive surgical approach needed to treat more fibrous types of gynaecomastia [6].

Systematic approach

A unifying approach, which seeks to maximise the strengths of the above treatment modalities, while minimising the drawbacks of each technique, has therefore been proposed [10]. The degree of the gynaecomastia is assessed clinically using a simplification of Simon's classification [7]. The starting point for all cases of gynaecomastia in our practice is liposuction [10]. This is undertaken even in those patients with firm sub-areolar discs in whom open excision is planned. This is because liposuction alone is often effective [10, 37-39, 48] as a single treatment modality (Figure 2). Additionally, even in patients who

pre-operatively need or are intra-operatively found to require open excision, the initial liposuction facilitates the subsequent resection [10, 55, 64] by pre-tunnelling, reducing bleeding and softening of the glandular tissue. It also allows contouring and feathering of the peripheries or surrounding areas, and therefore prevents saucerisation [10, 35, 36, 38] **(IV/C)**. It is technically easier to undertake liposuction at the beginning of the operation rather than after excision. Furthermore, liposuction stimulates postoperative skin contraction [34, 39, 46, 48], although this may be better with UAL [8, 10, 55, 58, 60, 63]. Webster's open excision technique via an inferior peri-areolar incision is indicated for firm/hard sub-areolar lumps and for residual glandular/stromal tissue following liposuction **(IV/C)**.

Patients in whom open excision is not mandated by the pre-operative appearance and consistency, are also routinely consented for open excision in case the liposuction leaves significant residual stromal tissue. This is best achieved by the inferior peri-areolar incision, as it is relatively inconspicuous if correctly positioned at the junction of the areola and chest wall skin [10] **(IV/C)**. Liposuction followed by open excision is very effective in most patients with grade I and II gynaecomastia [5, 32, 35, 36, 38] and has also been advocated for grade III [5] **(IV/C)**.

SAL is only used when UAL is not available because the latter is more efficacious [18, 55-58] and stimulates better skin contraction [10, 53, 55, 58, 60, 65] **(III/B)**. The overall clinical superiority of UAL has, however, yet to be proven by quantitative assessment [50, 63].

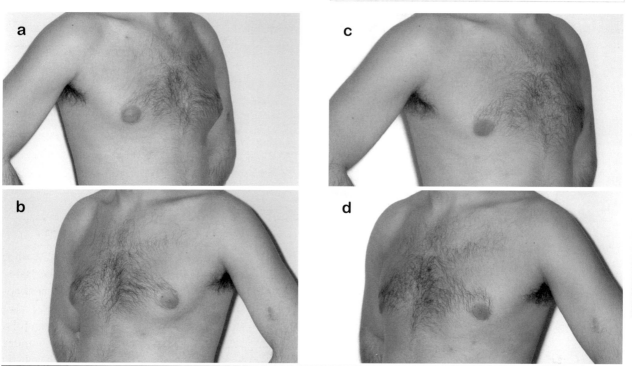

Figure 2. a) and b) A 23-year-old man with diffuse but moderate size gyneacomastia with excellent skin quality and no skin excess. c) and d) Six months following contouring with UAL.

Histologically and biochemically, UAL has been found to be superior to SAL or externally applied UAL [65-67] in terms of adipose cell disruption **(IIb/B)**. In animal models, UAL caused significantly less blood loss compared with traditional liposuction [68] **(IIa/B)**. This has been confirmed clinically by Kloehn [61] in a large series of 600 consecutive patients (30-50% reduction in blood loss compared with traditional or standard suction-assisted lipoplasty) and also by Fodor and Watson [50].

The incidence of intra-operative conversion to open excision is much less with UAL [58] (two out of 49 consecutive breasts over a five-year period) and we have noted a low revisional surgery rate (six out of 49 breasts) compared with a revisional rate of 26% with SAL. It is also less tiring for the surgeon [57, 61-63, 69], who is then 'free' to concentrate on the sculpting [58, 61]. UAL has, therefore, extended the role of liposuction in the management of gynaecomastia patients.

When there is skin excess with or without ptosis, we prefer to address the skin excess at the original operation [64, 70]. This is especially so in cases with poor or borderline skin elasticity. However, patients with large breasts and skin excess may sometimes not need skin resection or may refuse to accept the scars associated with it. These patients can be adequately treated by liposuction with or without open excision of any remaining breast parenchyma [27, 42] **(IV/C)**. In such patients the glandular resection needed after SAL is easily achieved via an inferior peri-areolar incision because the dissection is easier, bleeding is less and the amount of tissue to be removed is significantly less [5, 38, 39]. In the world's largest surgical series to date, Wiesman et al [5] have recommended that even for Grade III gynaecomastia a skin-sparing operation (SAL ± open glandular excision) should be the operation of choice **(III/B)**. If there is residual skin excess this can be excised in a second stage if needed, i.e. as a 'planned revision'. In cases with borderline skin elasticity, resection may occasionally be necessary after six months. Rohrich et al (2003) [8] contend that undertaking the delayed excision of the remaining ptotic breast skin and/or breast parenchyma six to nine months after UAL allows maximal skin retraction to occur.

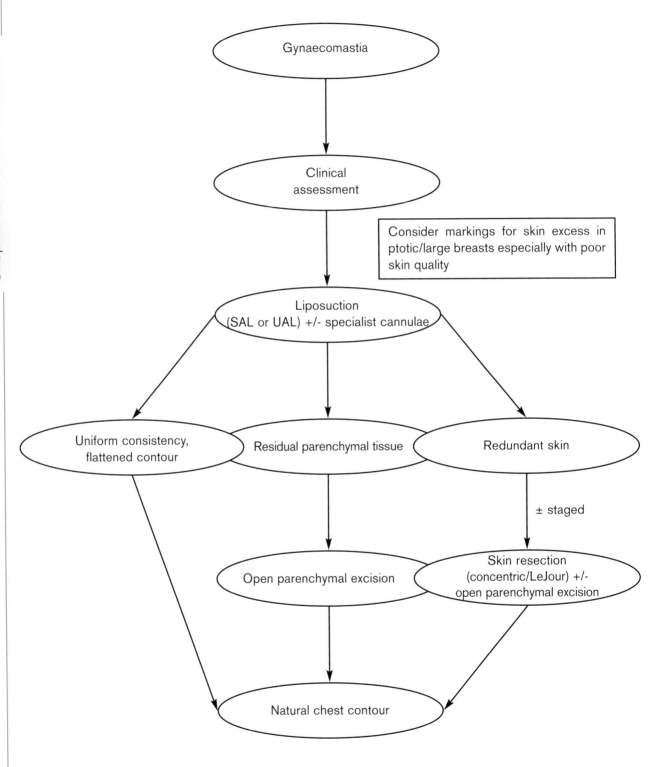

Figure 3. Diagrammatic algorithm for a systematic approach to the surgical management of gynaecomastia.

Patients needing skin reduction also benefit from initial liposuction as it reduces the bulk and initiates some skin retraction; these patients are often obese and therefore need tapering of the breast-fat junction. The peri-areolar concentric mastopexy-type reduction results in pleats or skin folds which settle down satisfactorily after 2-3 months [71, 72] (Figure 1). The peri-areolar Benelli suture is, however, sometimes palpable (not a major problem in men) and its knot needs to be buried deep to the dermis. The vertical component of the LeJour mammaplasty scar, like the lateral wedge excision, is noticeable but leads to dramatic improvement in contour. Surprisingly it is quite well accepted by patients [10]. A lateral gathering and resection of the excess skin has been suggested by some, but it may lead to nipples being positioned too laterally and thus rendering them unnatural.

Skin reduction with its resultant large visible scars is sometimes resisted by patients and thus another approach is to stage the surgery - starting with liposuction followed by subsequent skin resection six months or so later. This potentially reduces the extent of skin resection and hence minimises scarring. Occasionally patients planned for two-stage surgery accept the initial results (some skin redundancy) and decline the second skin reduction procedure. We prefer to reserve skin reduction/excisional techniques for severe gynaecomastia with significant skin excess after attempted UAL/SAL. Severe gynaecomastia (Rohrich grade III and IV) and patients whose glandular component is primarily fibrous tissue, have suboptimal results even with UAL and require staged excision [8].

Conclusions

Although many plastic surgeons can obtain excellent results using many treatment modalities, today's breast surgeon is faced with a plethora of techniques and a logical approach can lead to predictable results in the surgical management of gynaecomastia. The aim of a natural-looking chest can thereby be more consistently achieved.

A diagrammatic algorithm for a systematic approach to the surgical management of gynaecomastia is shown in Figure 3.

Recommendations	Evidence level
◆ In all grades of gynaecomastia, liposuction should always be the starting point.	IV/C
◆ SAL alone can be effective treatment, especially in soft/moderate diffuse gynaecomastia.	IV/C
◆ UAL alone has extended the role of liposuction in all grades of gynaecomastia and is more efficacious than SAL.	III/B
◆ Skin reduction is sometimes required whether SAL or UAL is used.	IV/C
◆ The most effective treatment for firm/hard sub-areolar discs and grade III/IV gynaecomastia remains open excision.	IV/C

References

1. Nydick M, Bustos J, Dale JH, *et al*. Gynecomastia in adolescent boys. *JAMA* 1961; 178: 449-54.

2. Nutall FQ. Gynecomastia as a physical finding in normal men. *J Clin Endocrinol Metab* 1979; 48: 338-40.

3. Hands LJ, Greenall MJ. Gynaecomastia. *Br J Surg* 1991; 78(8): 907-11.

4. Neuman. Evaluation and treatment of gynaecomastia. *American Fam Physician* 1997; 55 (5): 1835-49, 1849-50.

5. Wiesman IM, Lehman JA Jr, Parker MG, Tantri MD, Wagner DS, Pedersen JC. Gynecomastia: an outcome analysis. *Ann Plast Surg* 2004; 53(2): 97-101.

6. Ha RJ, Rohrich RJ, Kenkel JM. Treatment of gynaecomastia. In: *The Art of Aesthetic Surgery, Principles and Techniques.* Nahai F, Ed. St. Louis, Mo: Quality Medical Publishing, Inc., 2005; Chapter 54: 2076-101.

7. Simon BE, Hoffman S, Kahn S. Classification and surgical correction for gynecomastia. *Plast Reconstr Surg* 1973; 51: 48.

8. Rohrich RJ, Ha RY, Kenkel JM, Adams WP Jr. Classification and management of gynecomastia: defining the role of ultrasound-assisted liposuction. *Plast Reconstr Surg* 2003; 111(2): 909-23.

9. Fodor PB. Breast cancer in a patient with gynecomastia. *Plast Reconstr Surg* 1989; 84: 976-9.

10. Fruhstorfer BH, Malata CM. A systematic approach to the surgical treatment of gynaecomastia. *Br J Plast Surg* 2003; 56(3): 237-46.

11. Daniels IR, Layer GT. How should gynecomastia be managed? *ANZ J Surg* 2003; 73(4): 213-6.

12. Carlson HE. Gynecomastia. *N Engl J Med* 1980; 303(14): 795-9.

13. Di Lorenzo G, Perdona S, De Placido S, D'Armiento M, Gallo A, Damiano R, Pingitore D,Gallo L, De Sio M, Autorino R. Gynaecomastia and breast pain induced by adjuvant therapy with bicalutamide after prostatectomy in patients with prostate cancer: the role of tamoxifen and radiotherapy. *J Urol* 2005; 174(6): 2197-203.

14. Tyrrel CJ, Payne H, Tammela TL, Bakke A, Lodding P, Goedhals L, Van Erps P, Boon T, Van De Beek C, Andersson SO, Morris T, Carroll K. Prophylactic breast irradiation with a single dose of electron beam radiotherapy (10 Gy) significantly reduces the incidence of bicalutamide-induced gynaecomastia. *Int J Radiat Oncol Biol Phys* 2004; 60(2): 476-83.

15. Van Poppel H, Tyrrell CJ, Haustermans K, Cangh PV, Keuppens F, Colombeau P, Morris T, Garside L. Efficacy and tolerability of radiotherapy as treatment for bicalutamide-induced gynaecomastia and breast pain in prostate cancer. *Eur Urol* 2005; 47(5): 587-92.

16. Braunstein GD. Gynecomastia. *N Engl J Med* 1993; 328(7): 490-5.

17. Bannayan GA, Hajdu SI. Gynecomastia: clinicopathologic study of 351 cases. *Am J Clin Pathol* 1972; 57: 431-7.

18. Adams F. In the seven books of Paulus Aegineta, Trans. Vol 2. London: The Syndenham Society, 1846.

19. Aslan G, Tuncali D, Terzioglu A, Bingul F. Periareolar-transareolar-perithelial incision for the surgical treatment of gynecomastia. *Ann Plast Surg* 2005; 54(2): 130-4.

20. Webster JP. Mastectomy for gynecomastia through a semi-circular intra-areolar incision. *Ann Surg* 1946; 124: 557.

21. Davidson BA. Concentric circle operation for massive gynecomastia to excise the redundant skin. *Plast Reconstr Surg* 1979; 63(3): 350-4.

22. Smoot EC. Eccentric skin resection and purse-string closure for skin reduction with mastectomy for gynecomastia. *Ann Plast Surg* 1998; 41(4): 378-83.

24. Balch CR. A transaxillary incision for gynaecomastia. *Plast Reconstr Surg* 1978; 61: 13-6.

23. Wray RC, Hoopes JE, Davis GM. Correction of extreme gynaecomastia. *Br J Plast Surg* 1974; 27: 39-41.

25. Murphy TP, Ehrlichman RJ, Seckel BR. Nipple placement in simple mastectomy with free nipple grafting for severe gynecomastia. *Plast Reconstr Surg* 1994; 94: 818-23.

26. Letterman J, Schurter M. Surgical correction of massive gynecomastia. *Plast Reconstr Surg* 1972; 49: 259-62.

27. Aiache AE. Surgical treatment of gynecomastia in the body builder. *Plast Reconstr Surg* 1989; 83: 61-6.

28. Rosenberg GJ. A new cannula for suction removal of parenchymal tissue of gynaecomastia. *Plast Reconstr Surg* 1994; 94: 548-51.

29. Ohyama T, Takada A, Fujikawa M, Hosokawa K. Endoscope-assisted transaxillary removal of glandular tissue in gynecomastia. *Ann Plast Surg* 1998; 40(1): 62-4.

30. Prado AC, Castillo PF. Minimal surgical access to treat gynecomastia with the use of a power-assisted arthroscopic-endoscopic cartilage shaver. *Plast Reconstr Surg* 2005; 115(3): 939-42.

31. Bracaglia R, Fortunato R, Gentileschi S, Seccia A, Farallo E. Our experience with the so-called pull-through technique combined with liposuction for management of gynecomastia. *Ann Plast Surg* 2004; 53(1): 22-6.

32. Iwuagwu OC, Calvey TA, Ilsley D, Drew PJ. Ultrasound-guided minimally invasive breast surgery (UMIBS): a superior technique for gynecomastia. *Ann Plast Surg* 2004; 52(2): 131-3.

33. Steele SR, Martin MJ, Place RJ. Gynecomastia: complications of the subcutaneous mastectomy. *Am Surg* 2002; 68(2): 210-3.

34. Courtiss EH. Gynecomastia: analysis of 159 patients and current recommendations for treatment. *Plast Reconstr Surg* 1987; 79(5): 740-53.

35. Teimourian B, Perlman R. Surgery for gynecomastia. *Aesthetic Plast Surg* 1983; 7(3): 155-7.

36. Lewis CM. Lipoplasty: treatment for gynaecomastia. *Aesthetic Plast Surg* 1985; 9(4): 287-92.

37. Mladick RA, Morris RL. Sixteen months' experience with the Illouz technique of lipolysis. *Ann Plast Surg* 1986; 16: 220-32.

38. Mladick RA. Gynecomastia. Liposuction and excision. *Clin Plast Surg* 1991; 18(4): 815-22.

39. Rosenberg GJ. Gynecomastia: suction lipectomy as a contemporary solution. *Plast Reconstr Surg* 1987; 80(3): 379-86.

40. Rigg BM. Morselization suction: a modified technique for gynecomastia. *Plast Reconstr Surg* 1991; 88: 159-60.

41. Samdal F, Kleppe G, Amland PF, Abyholm F. Surgical treatment of gynaecomastia. Five years' experience with liposuction. *Scand J Plast Reconstr Surg Hand Surg* 1994; 28(2): 123-30.

42. Gasperoni C, Salgarello M, Gasperoni P. Technical refinements in the surgical treatment of gynaecomastia. *Ann Plast Surg* 2000; 44(4): 455-8.

43. Dolsky RL. Gynecomastia. Treatment by liposuction subcutaneous mastectomy. *Dermatol Clin* 1990; 8(3): 469-78.

44. Abramo AC. Axillary approach for gynaecomastia liposuction. *Aesthetic Plast Surg* 1994; 18: 265-8.

45. Stark GB, Grandel S, Spilker G. Tissue suction of the male and female breast. *Aesthetic Plast Surg* 1992; 16(4): 317-24.

46. Becker H. The treatment of gynaecomastia without sharp excision. *Ann Plast Surg* 1990; 24: 380-3.

47. Samdal F, Kleppe G, Aabyholm F. A new suction-assisted device for removing glandular gynecomastia. *Plast Reconstr Surg* 1991; 87(2): 383-5.

48. Rosenberg GJ. Gynecomastia. In: *Surgery of the Breast: Principles and Art*, 2nd Edition. Spear SL, Ed. Philadelphia, PA: Lippincott Williams & Wilkins, 2006; Chapter 87: 1210-9.

49. Botta SA. Alternatives for surgical correction of severe gynaecomastia. *Aesthetic Plast Surg* 1998; 22: 65-70.

50. Fodor PB, Watson J. Personal experience with ultrasound-assisted lipoplasty: a pilot study comparing ultrasound-assisted lipoplasty with traditional lipoplasty. *Plast Reconstr Surg* 1998; 101(4): 1103-16.

51. Zocchi ML. Basic physics for ultrasound-assisted lipoplasty. *Clin Plast Surg* 1999; 26(2): 209-20.

52. Zocchi ML. Ultrasonic-assisted lipoplasty. Technical refinements and clinical evaluations. *Clin Plast Surg* 1996; 23: 575-98.

53. Zocchi M. Ultrasonic liposculpturing. *Aesthetic Plast Surg* 1992; 16(4): 287-98.

54. Chang CC, Commons GW. A comparison of various ultrasound technologies. *Clin Plast Surg* 1999; 26(2): 261-8.

55. Rohrich RJ, Beran SJ, Kenkel JM, *et al*. Extending the role of liposuction in body contouring with ultrasound-assisted liposuction. *Plast Reconstr Surg* 1998; 101(4): 1090-102.

56. Gingrass MK, Shermack MA. The treatment of gynecomastia with ultrasound-assisted lipoplasty. *Perspect Plast Surg* 1999; 12: 101-12.

57. Tebbetts JB. Minimizing complications of ultrasound-assisted lipoplasty: an initial experience with no related complications. *Plast Reconstr Surg* 1998; 102(5): 1690-7.

58. Hodgson EL, Fruhstorfer BH, Malata CM. Ultrasonic liposuction in the treatment of gynaecomastia. *Plast Reconstr Surg* 2005; 116(2): 646-53.

59. Gingrass MK. Lipoplasty complications and their prevention. *Clin Plast Surg* 1999; 26(3): 341-54.

60. Beckenstein MS, Grotting JC. Ultrasound-assisted lipectomy using the solid probe: a retrospective review of 100 consecutive cases. *Plast Reconstr Surg* 2000; 105(6): 2161-74.

61. Kloehn RA. Commentary on ultrasound-assisted lipoplasty: Task Force, July 1996, report to the membership. *Plast Reconstr Surg* 1997; 4: 1198-9.

62. Maxwell GP, Gingrass MK. Ultrasound-assisted lipoplasty: a clinical study of 250 consecutive patients. *Plast Reconstr Surg* 1998; 101(1): 189-202.

63. Scuderi N, Paolini G, Grippaudo FR, Tenna S. Comparative evaluation of traditional, ultrasonic and pneumatic lipoplasty; analysis of local and systemic effects, efficacy and costs of these methods. *Aesthetic Plast Surg* 2000; 24(6): 395-400.

64. Mladick RA. [Discussion] Classification and management of gynecomastia: defining the role of ultrasound-assisted liposuction. *Plast Reconstr Surg* 2003; 111(2): 924-5.

65. Lee Y, Hong JJ, Bang C. Dual-plane lipoplasty for the superficial and deep layers. *Plast Reconstr Surg* 1999; 104(6): 1844-84, discussion 1885-6.

66. Walgenbach KJ, Riabikhin AW, Galla TJ, *et al*. Effects of ultrasonic-assisted lipectomy (UAL) on breast tissue: histological findings. *Aesthetic Plast Surg* 2001; 25(2): 85-8.

67. Rohrich R, Morales DE, Krueger JE, *et al*. Comparative lipoplasty analysis of *in vivo*-treated adipose tissue. *Plast Reconstr Surg* 2000; 105(6): 2152-8, discussion 2159-60.

68. Kenkel J, Gingrass MK, Rohrich RJ. Ultrasound-assisted lipoplasty. Basic science and clinical research. *Clin Plast Surg* 1999; 26(2): 221-34.

69. Gingrass MK, Kenkel JM. Comparing ultrasound-assisted lipoplasty with suction-assisted lipoplasty. *Clin Plast Surg* 1999; 26: 283-8.

70. Strasser EJ. Ultrasound aspiration for gynecomastia. *Plast Reconstr Surg* 2003; 112(7): 1967-8.

71. Filho DH, Arruda RG, Alonso N. Treatment of severe gynaecomastia (III) by resection of peri-areolar skin. *Aesthetic Surg J* 2006; 26(6): 669-73.

72. Tashkandi M, Al-Qattan MM, Hassanain JM, Hawary MB, Sultan M. The surgical management of high-grade gynaecomastia. *Ann Plast Surg* 2004; 53(1): 17-20.

Chapter 23

Chapter 23

Chapter 24

Trends in aesthetic facial surgery: the role of endoscopic brow and minimal access facial lifts

Gary L Ross MB ChB MRCS (Ed) MD FRCS (Plast.) 1
Consultant Plastic Surgeon
David J Whitby MB BS FRCS 2
Consultant Plastic Surgeon

1 CHRISTIE HOSPITAL NHS FOUNDATION TRUST, MANCHESTER, UK
2 UNIVERSITY HOSPITAL OF SOUTH MANCHESTER
NHS FOUNDATION TRUST, MANCHESTER, UK

Introduction

Facial rejuvenation surgery has undergone significant changes. The need for an optimal long-term result with a shorter recovery, fewer complications and reduced scarring has led to a more critical appraisal of traditional surgical techniques and the development of endoscopic, suture/threads and minimal access cranial suspension techniques. This chapter aims to address the roles of endoscopic brow lifting and minimal access facial lifts in facial rejuvenation surgery.

Methodology

A Medline search was employed to gather evidence, using the search terms 'brow lifts', 'rhytidectomy', 'endoscopic brow lifts', 'minimal access face lifts' and supplemented by a hand search of references from the articles obtained.

Endoscopic brow lifting

Anatomy of the forehead

A clear grasp of the anatomy of the forehead, scalp and peri-orbital area, particularly the transition between the tissue planes of the temple and the tissue planes of the forehead along the temporal fusion line, is the key to understanding the mechanism of aging in this area (Figure 1). This will guide the selection of an appropriate technique to reverse these changes. Traditionally we have been taught that the scalp is composed of five layers, skin, connective tissue, aponeurosis, loose areolar tissue and periosteum. Moving from scalp to forehead, the galea aponeurotica becomes contiguous with the superficial temporal fascia, and the periosteum of the frontal bone becomes contiguous with the temporalis fascia. The confluence of these tissue planes occurs just medial to the temporal fusion line of the skull and its continuation as the superior temporal line [1-2]. Near the junction between the temporal fusion line of the skull and the orbital rim is the orbital ligament, a fibrous band connecting superficial temporal fascia to the orbital rim. It limits cephalad superficial temporal fascial movement during forehead flap transposition

inserts into the skin beneath the medial head of the eyebrow. It is considered to be distinct from the orbicularis oculi.

Mobility of the frontalis muscle is essentially limited to its inferior 20%, under which exists the galeal fat pad enveloped by the deep galeal plane. The corrugator supercilii muscle passing through the galeal fat pad is incorporated into the roof of the subgaleal fat pad glide space, which then penetrates the frontalis and orbicularis muscles en route to its dermal insertion. Its smooth walls serve as a glide plane surface allowing the corrugator and inferior 20% of the frontalis muscles to move the overlying soft tissues with less resistance. The subgaleal fat pad glide space provides the greatest movement between surfaces [1, 2].

The deep division of the supra-orbital nerve innervating the frontoparietal scalp runs from the orbital rim between the deep galeal plane and periosteum under the glide plane space floor toward the superior temporal line of the skull. It then runs parallel with the superior temporal line and is always found from 0.5 to 1.5cm medial to the superior temporal line [3] until the nerve turns medially to enter the scalp. The superficial division of the supra-orbital nerve runs from the orbital rim over the frontalis muscle to terminate in the anterior scalp in most patients. The frontal branch of the facial nerve runs across the anterior temporal fossa within the superficial temporal fascia before entering the frontalis muscle.

Aging changes

A youthful eyebrow is one in which the medial brow is at or below the supra-orbital rim and the lateral two thirds of the eyebrow is arched or elevated. Aging in the upper face becomes evident with a descent in the level of the eyebrow and the appearance of wrinkles and furrows, sometimes from an early age. One of the earliest signs of facial aging starting is the descent or flattening of the lateral eyebrow [2-6].

Although partly attributable to the progressive laxity of scalp and forehead soft tissues, with age many other structures promoting mobility and gravitational descent of the eyebrow have been shown to be causative. An understanding of these complex interactions is required in order to surgically address these aging changes.

The lateral margin of the frontalis muscle almost always ends or abruptly attenuates along the temporal fusion line of the skull; therefore, the more medially the palpable temporal line intersects the eyebrow, the less lateral eyebrow support is available from the frontalis muscle [2]. Any lateral eyebrow segment not suspended by the frontalis muscle is pushed downward by the descending temporal fossa soft tissue mass and the depressor forces affecting the lateral brow from the orbicularis oris [7]. Unsupported soft tissues superficial to the plane of the temporalis fascia drift downward with aging. This explains, in part, why the lateral eyebrow segment almost always becomes more ptotic than the medial segment. The galeal fat pad over the superolateral orbital rim is relatively mobile and may act as a lubricating surface for lateral eyebrow descent, possibly complemented in this function by the lateral end of the preseptal fat pad [8] when it extends over the orbital rim. The glide plane space, located between the galeal fat pad and the deepest layer of the multi-layered deep galeal plane, also may facilitate lateral eyebrow ptosis through a glide plane effect from its smooth lining surfaces.

A dynamic equilibrium at the lateral eyebrow level exists between the force of descending temporal fossa soft tissue pushing the eyebrow down and the force of frontalis muscle action suspending it. Action of the corrugator and orbicularis oculi muscles may upset this equilibrium by promoting lateral eyebrow ptosis. The strength of orbicularis depression varies from patient to patient [7]. Action of the procerus muscle, the medial orbicularis oculi muscle and the depressor supercilii may promote medial eyebrow segment ptosis [1, 2]. With aging, attenuation of the facial muscles lead to increased wrinkles and furrows.

The goals of surgical rejuvenation of the forehead include reproducible and long-lasting brow manipulation, attenuation of transverse forehead rhytids, and reduction of glabellar frown lines [9].

History

For nearly a century, aesthetic improvements of the aging upper third of the face have remained a challenging problem [10, 11]. Since the earliest description of brow lifting by Passot in 1919 [12], brow ptosis management has undergone evolutionary changes from the classic coronal open brow and anterior hairline techniques to the more recently described, less invasive techniques, such as the minimal incision lateral brow and endoscopic brow lift [2, 4-11, 13-31].

The use of the endoscope in brow lifting was first introduced in 1992 [13, 14]. Elevation in the subperiosteal plane was subsequently described. This early experience was further developed over the next two years. Isse [14] and Chajchir [15] detailed their method of performing a brow lift through small incisions behind the anterior hairline. Isse noted that a dynamic functional lift could be achieved by modifying or weakening the corrugator supercilii and thus addressing the balance of muscular activity between the frontalis and the corrugator supercilii muscle. He also identified the need to vary techniques on the basis of the configuration of the skull, bony architecture, and soft tissue thickness and tightness.

Other elements of the endoscopic brow lift have subsequently been modified. These include placement of incisions, plane of dissection, muscle dissection and method of flap fixation.

Incisions

The number of incisions generally varies between two and five. The length of incisions generally varies between 1.5-2.5cm. The orientation of incisions may vary also [6, 7, 9, 10, 13-26]. Three triangular incisions are used by De Cordier [17], postulating that the triangular flaps will close in a transverse fashion and allow easy introduction of the endoscope with minimal trauma to the surrounding tissues. The centre of the triangle is in the midline and the other two above both pupils. Baker[18] advocates five incisions, a single vertical incision in the midline, bilateral 15mm incisions at the level of the lateral canthus and 25mm bilateral vertical incisions in the temporal area.

Placement of incisions have increasingly been more anteriorly. Frontal hairline incisions have allowed a more precise eyebrow positioning, improving visualisation with increased safety and accuracy. In patients with short foreheads, lifting is improved with incision sites closer to the structure requiring elevation. This is particularly important in patients with very convex foreheads. In patients with long foreheads or male receding patients positioning of the incisions can also be made in the forehead creases [13-26].

Plane of dissection

The main discussion regarding plane of dissection is between subgaleal and subperiosteal dissection or a combination of the two. The first description of subperiosteal dissection was introduced in 1994 [15, 16]. It has been postulated that the inherent rigidity of the tissues overlying the subperiosteal dissection mean that this technique is the most effective at lifting the brow and less likely to suffer from stress relaxation. Also, the scarring following subgaleal dissection produces variable adherence of the tissues to the pericranium with potentially unnatural forehead activity. Finally, the subperiosteal dissection preserves the areolar tissue at the galeal-periosteal interface, maintaining the normal gliding of the frontalis muscle complex over the periosteum [19].

A number of authors have advocated a subgaleal plane posteriorly and a subperiosteal plane for the anterior dissection with a change of planes in the central portion of the forehead. It is generally accepted that as long as the dissections continue down to the orbital rims and nasal bones, that if the galea is released from the periosteum at the supra-orbital rim, the difference in plane has minimal bearing on the overall result [9].

Ramirez [21, 22] has suggested a biplanar endoscopically-assisted forehead lift in patients with a very furrowed or high forehead or with pronounced brow ptosis or asymmetry. By undermining the skin of the superior 3-4cm of the forehead, a more direct impact can be made on the fibrous septae between the muscle and the dermis. This may benefit patients in whom the subgaleal or subperiosteal elevation may not address possible skin redundancy [17].

A US national survey showed that the most common plane of endoscopic dissection was subperiosteal followed by subgaleal and, finally, a combination of both [23] **(III/B)**.

Muscle dissection

Procedures dedicated to forehead rejuvenation address transverse forehead rhytids and reduction of glabellar frown lines, while maintaining long-term brow manipulation.

Action of the corrugator and orbicularis oculi muscles may promote lateral eyebrow ptosis while the procerus muscle, medial orbicularis oculi and depressor supercilii, may promote medial eyebrow segment ptosis. Individual patients must be assessed pre-operatively to determine which portions of the eyebrow are ptotic. The weakening of these muscles is determined by pre-operative function and the result the patient wishes to achieve. It is generally accepted that ablation of the brow depressors is an integral part of the endoscopic forehead lift [17] **(III/B)**. Modifications include muscular detachment, myotomies, myectomies and neurotomies to denervate the brow depressors [10]. Treatment of the corrugator, depressor supercilii and procerus will improve the transverse, oblique and vertical wrinkles of the glabella in addition to elevating the medial brow [17].

Deep transverse lines or furrows are a common complaint caused by contraction of the frontalis. Opinions remain divided on whether to incise/excise a portion of the frontalis to limit its contraction or rely on the transverse lines vanishing once the eyebrows are restored to their normal height and the frontalis relaxes. The need to treat being more apparent in those with thick skin.

Methods of fixation

Fixation of the endoscopic brow has proved difficult and many techniques have been advocated. The frontalis muscle is a powerful elevator medially and centrally but has limited attachments to the lateral third of the brow, and the orbicularis oculi is a stong lateral brow depressor. It is, therefore, difficult to overcome the dynamic depression of the orbicularis oculi, which produces recurrent lateral brow descent after any brow lifting technique with a static lift. The onus of the static lift is dependent upon obtaining secure intra-operative fixation [9].

Fixation devices may be either endogenous or exogenous. Endogenous methods include: extensive galea-frontalis-occipitalis release, lateral spanning suspension sutures, external bolster fixation, anterior port skin excision, galea-frontalis advancement, cortical tunnels, and tissue adhesives. Exogenous techniques include: internal screw or plate fixation, Mitek anchor fixation, external screw fixation, and absorbable K-wires [9].

Fixation should hold the brow tension free not pull or distract the brow. If the fixation is performed under tension, brow ptosis will recur and alopecia may develop from the vertex of scalp tension. Fixation must hold the brow position until enough healing has occurred to prevent recurrence. Romo *et al* [24] demonstrated in a rat model that it requires three months for the periosteum to completely heal after periosteal elevation in the frontal region.

Fixation must be simple, reproducible, safe and give long-term results, while being cost-effective. The ideal fixation device has yet to be defined (Table 1) **(III/B)**.

Other methods of forehead lifting

The main benefits of endoscopic brow lifting, as compared with the classical bicoronal open lift [30, 31], are related to the limited access incision and the associated decreased incidence of alopecia resulting from the shortened scar. There is also the advantage of not dividing the deep branch of the supra-orbital nerve producing a lower incidence of numbness and postoperative neuralgia after endoscopic techniques. From an aesthetic standpoint the long incision of the coronal brow lift has several disadvantages. It is situated distant to the eyebrow and thus long-term fixation is more difficult. A 2:1 ratio of scalp resection to eyebrow elevation is required via the coronal

Table 1. Comparative factors in fixation devices for endoscopic brow lifts.

	Effectiveness	Technical complexity	Risk of complications	Cost
Suture fixation	+	+	+	+
Cortical bone tunnels	+++	+++	+++	+
Internal screw fixation	++	++	++	++
External screw fixation	++	++	++	++
Tissue adhesives	+	+	+	++

approach accounting for the significant hairline shift commonly associated with this procedure. The long-term fixation is also achieved by scalp excision only, which is less stable compared with the more rigid fixation of securing scalp to calvarium as seen in the endoscopic lifts. As the posterior scalp is a mobile structure there is a tendency for the posterior scalp to re-descend. Controlling brow shape is more difficult with long scar techniques with the tension of fixation distributed along the incision. It cannot address individual portions of the brow. Endoscopic techniques allow access incision placement directly superior to the region that requires elevation [25].

Complications, however, of endoscopic brow lifting include alopecia, hairline position change, asymmetry, prolonged paraesthesia over the forehead/brow area, scalp dysaesthesia and frontal nerve paralysis [23, 26]. It would seem that the initial surge of enthusiasm for the endoscopic technique has since tailed off with a decrease in the number of procedures performed. Possible reasons include more stringent criteria for patient selection and the use of other equally or effective medical and surgical techniques [23]. These include surgery through the upper eyelid, minimal incision brow lift/foreheadplasty [2-6, 29], minimally invasive thread/mesh/suture suspension [27, 28], botulinum toxin injections and laser resurfacing [10, 11].

Minimal access facial surgery

Facial rejuvenation surgery continues to evolve with more consideration given to minimal downtime while providing instant results, which are longer lasting. This has become especially important for younger patients or for those wishing for minimal changes in appearance. The introduction of minimal access face lifts will be discussed in the remainder of this chapter [32-50].

Anatomy

In the midface, the superficial musculo-aponeurotic system (SMAS) is a fascial layer separating the subcutaneous fat from the fascia enveloping the parotid gland, the mimetic muscles, and facial nerve branches. The SMAS is an extension of the superficial cervical fascia into the face and is continuous with the temporoparietal fascia in the temporal region. The SMAS is thickest over the parotid region and becomes thin in its anterior extent over the malar region. The malar fat pad, a triangular subcutaneous structure based at the nasolabial fold with its apex at the malar eminence, lies superficial to the SMAS in the anterior midface. Ligaments from the periosteum of the zygoma run through the subcutaneous portion of the malar pad and insert directly into the dermis [32]. The SMAS extension (the temporoparietal fascia) invests the frontal (temporal) branch of the facial nerve (cranial

VII) and the branches of the superficial temporal artery. This superficial fascia is separated from the deep temporal fascia by loose areolar tissue [34]. The deep temporal fascia covers the temporalis muscle and splits to envelop the periosteum of the zygomatic arch [33]. Both subcutaneous dissection planes and that immediately above the deep temporal fascia will avoid damage to the frontal branch of the facial nerve.

Aging

The malar fat pad is the focus of the central third of the face whose borders include the nasolabial fold, the infra-orbital rim, and the zygomatic prominence. It is fixed by fibrous septae or suspensory ligaments and attached to the mimetic muscles below and to the dermis superficially.

With age, characteristic changes occur in the central third of the face. Gravity and the repeated actions of facial animation stretch the suspensory ligaments, resulting in a gradual descent of the malar fat pad and the overlying soft tissues. As the pad descends, the malar eminence becomes flatter, the nasolabial fold becomes deeper and more prominent, progressive jowl formation disrupts the smooth line of the mandible, and loss of tissue in the infra-orbital region creates a tired, hollow appearance that characterises the aging face. Correction requires proper identification and mobilisation of the malar fat pad to reposition the architecture and recreate a youthful appearance [32-35]. Traction on the malar fat pad in a supero-oblique direction, along a line from the midportion of the nasolabial crease to the junction of the zygoma and temporal bones, elevates the skin of the medial cheek and flattens the nasolabial fold.

Surgical goals for midface rejuvenation include elevation of the corner of the mouth, restoration of the prominence of the cheek, and improvement of the nasolabial fold.

Unlike the midface, the aging changes of the lower face and neck occur at a plane of descent deep to the SMAS, at the fascial cleft between the superficial and deep facial fascia layers. The platysma has a single small bony attachment at the anterior mandible and is chiefly supported by the midcheek SMAS. The SMAS has been shown to develop aging changes characterised by conversion of elastic connective tissue to fibrous connective tissue, with loss of elasticity and tone, similar to that seen occurring in skin. These changes in the skin and SMAS result in decreased support for the skin, platysma, and subcutaneous fat in the lower face and neck, which undergo gravitational descent at the plane between the SMAS and the underlying deep cervicofacial fascia [36, 37].

History

Almost three decades ago the SMAS was described by Mitz and Peyronie [38], and Skoog [39] demonstrated that dissection could be performed beneath the SMAS, and a new era in face-lift surgery began. In 1977, Owsley [32] reported plicating the SMAS tissue, which gave an optimal traction of the lower facial tissues. During the following years, different surgeons chose to use the SMAS in different ways, but typically, a single large flap was elevated over the lower cheek. In the early 1980s, Jost and Lamouche [40] published articles on resection and even segmentation of the SMAS flaps pulling in different directions. Recently, Baker [41] published his work on short scar face lifts with a lateral SMASectomy. Saylan [42, 43] described a technique that required a modified SMAS plication in purse-string form with the soft tissue (the SMAS, the parotid fascia, and the extension of the platysma of the submandibular region) being pulled together by means of U- and O-shaped purse-string sutures with multiple small bites and fixed to the periosteum of the zygomatic bone [42, 43]. This was performed via an S lift which Tonnard subsequently modified as the MACS lift (minimal access cranial suspension lift) combining the U- and O-suture techniques with a malar fat pad hitching suture (extended MACS) [44, 45]. Various other midface suspension techniques have been described using sutures [33, 46, 47] in different planes [33, 46, 47]. Subperiosteal undermining and repositioning with sutures *en bloc* have been incorporated into minimally invasive endoscopic-assisted mid and lower face-lift procedures. In 2000, the use of threads and barbed sutures was introduced into facial cosmetic surgery as a no downtime facial rejuvenation procedure either on their own or as an adjunct to other surgical procedures [48-51].

Minimal access cranial suspension

The MACS lift is a facial rejuvenation procedure used to correct the aging neck and lower third of the face, and can be extended to address the middle third of the face (extended SMAS). The technique is a pure antigravitational facial rejuvenation achieved by acting on the deep facial soft tissues and the skin in the same vertical direction. Strong purse-string sutures are anchored to the deep temporal fascia and zygomatic arch following minimal skin undermining through a pre-auricular and temporal prehairline incision [44, 45].

With a simple MACS, two purse-string sutures are used for correction of the neck, the jowls and the marionette grooves. They both are anchored to the deep temporal fascia above the zygomatic arch 1cm in front of the auricular helix. The first suture runs as a narrow vertical U-shaped purse string to the region of the mandibular angle. Tying of this suture under maximal tension produces a strong vertical pull on the lateral part of the platysma muscle correcting the cervicomental angle of the neck region, which has been liposuctioned previously. The second purse-string suture starts from the same anchoring point above the zygomatic arch and runs obliquely in the direction of the jowls as a wider O-shaped loop. This suture corrects the jowls, the marionette grooves, and the downward slanting of the corners of the mouth. With the extended MACS, an additional undermining of the skin over the malar region is performed. A point marked 2cm below the lateral canthus is marked, with the patient in the standing position and is the inferior limit of the third purse-string suture. This suture also originates from the deep temporal fascia, but in its anterior part, lateral to the lateral orbital rim. It provides a strong correction of the nasolabial fold, an enhancement of the malar region, a lifting of the midface, and a shortening of the vertical height of the lower eyelid [44, 45].

With both the MACS and extended MACS, the skin redraping is in a pure vertical direction and the skin excess tailored at the temporal incision. The malar stitch leads to an excess of skin at the lateral lower eyelid which can be adjusted via a lower lid blepharoplasty incision [44, 45].

Early results of this technique have shown satisfactory results of almost 95%, with the remaining patients undergoing subsequent additional procedures to the neck, either anterior or posterior cervicoplasty. However, long-term results of this technique are not yet available [44, 45].

Threads and sutures

Threads/sutures can be used as the sole means of tissue repositioning in a closed approach, or as part of an open facial rejuvenation approach that may incorporate an endoscopic, supraperiosteal or subperiosteal face lift [46-51]. The cephalad reposition of the cheek tissues brings about a series of effects on the surrounding adjacent tissues. Therefore, in addition to elevation of the malar area, results may include shortening of the lower eyelid distance, flattening of the nasolabial fold, elevation of the submalar tissue, improvement of jowling, and a decrease in fullness of the submalar area.

Indications for the procedures include descent of mid and lower face fatty tissues, palpable fatty tissue of good volume, unwillingness to undergo conventional face-lift surgery, contraindications for more invasive facial surgery (hypertension, previous cardiac surgery, diabetes, heart problems), a facial configuration characterised by voluminous facial fatty tissue in a round face so that the conventional face lift would likely not yield sufficient results, no excess skin flaccidity, a secondary lift with insufficient result in the centre oval of the face, and late or congenital facial paralysis [46-51].

Contraindications to use of threads/sutures as the sole procedure include insufficient facial fat volume, presence of marked wrinkles, excess skin, a positive HIV test, medication that causes fat atrophy and skin with cystic acne [46-51].

Chapter 24

Various threads and sutures have been described. They vary in terms of positioning and the tissues being elevated, the number/length of the sutures/threads and the composition of the threads/sutures themselves [46-51].

Many of these procedures utilise non-absorbable sutures in the dermis and subcutis to lift lax skin. Sasaki [46] found that non-absorbable sutures allowed a longer-term result than absorbable sutures and elevation of the malar fat pad was better with two sutures rather than [1]. More recently, he utilised Goretex grafts with improved results.

If threads/sutures are incorrectly placed, the skin becomes merely puckered or may even become depressed. The threads/sutures may be placed too superficially and cause visible dimpling and tethering, or may be placed too deeply and have little effect. Complications of 25-30% with barbed sutures have been described with palpability, migration, infection, skin dimpling, extrusion, and hyperalgia being the commonest [50, 51]. Suture fixation has shown complications of 10% in larger series [46].

The durability of threads/sutures in facial rejuvenation is unknown long term and asymmetry of cosmetic effect may require correction with additional sutures [46-51].

Conclusions

Endoscopic brow and minimal access facial lifts provide facial rejuvenation with limited scarring. They can provide long-term results with a shorter downtime, when compared with more traditional surgical techniques, in a carefully selected patient population.

Recommendations	Evidence level
◆ The most common plane of endoscopic dissection is subperiosteal, followed by subgaleal and, finally, a combination of both.	III/B
◆ Action of the corrugator and orbicularis oculi muscles promote lateral eyebrow ptosis, while action of the procerus muscle, medial orbicularis oculi and depressor supercilii promote medial eyebrow segment ptosis. Treatment of the corrugator, depressor supercilii and procerus improve the transverse, oblique and vertical wrinkles of the glabella in addition to elevating the medial brow.	III/B
◆ The ideal endoscopic forehead fixation device has yet to be defined.	III/B
◆ Minimal access cranial suspension face lifts result in shortened scars.	III/B
◆ Minimal access cranial suspension is an antigravitational facial rejuvenation achieved by acting on the deep facial soft tissues and the skin in the same vertical direction.	III/B
◆ Thread/suture-only facial rejuvenation surgery has been associated with increased complications.	III/B

References

1. Knize DM. An anatomically-based study of the mechanism of eyebrow ptosis. *Plast Reconstr Surg* 1996; 97: 1321-33.

2. Knize DM. Limited-incision forehead lift for eyebrow elevation to enhance upper blepharoplasty. *Plast Reconstr Surg* 1996; 97: 1334-42.

3. Knize DM. A study of the supra-orbital nerve. *Plast Reconstr Surg* 1995; 96: 564-9.

4. Knize DM. Limited incision foreheadplasty. *Plast Reconstr Surg* 1999: 103: 271-84.

5. Knize DM. Limited incision forehead lift for eyebrow elevation to enhance upper blepharoplasty. *Plast Reconstr Surg* 2001; 108: 564-7.

6. Strauch B, Baum T. Correction of lateral brow ptosis: a nonendoscopic subgaleal approach. *Plast Reconstr Surg* 2002; 109: 1164-7.

7. Stuzin JM, Rohrich RJ. A comparison between subgaleal and subperiosteal brow lifts. *Plast Reconstr Surg* 1999; 104: 1091-2.

8. Meyer DR, Linberg JV, Wobig JL, McCormick SA. Anatomy of the orbital septum and associated eyelid connective tissues. Implications for ptosis surgery. *Ophthal Plast Reconstr Surg* 1991; 7: 104-13.

9. Rohrich RJ, Beran SJ. Evolving fixation methods in endoscopically-assisted forehead rejuvenation: controversies and rationale. *Plast Reconstr Surg* 1997; 100: 1575-82.

10. Paul MD. The evolution of the brow lift in aesthetic plastic surgery. *Plast Reconstr Surg* 2001; 108: 1409-24.

11. Matarasso A, Hutchinson O. Evaluating rejuvenation of the forehead and brow: an algorithm for selecting the appropriate technique. *Plast Reconstr Surg* 2003; 12: 1467-9.

12. Passot, R. La chururgie esthetique des rides du visage. *Presse Med* 1919; 27: 258.

13. Vasconez, L. O. The use of the endoscope in brow lifting. A video presentation at the Annual Meeting of the American Society of Plastic and Reconstructive Surgeons, Washington, DC, 1992.

14. Isse NG. Endoscopic forehead lift. Presented at the Annual Meeting of the Los Angeles County Society of Plastic Surgeons, Los Angeles, September 12, 1992.

15. Chajchir A. Endoscopic subperiosteal forehead lift. *Aesthetic Plast Surg* 1994; 18: 269-74.

16. Isse NG. Endoscopic facial rejuvenation: endoforehead, the functional lift. *Aesthetic Plast Surg* 1994; 18: 21.

17. De Cordier BC, de la Torre JI, Al-Hakeem MS, *et al.* Endoscopic forehead lift: review of technique, cases, and complications. *Plast Reconstr Surg* 2002; 110: 1558-68.

18. Daniel RK, Tirkanitis B. Endoscopic forehead lift: an operative technique. *Plast Reconstr Surg* 1996; 98: 1148-57.

19. Ramirez OM. Endoscopic techniques in facial rejuvenation: an overview. Part 1. *Aesthetic Plast Surg* 1994; 18: 141-7.

20. Withey S, Witherow H, Waterhouse N. One hundred cases of endoscopic brow lift. *Br J Plast Surg* 2002; 55: 20-4.

21. Ramirez OM. Endoscopically-assisted biplanar forehead lift. *Plast Reconstr Surg* 1995; 96: 323-33.

22. Ramirez OM. The anchor subperiosteal forehead lift. *Plast Reconstr Surg* 1995; 95: 993-1003.

23. Elkwood A, Matarasso A, Rankin M, *et al.* National plastic surgery survey: brow lifting techniques and complications. *Plast Reconstr Surg* 2001; 108: 2143-50.

24. Romo T, Sclafani AP, Yung RT, *et al.* Endoscopic foreheadplasty: a histologic comparison of periosteal refixation after endoscopic versus bicoronal lift. *Plast Reconstr Surg* 1999; 105: 1111-7.

25. Ramirez OM. Anchor subperiosteal forehead lift: from open to endoscopic. *Plast Reconstr Surg* 2001; 107: 868-71.

26. Chiu ES, Baker DC. Endoscopic brow lift: a retrospective review of 628 consecutive cases over 5 years. *Plast Reconstr Surg* 2003; 112: 628-33.

27. Erol OO, Sozer SO, Velidedeoglu HV. Brow suspension, a minimally invasive technique in facial rejuvenation. *Plast Reconstr Surg* 2002; 109: 2521-32.

28. Mutaf M. Mesh lift: a new procedure for long-lasting results in brow lift surgery. *Plast Reconstr Surg* 2005; 116: 1490-9.

29. Miller TA, Rudkin G, Honig M, *et al.* Lateral subcutaneous brow lift and interbrow muscle resection: clinical experience and anatomic studies. *Plast Reconstr Surg* 2000; 105: 1120-7.

30. Wolfe SA, Baird WL. The subcutaneous forehead lift. *Plast Reconstr Surg* 1989; 83: 251-6.

31. Ellenbogen R. Transcoronal eyebrow lift with concomitant upper blepharoplasty. *Plast Reconstr Surg* 1983; 71: 490-9.

32. Owsley JQ, Fiala TG. Update: lifting the malar fat pad for correction of prominent nasolabial folds. *Plast Reconstr Surg* 1997; 100: 715-22.

33. Noone RB. Suture suspension malarplasty with SMAS plication and modified SMASectomy: a simplified approach to midface lifting. *Plast Reconstr Surg* 2006; 117: 792-803.

34. Anderson RD, Lo MW. Endoscopic malar/midface suspension procedure. *Plast Reconstr Surg* 1998; 102: 2196-208.

35. De Cordier BC, Vasconez LO. Rejuvenation of the midface by elevating the malar fat pad: review of technique cases and complications. *Plast Reconstr Surg* 2002; 110: 1526-36.

36. Ruess W, Owsley JQ. The anatomy of the skin and fascial layers of the face in aesthetic surgery. *Clin Plast Surg* 1987; 14: 677-82.

37. Stuzin JM, Baker TJ, Gordon HL. The relationship of the superficial and deep facial fascias: relevance to rhytidectomy and aging. *Plast Reconstr Surg* 1992; 89: 441-9.

38. Mitz V, Peyronie M. The superficial musculo-aponeurotic system (SMAS) in the parotid and cheek area. *Plast Reconstr Surg* 1976; 58: 80-8.

39. Skoog T. Plastic surgery: the aging face. In: *Plastic Surgery: New Methods and Refinements*. Skoog TG, Ed. Philadelphia: WB Saunders, 1974: 300-30.

40. Jost G, Lamouche G. SMAS in rhytidectomy. *Aesthetic Plast Surg* 1982; 6: 69-74.

41. Baker DC. Minimal incision rhytidectomy (short scar face lift) with lateral SMASectomy. *Aesthetic Surg J* 2001; 21: 68-80.

42. Saylan Z Purse string-formed plication of the SMAS with fixation to the zygomatic bone. *Plast Reconstr Surg* 2002; 110: 667-71.

Chapter 24

Chapter 24

43. Saylan Z. The S-lift: less is more. *Aesthetic Surg J* 1999; 19: 406.

44. Tonnard P, Verpaele A, Monstrey S, *et al.* Minimal access cranial suspension lift: a modified S-lift. *Plast Reconstr Surg* 2002; 109: 2074-86.

45. Tonnard PL, Verpaele A, Gaia S. Optimising results from minimal access cranial suspension lifting (MACS-lift). *Aesthetic Plast Surg* 2005; 29: 213-20.

46. Sasaki GH, Cohen AT. Meloplication of the malar fat pads by percutaneous cable-suture technique for midface rejuvenation: outcome study (392 cases, 6 years experience). *Plast Reconstr Surg* 2002; 110: 635-54.

47. Keller GS, *et al.* Elevation of the malar fat pad with a percutaneous technique. *Arch Facial Plast Surg* 2002; 4: 20-5.

48. Sulamanidze MA, Fournier PF, Paikidze TG, Sulamanidze G. Removal of facial soft tissue ptosis with special threads. *Dermatol Surg* 2000; 28: 367-71.

49. Isse GN, Fodor PB. Elevating the midface with barbed polypropylene sutures. *Aesthetic Surg J* 2005; 25: 301-3.

50. Badini AZED, Forte MRC, Silva OL. Scarless mid and lower face lift. *Aesthetic Surg J* 2005; 25: 340-7.

51. Wu WTL. Barbed sutures in facial rejuvenation. *Aesthetic Surg J* 2004; 24: 582-7.

Chapter 25

Surgical rejuvenation of the aging neck

Ahid Abood MB BS MA MSc MRCS
Research Fellow, Plastic Surgery

Charles Malata BSc (HB) MB ChB LRCP MRCS FRCS (Glasg) FRCS (Plast.)
Consultant Plastic and Reconstructive Surgeon

ADDENBROOKE'S UNIVERSITY HOSPITAL
CAMBRIDGE UNIVERSITY HOSPITALS NHS TRUST, CAMBRIDGE, UK

Introduction

A variety of procedures have been described for rejuvenation of the aging neck, which is often, but not invariably, performed in conjunction with that of the face [1]. This chapter focuses primarily on the surgical options available for neck contour restoration and puts it in the overall context of cervicofacial rejuvenation.

Numerous non-surgical treatments have been advocated for neck lifting including the use of Botulinum toxins [2], injectable fillers [3, 4], photodynamic therapy, pulsed light and lasers [5-7]. Although a discussion of these alternatives is beyond the scope of this chapter, occasionally they are combined with surgery.

Methodology

This chapter is a review of the literature on the surgical aspects of neck rejuvenation, of which there are numerous techniques. Lists of articles were accessed through the PubMed search engine using the following key words and terms: 'neck

rejuvenation', 'cervical rejuvenation', 'platysmaplasty', 'neck lift', 'face lift' and 'cervicoplasty'. The relevant articles, along with the senior author's own experience, were then compiled into a review of this common aesthetic challenge.

The aging neck and an aesthetic 'ideal'

Numerous factors contribute to the loss of shape and contour which are characteristic of the aging neck [8]. The anatomical appearances are a consequence of changes occurring in all tissue layers of the neck, from skin through to the bone of the cervical spine. These changes include loss of collagen and dermal elastic fibres with subsequent sagging of the skin and ptosis of the soft tissues in the neck and chin. Attenuation of Stuzin's retaining ligaments, which hold the platysma against the deep cervical fascia, causes the appearance of platysmal bands and obliquity of the cervicomental angle [9] **(III/B)**. In addition to the banding of the platysma muscles, there is elimination of the anterior sternocleidomastoid border. With age there is also increased fat deposition and submandibular gland

Table 1. Options for surgical rejuvenation of the neck. *Adapted from Nahai F. The Art of Aesthetic Surgery, Principles & Techniques, 2005* [12].

Liposuction alone	a) Suction-assisted lipectomy (SAL)
	b) Ultrasound-assisted liposuction (UAL)
Submental lift (open neck lift)	
Endoscopic neck lift	
Short scar face and neck lift	a) With a submental incision
	b) Without a submental incision
As part of a full face lift	a) With a submental incison:
	i) through and through dissection
	ii) unconnected/interrupted
	b) Without a submental incision

Chapter 25

protrusion. Furthermore osteoporosis causes bone resorption of the mandible and cervical spine. The latter causes shortening of the cervical spine [10].

It is important to pay special attention to specific external anatomical areas in order to optimise the surgical outcome from neck rejuvenation. These are the cervicomental angle, definition of the mandibular border, prominence of the labiomandibular fold (jowling), mental prominence and neck width. Changes to these areas can have significant effects on the appearance of the neck. In 1980, Ellenbogen and Karlin described the visual criteria that have been widely adopted as a means of focusing the surgeon's attention upon attaining specific anatomical features of the youthful neck **(III/B)**. These criteria are:

- A distinct mandibular border.
- A visible subhyoid depression.
- A visible thyroid cartilage bulge.
- A visible anterior sternocleidomastoid.
- A submental sternocleidomastoid line angle of 90° or a cervicomental angle of 105-120° [11].

Options for surgical rejuvenation of the neck (Table 1)

There are many surgical procedures used in rejuvenating and recontouring the neck. Each patient must be assessed carefully and the correct technique(s) selected in order to optimise the outcome.

Liposuction

Cervicofacial rejuvenation using liposuction is well described [13-24]. This technique is best suited to patients with excessive adipose tissue in the lower face and neck and normal skin quality (usually younger patients). It improves the contour by removal of the fat, skin redraping to the altered underlying framework, and skin contraction. Excellent skin quality is therefore essential for optimal results. The ideal candidate for liposuction alone has good skin elasticity and general skin quality [21] **(IV/C)**, may manifest early signs of facial aging in the lower face, but with minimal skin redundancy, and no platysmal banding (Figure 1). The midface should not show evidence of significant signs of facial aging that would warrant a rhytidectomy. One way to determine

Chapter 25

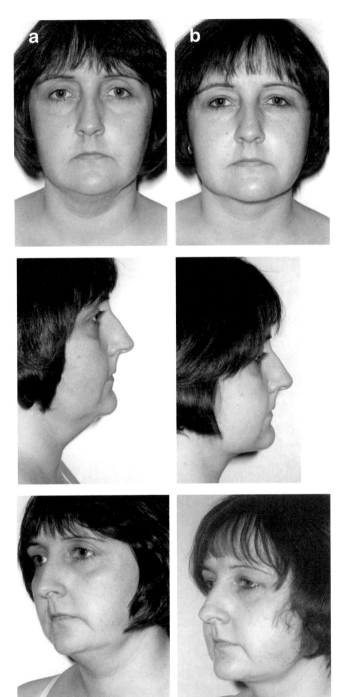

Figure 1. A 39-year-old woman with a fatty neck and good skin quality. Note the obtuse cervicomental angle and generalised pre-operative adiposity. Rejuvenation of the neck was achieved by UAL alone, to the neck and submental area. There is significant improvement of the neck-jaw angle and reduction of early jowling. Note that excellent skin quality was essential for redraping. The jowls are reduced and the patient looks thinner.

whether there is excess skin redundancy and poor elasticity is to perform the Ilouz test. The distance between the earlobe and chin tip is measured, the skin is then pulled away from the face, and a second measurement of the distracted distance is made. If the distraction distance exceeds the initial measurement by 15% or less, a lipectomy technique should suffice; if it is 20% or more, a rhytidectomy is indicated. Neck skin is more amenable to redraping and redistribution than facial skin. Hence, skin excision is not necessary in most cases to achieve excellent cosmetic results.

The effect of volume reduction in patients with an obtuse cervicomental angle will be to sharpen this angle (Figure 1). It is possible that removal of excess adipose tissue may subsequently reveal significant signs of facial aging that were being masked, such as platysmal bands, prominent digastric muscles, redundant skin or ptotic submandibular glands. This highlights the importance of very careful pre-operative surgical assessment and planning. Patients with obtuse cervicomental angles must, therefore, be warned of the possibility of having a staged rejuvenation procedure. Alternatively they should be advised pre-operatively that an open neck lift or face lift is more appropriate. In general terms, younger patents with good skin elasticity are excellent candidates for this technique. Liposuction of the neck can either be undertaken with suction-assisted lipectomy (SAL) or ultrasound-assisted liposuction (UAL).

Suction-assisted lipectomy (SAL) [13-23]

Courtiss demonstrated that following submental liposuction there was sufficient redraping and recontouring of the submental skin without redundancy. The patients, however, had to have normal skin quality and elasticity [20] **(III/B)**.

Technique
Cervical contouring by liposuction involves the removal of pre-platysmal fat while relying on skin contraction to tighten the neck skin. It is important to leave at least 5mm of fat on the skin flaps in order to disguise any underlying irregularities. Liposuction cannot reliably or safely deal with subplatysmal fat and this needs to be dealt with by open fat excision via a submental incision.

Liposuction can be performed either under local or general anaesthesia. Stab access incisions are made in the submental area and occasionally behind each ear lobe (for jaw line and lateral neck). The area is infiltrated with a standard liposuction solution. The suction is then undertaken using either a flat 2-3mm cannula (with the holes always facing the deep tissues) or a 2.3 or 3mm Mercedes cannula staying at least 5mm deep to the skin. The suction should be judicious with only 1-2 passes per tunnel to avoid over-suction and postoperative irregularities.

Mechanism of action

Liposuction exerts some of its effect via a simple volume reduction through extraction of fat. Another important mechanism is the creation of tunnels in the subcutaneous plane. The tunnels heal through a fibrous contractile process, which, in effect, retracts the subcutaneous tissue. The elastic properties of the overlying skin allow it to redrape over the subcutaneous framework with a net result of skin retraction [25-32] and skin redraping, reducing the ptotic appearance. The removal of this superficial layer has been described as being more evenly accomplished through emulsification with ultrasound-assisted lipectomy, compared with suction-assisted lipectomy [12, 24] **(IV/C)**.

Ultrasound-assisted liposuction (UAL) [12, 24]

Ultrasound-assisted liposuction has been found to be effective in neck rejuvenation [24] (Figure 1). It emulsifies the supraplatysmal fat making it easy for evacuation and contouring. Ultrasonic energy itself stimulates skin retraction through a different mechanism. It seems that the fibrous framework supporting the skin undergoes an inflammatory reaction in response to the exposure to ultrasonic energy. This framework subsequently contracts, resulting in retraction of the skin. The use of ultrasound-assisted liposuction carries with it a potential risk of thermal injury. In order to avoid this risk it is important that the probe is in constant motion, and a wet environment is necessary. It is also important to lower the amplitude (25-50%) and the emulsification time (2-3 minutes) in order to avoid marginal mandibular nerve palsy [12, 24].

Lipectomy (open fat excision): en bloc/piecemeal

Despite the popularity of suction-assisted lipectomy for removal of cervical fat, some authors advocate an alternative excisional approach, that can either be en bloc or piecemeal [33, 34]. Proponents of this approach describe a more anatomical dissection that facilitates removal of greater amounts of fat with superior redraping of the cervical skin. Unlike liposuction this approach can be used to deal with the subplatysmal fat.

The fat excision can, therefore, be supraplatysmal and/or subplatysmal. It is performed under direct vision and therefore can be more precise. In contrast to liposuction, excisional lipectomy is usually undertaken in conjunction with rhytidectomy [35]. It facilitates management of the platysma muscle and therefore overlaps with the submental/open neck lift. Open fat excision is indicated in the difficult neck [33, 34], but as an isolated procedure has largely been superceded by liposuction or the submental lift as part of a face-lift procedure.

Submental neck lift

This procedure involves a submental incision, undermining of the neck skin, followed by modifications of the fat (supra, inter, and sub-platysmal), platysma muscle and sometimes deeper structures under direct vision. Adequate visualisation is possible using a lighted retractor or a headlight and narrow Deaver retractor.

It is rarely undertaken in isolation (Figure 2), usually preceded by liposuction or pre-tunnelling, and often in conjunction with a face lift (short scar or long scar). It is indicated in patients with platysmal bands at rest, or bands visible on animation. In an isolated submental lift the extent of lateral undermining depends upon whether or not any skin redundancy persists or not. Any remaining contour irregularities are smoothed out either by liposuction or by direct fat excision. Drains are routinely used for this procedure.

Managing the platysma (platysma modification)

Open surgical rejuvenation of the aging neck usually includes some form of platysma modification. The numerous methods by which the platysma muscle is dealt with in neck rejuvenation [36-47] suggest that no one single approach suits all cases.

Aging causes attenuation of the cervical support for the platysma allowing the anterior borders of the platysma to descend inferiorly thus causing prominence of the platysmal bands [36, 37]. Other contributory factors to platysmal band prominence include muscle hypertrophy with age and shortening of the bow-stringed platysma [9]. Descent of the platysma muscle also contributes to the obliquity of the neck and creation of an obtuse cervicomental angle. The central or medial aspects of the platysma muscles separate in the midline, and frequently, medial bands appear, perhaps owing to vertical shortening of the corresponding muscular fibres [9].

The platysma needs to be approximated in the midline (anterior edge to edge approximation with or without trimming of any excess) and occasionally division of the bands. This inferior transection myotomy is designed to release and lengthen the muscle and allow superior redraping of muscle, better definition of the neck and recreation of the youthful acute cervicomental angle (Figure 2). Platysmaplasty has taken on many forms, including lateral plication [42], sectioning and flap rotation [43], simple midline suturing [44, 45], progressively tensioned midline sutures [44], muscular Z-plasty [45], resection of muscular 'bridles' [46], and suspension sutures. Other descriptions which incorporate a combination of these principles, include Feldman's 'corset platysmaplasty' [46] and the 'hammock platysmaplasty' as described by Fuente del Campo [38] (III/B). Feldman's corset platysmaplasty not only improves the submental contour and jawline but also eliminates platysmal bands [46]. Del Campo's double breasting of the platysma muscles in the midline, entirely through a submental approach, enables excellent platysmal suspension and neck recontouring with no need for posterior traction of the platysma muscle or peri-auricular incisions.

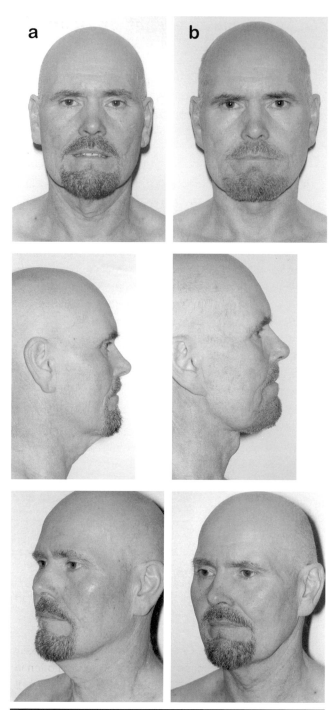

Figure 2. A 57-year-old man with isolated aging of the neck. He has heavy skin with true skin excess. An open submental necklift with minimal liposuction, midline platysma plication and short scars around the ear lobes for skin excision were used to rejuvenate the neck. Note the well redraped skin, acute cervicomental angle and visible thyroid cartilage bulge postoperatively [11].

Suspension sutures designed to improve the jaw line and neck-jaw angle were first described by Guerrero-Santos in 1983 [37] and have since been popularized by Giampapa and Di Bernardo [17]. The principle behind this method is to create a permanent artificial 'ligament' under the mandible, thereby correcting the deformities of the aging neck. The procedure is carried out through submental and post-auricular incisions. The neck is undermined (varied depending on the degree of ptosis and laxity), followed by plication of the platysmal edges medially. Subsequently, an interlocking, permanent suture is secured under the angle of the mandible before it is sutured onto the mastoid fascia. Specifically, one end of the interlocking suture creates the loop, and the other end passes through the loop. Only the first end is secured on the sternocleidomastoid muscle with two 'bites' on its fascia (less than 1cm apart). They then both get secured to the mastoid area. The long-term efficacy of suture suspension techniques in improving and masking abnormalities deep to the platysma has been questioned by Nahai [48].

Commonly used platysmaplasty techniques are shown in Table 2.

Endoscopically-assisted neck lift

The Emory University Hospital group has demonstrated that all the steps of a neck lift can be accomplished through minimal-access incisions. The incision behind the ear can be avoided if no skin excision is required [49]. The endoscope facilitates wide undermining of the neck skin and achievement of haemostasis. It has no particular advantages over the submental neck lift [12].

Neck lift as part of a face lift

Almost all face lifts have a rejuvenating effect on the neck, in particular the jaw line (and the jowls). This is especially so with face lifts incorporating the superficial musculo-aponeurotic system (SMAS) lift or plication. In the senior author's experience only a minority of face lifts achieve effective improvement of the neck without submental liposuction or without opening the neck **(IV/C)**. Most face-lift patients' necks are rejuvenated with an open neck lift (involving a submental incision) and modification of the platysma.

Table 2. Commonly used platysmaplasty techniques.

Platysmaplasty	Technique	Advantages	Disadvantages
Standard plication [37]	Lateral or medial edge of platysma sutured to SCM* or to itself (medial)	Technically simple	Could result in 'bunching' effect
Corset platysmaplasty [46]	Suture down, up and down the full length of platysma	Contour definition	
Suture-suspension methods [17, 37]	Numerous methods using absorbable or non-absorbable sutures	Allow careful adjustment of the desired outcome	Scarring could result in tethering of skin to platysma. Requires very careful skin redraping
'Anterior only' approach [50]	Direct anterior skin excision with platysma and Z-plasty	Good if elderly and wouldn't tolerate a big operation	Scarring of anterior neck

* Sternocleidomastoid muscle

The results are more spectacular with through and through subcutaneous dissection of the neck. The face lift's retro and pre-auricular incisions allow better or more excision of the loose cervical skin, better redraping of the neck, in addition to very wide access for platysma plication, SMAS-platysma lift/ suspension and elimination of the jowls.

Short scar face and neck lift

This is indicated in patients with no excess neck skin with jowls and aging of the neck-face interface. The incision is entirely in front of the ear (pre-auricular) and extends superiorly below the side burn (pre-hairline). The MACS lift and the short scar lateral SMASectomy are such examples [51, 52].

Full scar face and neck lift

This is similar to the short scar technique but includes retro-auricular incisions. It is indicated in patients with aging changes of the face and neck, especially the neck-face interface, with inelastic skin and excess lower and posterior neck skin [12]. True skin excess is present if the neck wrinkles extend below the thyroid cartilage or laterally beyond the sternocleidomastoid muscles. Poor quality or sun-damaged skin is inelastic and will not contract sufficiently postoperatively; it thus requires excision (Figure 3).

Skin excision

In patients with significant skin laxity and redundancy, excision of skin is mandatory. This is usually incorporated into the standard peri-auricular face-lift incisions; however, numerous authors have described a direct skin excision from an 'anterior only' procedure [53, 54]. The anterior incision is usually incorporated into a Z-plasty [55]. This approach is probably only acceptable in the elderly population that would be willing to accept the scar trade off for a less involved operation and faster recovery.

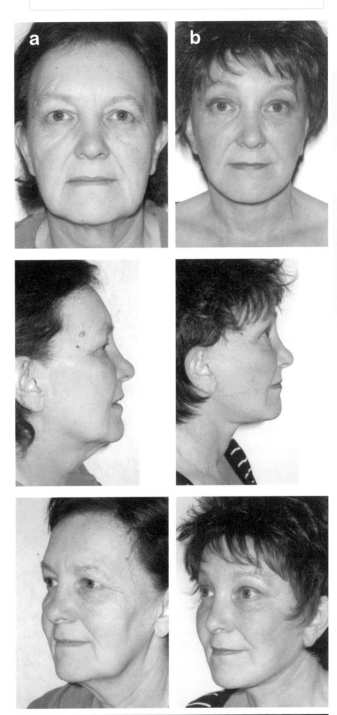

Figure 3. A 63-year-old lady with severe aging of the neck and face underwent a full face lift including endoscopic brow lift, open cervicoplasty and through and through submental dissection.

Table 3. Procedures deep to the platysma.

- Fat excision: open excision

- Tangential excision of the anterior bellies of the digastric muscles

- Intracapsular removal of the superficial lobe of the submandibular gland

- Release of the suprahyoid fascia (indicated for high hyoid)

Technical fine points

As previously mentioned there are specific anatomical sites that warrant special consideration. These areas have undergone further refinement over the years following improvement in surgical techniques, contributing to better aesthetic outcomes. Giampapa *et al*, in 2005, recently provided an excellent approach to the technical fine points involved in improving outcomes [10].

Depth of cervicomental angle

A number of options exist for enhancing this point. Firstly, if an interlocking suture method has been used (Giampapa) [17], then careful adjustment of the tension on this suture allows for adjustment of the depth of the angle. Additionally, defatting of the supra- and subplatysmal fat can also enhance the angle or help it remain soft. It is vital not to 'over correct' the neck, which occurs if too much tension is applied to the suspension sutures or if too much fat is removed from the supraplatysmal or subplatysmal plane.

Suturing of the digastric muscles together can further enhance the angle and help create a more concave or flat submental triangle [56, 57]. Finally, transection of the platysmal muscle borders has been popular; however, this is usually reserved for those with extremely thick platysmal bands or severe medial redundancy.

Modification of subplatysmal structures [12, 48, 57]

Connell demonstrated that even better neck contour (beyond that achieved with submental liposuction and corset platysmaplasty) could be obtained by removing the bulging caused by fat, the digastric muscles and the submandibular glands **(III/B)** (Table 3).

The fat between the platysma (interplatysmal) and deep to it (subplatysmal) cannot be dealt with by liposuction as it is difficult to access blindly, and it is dangerous to attempt to do so. Therefore, this is done by direct/open excision under direct vision. The anterior bellies of the digastric muscles can be excised tangentially [57] or totally. Rarely, they may be plicated in the midline.

Mandibular border definition

Liposuction both above and below the border of the mandible while leaving a strip of subcutaneous fat along the bony mandibular border for highlighting of the border itself will contribute significantly to defining this border.

Additional techniques that can be used with good effect here are fat grafting along the border of the mandible during the primary platysmaplasty, or the use of long-term fillers. Finally, some have utilised alloplastic implants with good results [58]. However, the risks associated with alloplastic implants discourage their widespread use.

Mandibular angle definition

If the suture suspension method is used, correct placement and tensioning will help enhance this angle. Additionally, fat grafting into the masseter muscle has resulted in even more defined mandibular angles. Similar results have been reported with the use of long-term fillers and with alloplastic augmentation.

Labial mandibular fold prominence

The labial mandibular fold is considered above the neck proper; however, it contributes directly to an overall youthful appearance of the neck. Suctioning of this area from below via a submental incision and/or from a postauricular incision flattens the labiomandibular fold. Camouflage fat grafting around the labiomandibular area can also markedly help to decrease the deformity. Dissection of the depressor labii muscle through a small intra-oral incision and subperiosteal dissection allows the muscle component of the fold to be released and helps to alleviate the downward turned corners of the mouth. Finally, an extended skin ellipse with a postauricular skin excision can further correct skin redundancy when prominent jowling is present.

Mental prominence

A naturally prominent chin projection adds considerably to the overall length and beauty of an aesthetically balanced neck. It also helps keep skin from becoming redundant in the submental area, but can easily be overlooked. A number of techniques for augmenting a deficient chin prominence exist and predominantly focus upon alloplastic implants and the use of sliding genioplasties with or without wire/plate fixation. The latter can be technically challenging and require significantly more time and effort with more potential complications. Fat grafting and long-term fillers have also been used, but results with them are more modest and await validation.

Anterior neck width

In many patients, the neck width is markedly increased with aging. As discussed earlier, this increase is mainly attributable to muscle laxity, collapse of the cervical spine, and an increase in subcutaneous and submental fat deposits. The creation of an aesthetically pleasing, thin neck can be accomplished by a number of techniques including resection of the redundant midline platysmal muscle and reconstitution of the muscle at the midline, by imbrication, or by a combination of both [59].

Algorithmic approach to surgical rejuvenation of the aging neck (Figure 4)

Categorising the problem and choosing the right technique

The ideal procedure for patients with aging of the lower face and neck is a cervicofacial rhytidectomy. However, within this population is a subgroup whose goals can be met by a lesser procedure that focuses solely upon the neck, with no change in the midface. This sub-group of patients has been described as falling into three broad categories:

- Patients with an obtuse cervicomental angle and good skin elasticity (who may be treated with liposuction alone).
- Patients with subplatysmal fat or mild to moderate skin and muscle laxity (these patients may be best treated by anterior lipectomy/liposuction and platysmaplasty).
- Patients with marked skin excess or severe skin laxity (best treated by procedures which excise skin).

Simply put, the young, the middle-aged and the elderly require different surgical techniques or approaches [50].

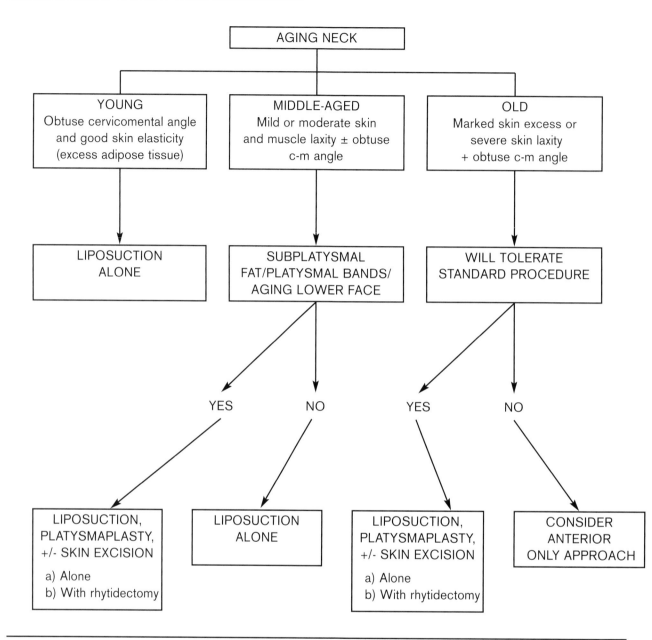

Figure 4. Algorithm for surgical rejuvenation of the aging neck.

Conclusions

Rejuvenation of the aging neck highlights a frequently recurring principle in surgery that no single approach suits all. It presents the plastic surgeon with an aesthetic and technical challenge that requires a structured approach in order to achieve a successful outcome. The evidence base outlined here aims to provide a framework through which consistent results can be achieved (Figure 4).

Recommendations

	Evidence level
◆ Attention to specific anatomical landmarks improves the surgical outcome from neck rejuvenation.	III/C
◆ SAL alone can be effective treatment in the young patient with excellent skin quality.	III/B
◆ UAL has extended the role of SAL and is more efficacious.	IV/C
◆ Numerous techniques are described in managing platysma, the utilisation of which depends upon the patient's requirements and the surgeon's skill and familiarity with each.	IV/C
◆ In patients with significant skin laxity and redundancy, excision of skin is mandatory.	IV/C

References

1. Rohrich RJ, Rios JL, Smith PD, Gutowski KA. Neck rejuvenation revisited. *Plast Reconstr Surg* 2006; 118(5): 1251-63.

2. Brandt FS, Boker A. Botulinum toxin for rejuvenation of the neck. *Clin Dermatol* 2003; 21: 513-20.

3. Agrawal A, Dejoseph L, Silver W. Anatomy of the jawline, neck and perioral area with clinical correlations. *Facial Plast Surg* 2005; 21(1): 3-10.

4. Scalfani AP. Soft tissue fillers for management of the aging perioral complex. *Facial Plast Surg* 2005; 21(1): 74-8.

5. Weiss RA, Weiss MA, Geronemus RG, *et al*. A novel non-thermal non-ablative full panel LED photomodulation device for reversal of photoaging; digital microscopic and clinical results in various skin types. *J Drugs Dermatol* 2004; 3: 605-10.

6. Weiss RA, Weiss MA, Beasley KL. Rejuvenation of photoaged skin: 5 years results with intense pulsed light of the face, neck and chest. *Dermatol Surg* 2002; 28: 1115-9.

7. Goldman MP, Marchell NL. Laser resurfacing of the neck with combined CO_2/Er: YAG laser. *Dermatol Surg* 1999; 25: 923-5.

8. Giampapa VC, Fuente del Campo A, Ramirez OM. Anti-aging medicine and the aesthetic surgeon: a new perspective for our specialty. *Aesthetic Plast Surg* 2004; 27: 493-501.

9. Stuzin JM, Baker TJ, Gordon HL. The relationship of the superficial and deep facial fascias: relevance to rhytidectomy and aging. *Plast Reconstr Surg* 1992; 89(3): 441-9; discussion 450-1.

10. Giampapa VC, Bitzos I, Ramirez O, Granick M. Suture suspension platysmaplasty for neck rejuvenation revisited: technical fine points for improving outcomes. *Aesthetic Plast Surg* 2005; 29(5): 341-50; discussion 351-2.

11. Ellenbogen R, Karlin JV. Visual criteria for success in restoring the youthful neck. *Plast Reconstr Surg* 1980; 66(6): 826-37.

12. Nahai F. Neck Lift. In: *The Art of Aesthetic Surgery, Principles & Techniques*. Nahai F, Ed. St. Louis, Missouri: Quality Medical Publishing, Inc,. 2005; Chapter 33: 1240-83.

13. Flageul G, Ilouz YG. Isolated cervicofacial liposuction in facial rejuvenation. *Ann Chir Plast Esthet* 1996; 41(6): 620-30.

14. Gasparotti M. Superficial liposuction: a new application of the technique for aged and flaccid skin. *Aesthetic Plast Surg* 1992; 16(2): 141-53.

15. Goodstein WA. Superficial liposculpture of the face and neck. *Plast Reconstr Surg* 1997; 100(1): 284.

16. Toledo LS. Facial rejuvenation: the role of skin retraction. In: Annals of the International Symposium: Recent Advances in Plastic Surgery. Sao Paulo, Brazil, March, 1992.

17. Giampapa VC, Di Bernardo BE. Neck recontouring with suture suspension and liposuction: an alternative for the early rhytidectomy candidate. *Ann Plast Surg* 1993; 30(6): 500-2.

18. Prabhat A, Dyer WK II. Improving surgery on the aging neck with an adjustable expanded polytetrafluoroethylene cervical sling. *Arch Facial Plast Surg* 2003; 5: 491-501.

19. Kamer FM, Minoli JJ. Postoperative platysmal band deformity: a pitfall of submental liposuction. *Arch Otolaryngol Head Neck Surg* 1993; 119(2): 193-6.

20. Pinto EB, Rocha RP, Queiroz W Jr, *et al*. Submental skin: morphohistological study of interest to liposuction. *Aesthetic Plast Surg* 1997; 21(6): 388-94.

21. Courtiss EH. Suction lipectomy of the neck. *Plast Reconstr Surg* 1985; 76(6): 882-9.

22. Gryskiewicz JM. Submental suction-assisted lipectomy without platysmaplasty: pushing the (skin) envelope to avoid a face lift for unsuitable candidates. *Plast Reconstr Surg* 2003; 112(5): 1393-405; discussion 1406-7.

23. Morrison W, Salisbury M, Beckham P, *et al*. The minimal face lift: liposuction of the neck and jowls. *Aesthetic Plast Surg* 2001; 25: 94.

24. Grotting JC, Beckenstein MS. Cervicofacial rejuvenation using ultrasound-assisted lipectomy. *Plast Reconstr Surg* 2001; 107(3): 847-55.

25. Zocchi M. Clinical aspects of ultrasonic liposculpture. *Perspect Plast Surg* 1993; 7:153.

26. Zocchi M. Ultrasonic-assisted lipoplasty. *Adv Plast Reconstr Surg* 1995; 11: 197.

27. Scheflan M, Tazi H. Ultrasound-assisted body contouring. *Aesthetic Surg Q* 1996; 16: 117.

28. Becker H. Subdermal liposuction to enhance skin contraction. A preliminary report. *Ann Plast Surg* 1992; 28(5): 479-84.

29. Gasperoni C, Salgarello M. Rationale for subdermal liposuction related to the anatomy of subcutaneous fat and the superficial fascial system. *Ann Plast Surg* 2000; 45(4): 369-73.

30. Rohrich RJ. Superficial liposculpture of the face and neck (Discussion). *Plast Reconstr Surg* 1996; 98(6): 988-96; discussion 997-8.

31. Shiffman MA. Superficial liposculpture of the face and neck (letter). *Plast Reconstr Surg* 1997; 100(2): 552-3.

32. Rohrich RJ, Beran SJ, Kenkel JM, *et al.* Extending the role of liposuction in body contouring with ultrasound-assisted liposuction. *Plast Reconstr Surg* 1998; 101(4): 1090-102; discussion 1117-9.

33. Robbins LB, Shaw KE. *En bloc* cervical lipectomy for treatment of the problem neck in facial rejuvenation surgery. *Plast Reconstr Surg* 1989; 83(1): 53-60.

34. Singer R. Improvement of the young fatty neck. *Plast Reconstr Surg* 1984; 73(4): 582-9.

35. Millard DR Jr, Beck RL, *et al.* Submental and submandibular lipectomy in conjunction with a face lift in the male or female. *Plast Reconstr Surg* 1972; 49(4): 385-91.

36. McKinney P. Management of platysmal bands. *Plast Reconstr Surg* 2002; 110(3): 982-4.

37. Guerrero-Santos J. Neck lift: simplified surgical techniques, refinements, and clinical classification. *Clin Plast Surg* 1983; 10: 379.

38. Fuente del Campo A. Midline plastysma muscular overlap for neck restoration. *Plast Reconstr Surg* 1998; 102 (5): 1710-4; discussion 1715.

39. Connell BF, Gaon A. Surgical correction of aesthetic contour problems of the neck. *Clin Plast Surg* 1983; 10 (3): 491-505.

40. Guerrero-Santos J. Surgical correction of the fatty fallen neck. *Ann Plast Surg* 1979; 2(5): 491-505.

41. Guerrero-Santos J. The role of the platysma muscle in rhytidoplasty. *Clin Plast Surg* 1978; 5(1): 29-49.

42. Guerrero-Santos J, Espillat G, Morales F. Muscular lift in cervical rhytidoplasty. *Plast Reconstr Surg* 1974; 54(2): 127-30.

43. Connell BF. Contouring the neck in rhytidectomy by lipectomy and muscle sling. *Plast Reconstr Surg* 1978; 61(3): 376-83.

44. Souther SG, Vistnes LM. Medial approximation of the platysma muscle in the treatment of neck deformities. *Plast Reconstr Surg* 1981; 67(5): 607-13.

45. Cardoso de Castro C. The value of the anatomical classification of the medial fibres of platysma muscle in cervical lifting. In: Transactions of the 8th International Congress of Plastic and Reconstructive Surgery. Montreal: McGill University, 1983: 515-6.

46. Feldman JJ. Corset platysmaplasty. *Plast Reconstr Surg* 1990; 85(3): 333-43.

47. Weisman PA. One surgeon's experience with surgical contouring of the neck. *Clin Plast Surg* 1983; 10(3): 521-41.

48. Nahai F. Reconsidering neck suspension sutures. *Aesthetic Surg J* 2004; 24: 365.

49. Eaves FE, Nahai F, Bostwick J III. The endoscopic neck lift. *Op Tech Plast Reconstr Surg* 1995; 2: 499-603.

50. Zins JE, Fardo D. The 'anterior only' approach to neck rejuvenation: an alternative to face lift surgery. *Plast Recostr Surg* 2005; 115 (6): 1761-8.

51. Tonnard PL, Verpaele A, Gaia S. Optimising results from minimal access cranial suspension lifting (MACS-lift). *Aesthetic Plast Surg* 2005; 29(4): 213-20; discussion 221.

52. Baker DC. Minimal incision rhytidectomy (short scar face lift) with lateral SMASectomy: evolution and application. *Aesthetic Surg J* 2001; 21: 14.

53. Biggs TM, Koplin L. Direct alternatives for neck skin redundancy in males. *Clin Plast Surg* 1983; 10(3): 423-8.

54. Gradinger GP. Anterior cervicoplasty in the male patient. *Plast Reconstr Surg* 2000; 106(5): 1146-54; discussion 1155.

55. Cronin TD, Biggs TM. The T-Z-plasty for the male 'turkey gobbler' neck. *Plast Reconstr Surg* 1971; 47(6): 534-8.

56. Ramirez OM. Cervicoplasty: nonexcisional anterior approach. *Plast Reconstr Surg* 2003; 111(3): 1342-5; discussion 1346-7.

57. Connell BF, Shamoun JM. The significance of digastric muscle contouring for rejuvenation of the submental area of the face. *Plast Reconstr Surg* 1997; 99(6): 1586-90.

58. Ramirez OM. Mandibular matrix implant system: a method to restore skeletal support to the lower face. *Plast Reconstr Surg* 2000; 106(1): 176-89.

59. Kipper P, Mitz V, Maladry D, Saad G. Is it necessary to suture the platysma muscles on the midline to improve the cervical profile? An anatomic study using 20 cadavers. *Ann Plast Surg* 1997; 39(6): 566-72.

Chapter 25

Chapter 26

Trends in aesthetic facial surgery: the Hamra lower lid blepharoplasty

Gary L Ross MB ChB MRCS (Ed) MD FRCS (Plast.) 1
Consultant Plastic Surgeon

David J Whitby MB BS FRCS 2
Consultant Plastic Surgeon

1 CHRISTIE HOSPITAL NHS FOUNDATION TRUST, MANCHESTER, UK
2 UNIVERSITY HOSPITAL OF SOUTH MANCHESTER
NHS FOUNDATION TRUST, MANCHESTER, UK

Introduction

The alterations caused by aging are noticeable first around the eyes and then on the neck and lower face. Peri-orbital rejuvenation techniques continue to evolve with a more detailed understanding of eyelid anatomy and the effects of aging on the eyelid and peri-orbital tissues.

Procedures have developed with time, with surgeons striving for a more youthful appearance. The Hamra technique for lower lid blepharoplasty is an example of one such procedure that has evolved over a 30-year period [1-13].

Methodology

A Medline search was employed to gather evidence, using the search terms 'lower lid blepharoplasty', 'Hamra technique' and supplemented by a hand search of references from the articles obtained.

Anatomy of the lower eyelid

The anterior lamella consists of the skin and orbicularis muscle. The middle lamella consists of the orbital septum, which originates from the arcus marginalis and inserts into the inferior tarsal margin. The posterior lamella includes the conjunctiva and lower eyelid retractors [14].

The orbicularis oculi muscle is immediately deep to the skin of the lower lid and extends from close to the ciliary margin past the infra-orbital rim to the cheek. It has both pretarsal and preseptal components. Pretarsally, the orbicularis is tightly adherent to the underlying tarsus. The pre-orbital portion of the orbicularis oculi has cephalad attachments to the orbital rim along the orbicularis retaining ligament and along its caudal margin to the fascia enveloping the origin of the elevators of the upper lip (zygomaticus muscles). The retaining ligaments that support the orbicularis oculi to the underlying orbital rim and cheek serve to fixate this muscle tightly against the underlying facial framework [15-16].

The orbital septum lies deep to the orbicularis. A plane of loose connective tissue, the suborbicularis fascia, lies between the orbicularis and orbital septum. The suborbicularis oculi fat (SOOF) lies in this plane and is the continuum of the malar fat pad [14]. The triangular malar fat pad has its base at the nasolabial fold and its apex at the malar eminence, and is situated between the skin and the superficial musculo-aponeurotic system (SMAS) [17, 18]. It is loosely connected to the SMAS and firmly attached to the skin.

The orbital septum fuses superiorly with the tarsal plate and inferiorly with the periosteum of the infra-orbital rim; this inferior attachment of the septum is termed the arcus marginalis. The arcus marginalis attaches medially to the anterior lacrimal crest and thins as it extends laterally attaching approximately 2mm inferior to the rim on the facial aspect of the zygomatic bone. The orbital septum serves to retain orbital fat within the orbit. The fat mass, as it encircles the extra-ocular muscles, causes it to be divided into three pads: medial, central and lateral.

Aging of the lower eyelid-cheek complex

The pathogenesis of herniation of lower orbital fat has been debated for decades [19, 20]. Whether excess fat appears in older age or whether this represents shifting of intra-orbital contents is unclear. The concepts of Manson *et al* [21] and Camirand *et al* [22] attributed lower fat extrusion to a weakening of Lockwood's suspensory ligament with the presence of intra-orbital septation within the fat compartments limiting the degree of protrusion. De la Plaza and Arroyo [23] first proposed the theory that fat protrusion is related to the weakness of the support system of the globe, allowing it to descend and causing enophthalmos and lower lid pseudoherniation (bags).

The most poorly supported part of the orbicularis oculi is the preseptal portion and it is this that shows the greatest tendency toward descent. As the retaining ligaments relax with aging, the herniated lower lid fat becomes situated not only anteriorly but also inferiorly below the orbital rim. This is most apparent along the central fat pad but may be noted medially as well. It is uncommon to note a lateral fat pad inferior to the infra-orbital rim. In youth, there is no herniation of orbital fat; the lateral orbicularis oculi blends with the malar pad. Malar bags are rarely apparent and there is a smooth contour between the preseptal and pre-orbital orbicularis. In youth, there is relatively more SOOF in the lower lid and more subcutaneous cheek fat. This helps to make the lower lid appear soft and smooth without the sharp demarcation between eyelid and cheek that become obvious with aging.

Hamra noted that in youth, the eyelid-cheek complex is a single mildly convex line on profile, running from the tarsus inferiorly over the young cheek. Aging causes descent of the globe and subsequent pseudoherniation of intra-orbital fat. The inferior and lateral descent of these structures produces an orbit that appears deeper with a wider diameter. This progressive ptosis and attenuation of soft tissue coverage produce skeletonisation of the entire orbital area to reveal the topographical contours of the inferior bony orbital rim. A youthful midface is characterised by a malar fat pad seated over the zygomatic arch, its upper border covering the orbital part of the orbicularis oculi and its inferior border located along the nasolabial fold. With advancing age, the malar fat pad, along with the SOOF, slides in an inferonasal direction and anteriorly over the SMAS. It bulges against the fixed nasolabial crease and exacerbates the appearance of the nasolabial fold.

The combination of descent of the orbicularis oculi, SOOF and malar fat with aging transforms the youthful single convexity to an aging double convex pattern.

Historical correction of lower lid aging

Historically, lower lid blepharoplasty was viewed as an operation to remove skin and fat in the lower eyelid [19, 20]. The traditional open blepharoplasty redraped the skin or the skin-muscle flap between the infra-orbital rim and the subciliary incision. Orbital fat that appeared excessive was removed, but the 'malar crescent' or inferior border of the orbicularis muscle remained undisturbed from its position over the malar eminence [8, 13].

Postoperatively, the appearance of the lower eyelid became smoother and usually deeper, particularly in patients with a negative vector. The appearance of the malar crescent or inferior orbicularis border, if present before surgery, remained unchanged. Removal of orbital fat caused eventual collapse of the existing skin cover, which created more wrinkling than before. With continuing aging, ptosis and attenuation of the orbicularis oculi led to a typical sunken appearance with possible scleral show [8, 13].

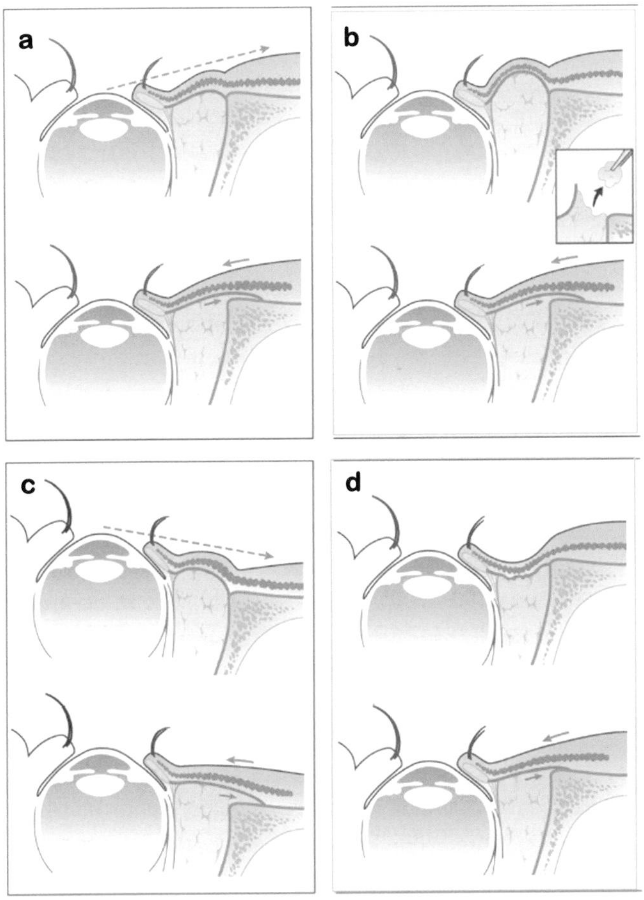

Hamra technique (Figures 1 and 2)

This technique aimed to address both the changes in the orbicularis muscle and the orbital fat changes contributing to aging contours.

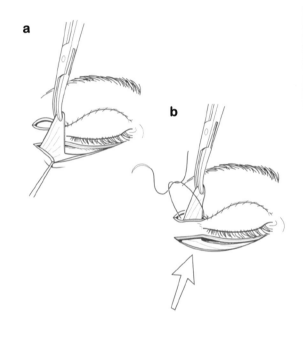

Figure 2. a) A laterally-based flap of orbicularis muscle is created and passed under the lateral raphe. b) The pedicle is attached with two sutures to the lateral orbital periosteum. Extraordinary tension is necessary to effectively elevate and suspend the cheek tissues. *Reproduced with permission from Lippincott Williams and Wilkins © 2004* [13].

Figure 1. a) In patients with a positive vector eye and a normal amount of fat, all fat is preserved when performing the septal reset. The axis drops anterior to the cheek. b) In the event that there is a congenital excess of fat, a certain amount must be excised to prevent postoperative bulging. c) In patients with a negative vector eye, one usually needs to utilise all of the orbital fat to create a smooth transition between eyelid and cheek. The axis drops in a posterior line to the cheek. d) In the hollow lower eyelid, one can always find adequate fat to be recruited from the subseptal space to give an adequate correction. *Reproduced with permission from Lippincott Williams and Wilkins © 2004* [13].

Repositioning of the orbicularis muscle

The use of the orbicularis muscle as a flap in surgery of the lower eyelid was first described by Adamson *et al* [24], Courtiss [25] and Furnas [26], and was first used to treat malar bags/festoons by Furnas [26] advocating lateral tensioning of the orbicularis muscle.

Hamra [6, 13] noted that by elevating the orbicularis muscle off the malar eminence, in a suborbicularis oculi plane, and repositioning it, the axis of the muscle from the medial orbital rim to the lateral raphe could be changed and the muscular ring around the bony orbit could be tightened. Hamra postulated that to negate the vector of aging in the orbicularis oculi (an inferolateral direction off the malar eminence), the vector of repair should be superomedial [6, 9, 13]. This superomedial vector could either be obtained by a composite rhytidectomy or by using a laterally-based orbicularis muscle flap. The laterally-based orbicularis muscle flap was turned superiorly under the raphe and sutured under extreme tension to the periosteum of the lateral orbital rim [6, 9, 13].

Hamra [9, 13] noticed limitations of this procedure, which included occasional prolonged malar oedema and an inability to exert sufficient tension on this skin muscle flap owing to the fear of lower eyelid retraction. He thus adapted the plane of dissection to continue the suborbicularis dissection under the medial portions of the zygomaticus minor and major muscles while maintaining an adequate soft tissue cover over the periosteum. With this level of dissection there was no need to disrupt the origins of the zygomaticus musculature while the orbicularis could still be repositioned with even more tension than before [9, 13]. This zygo-orbicular (zygomaticus-orbicularis) plane offered many advantages (Table 1) **(III/B)**. Hamra believes that this zygo-orbicular dissection plane is preferable to the subperiosteal plane as introduced by Tessier [27] and recommended by Hester [28].

Table 1. Advantages of zygo-orbicular dissection plane.

- Recovery time is shortened with minimal malar oedema and chemosis
- There is no flap retraction
- Rapid postoperative adherence between soft tissue and periosteum
- No temporary orbicularis dystonia
- No need for a formal canthoplasty
- The intermalar distance remained the same
- An arcus marginalis release and septal reset is still possible

Following dissection of the zygo-orbicular flap a 4-0 nylon suture is passed through the longitudinal axis of the lateral canthal tendon which is sutured to the inner wall of the lateral orbital periosteum. This suture stabilises the lower eyelid in yet a higher position, ensuring stability of the eyelid when suturing the septum with adequate tension over the orbital rim. Hamra called this a 'transcanthal' canthopexy, which requires neither detachment of the lateral canthal tendon nor a canthotomy [9, 13].

Preservation of orbital fat/septal reset

Loeb [29-31] was first to describe the technique of mobilising intra-orbital fat across the medial infra-orbital rim. He used it to fill and thus camouflage the nasojugal groove. Hamra [8] expanded this concept by advocating complete release of the arcus marginalis allowing the subseptal fat to be elevated to the level of the orbital rim. He extended Loeb's concept to include advancement of all of the lower lid fat pads in an effort to conceal the infra-orbital rim and to recreate the youthful fullness of the lower lid. As originally described, the arcus marginalis was incised and the orbital fat alone was advanced and sutured to the pre-periosteal fat of the upper cheek. Subsequently, Hamra [13] refined his technique leaving the septum orbitale that he once excised intact and resetting the inferior border of the septum after arcus marginalis release over the orbital rim. The septal flap included orbital fat creating a smoother transition of soft tissue covering the bony rim and a firm smooth convex surface for the redraped overlying skin-muscle flap, thus diminishing the rhytids. Hamra termed this procedure a septal reset. Hamra observed a marked improvement with the repositioned orbicularis now resting on a firm undersurface of septum, rather than on the concavity created by fat removal, or the soft fullness of fat only **(III/B)**.

Surgical technique

Peri-operatively, the dermis of the subciliary incision line is injected with local anaesthesia along with percutaneous injections of a few drops of local anaesthesia with adrenalin layered over the periosteum of the maxilla and zygoma.

The subciliary skin incision is followed by a skin flap dissection to the junction of the preseptal and peri-orbital portions of the orbicularis oculi muscle. The preseptal orbicularis is opened, leaving the pretarsal muscle undisturbed. After dissecting down to the orbital rim over the septum orbitale, the suborbicularis dissection is continued under the zygomaticus muscles. The origins of the zygomaticus major and minor muscles are left intact and an adequate layer of soft tissue is left overlying the periosteum. Dissection is started with cutting cautery and continued with scissors. This dissection prevents potential nerve injury, and pushes the dissection boundary under the midportion of the zygomaticus minor and major, and laterally to the zygomatic arch. The arcus marginalis is released by incising the junction of the septum orbitale and the periosteum of the inferior orbital rim with cutting cautery after the zygo-orbicular dissection has been accomplished. Decisions regarding fat removal or repositioning over the orbital rim are made pre-operatively.

Some medial and central fat may be resected, whereas lateral fat is in most cases used for repositioning. Before the septal reset is completed, a transcanthal canthopexy, with a 4.0 nylon, is undertaken fixing the lower eyelid position so that the septal reset can then be completed without tension. The inferior edge of the septum is then reset over the orbital rim with multiple 5-0 Vicryl sutures. Usually eight to 12 sutures are required for the septal reset to create a smooth transition, ensuring that tension is sufficient to create a firm undersurface for the orbicularis to rest upon.

After the reset is completed, the zygo-orbicular midface flap is advanced. Several 3-0 Vicryl sutures are placed between the zygo-orbicular flap and the pre-periosteal tissue to reduce dead space and serum collection. A laterally-based orbicularis pedicle is created from the lateral extension of the blepharoplasty incision. This pedicle is passed under the skin and muscle raphe to be secured with two sutures of 4-0 Monocryl to the periosteum of the lateral orbital rim. The very last manoeuvre is the trimming of skin, in the event that an adjustment needs to be made.

Fat removal

Before surgery, the surgeon must decide whether fat must be resected or not, and if so, how much. This is a pre-operative judgement dictated by the anatomy of each individual patient, which is difficult to assess when the patient is anaesthetised. Positive and negative vector eyelids refer to the axis dropped from the most anterior point of the globe to the cheek. The positive vector eyelid is usually the easiest for achieving a good result when using conventional blepharoplasty, and the negative vector eyelid presents a challenge when using conventional blepharoplasty. Hamra defined five groups of patients as illustrated in Table 2 [13].

Table 2. The five lower eyelid variable types.

Type	Anatomical variation	Orbital changes	Amount of fat
Type 1	Positive vector	Short vertical height or narrow convex orbit	Normal amount of septal fat
Type 2	Negative vector	Elongated vertical height, or wide concave orbit	Congential excessive subseptal fat
Type 3	Negative vector	Wide orbit	Normal amount of orbital fat
Type 4	Malar crescent deformity	Wide orbit. Elongated orbicularis	Excess fat
Type 5	The hollow eyelid	Wide orbit	Decrease of orbital fat

For significant scleral show/ectropion, Hester recommends canthoplasty. For recalcitrant lower lid malposition, usually with dry eye symptoms not corrected by repeated canthoplasty and re-elevation of the lower lid, Hester *et al* [42] recommended the use of lower lid spacers such as ear cartilage and hard palate mucosa. Hamra recommends alloderm as an alternative [43].

Conclusions

The Hamra technique for lower lid blapharoplasty is a personal technique that has evolved over a 30-year period. Adoption of the technique has not been widespread, although it has been shown to be reliable and reproducible. The varying aspects of the technique have been discussed in this review and many individual components of the technique have been widely adopted.

Recommendations	Evidence level
◆ Fat repositioning/septal reset creates a smoother transition of soft tissue covering the bony rim and is required to create an optimal result.	III/B
◆ Fat removal may be appropriate only in carefully selected patients, such as those with a negative vector and a congenital excess of fat.	III/B
◆ Repositioning of the orbicularis muscle allows a more appropriate vector and prevents the need for a formal canthoplasty.	III/B
◆ Use of the orbicularis flap does not result in impaired lower lid function.	III/B
◆ Transcanthal canthopexy rather than canthoplasty is recommended for patients requiring lower lid support.	III/B

References

1. Hamra ST. Composite rhytidectomy. *Plast Reconstr Surg* 1992; 90: 1-13.
2. Lemmon ML, Hamra ST. Skoog rhytidectomy: a five-year experience with 577 patients. *Plast Reconstr Surg* 1980; 65: 283-97.
3. Hamra ST. The tri-plane facelift dissection. *Ann Plast Surg* 1984; 12: 268-74.
4. Hamra ST. The deep plane rhytidectomy. *Plast Reconstr Surg* 1990; 86: 53-61.
5. Hamra ST. A study of the long-term effect of malar fat repositioning in face lift surgery: short-term success but long-term failure. *Plast Reconstr Surg* 2002; 110: 940-51.
6. Hamra ST. Repositioning of the orbicularis oculi in composite rhytidectomy. *Plast Reconstr Surg* 1992; 90: 14-22.
7. Hamra ST. *Composite Rhytidectomy*. St. Louis, Mo.: Quality Medical Publishing, 1993.
8. Hamra ST. Arcus marginalis release and orbital fat preservation in midface rejuvenation. *Plast Reconstr Surg* 1995; 96: 354-62.
9. Hamra ST. The zygorbicular dissection in composite rhytidectomy: an ideal midface plane. *Plast Reconstr Surg* 1998; 102: 1646-57.
10. Hamra ST. Frequent facelift sequelae: hollow eyes and the lateral sweep: cause and repair. *Plast Reconstr Surg* 1998; 102: 1658-66.
11. Hamra ST. Surgical anatomy of the midface and malar mounds. *Plast Reconstr Surg* 2002; 110: 900-5.
12. Hamra ST. Correcting the unfavorable outcomes following facelift surgery. *Clin Plast Surg* 2001; 28: 621-38.
13. Hamra ST. The role of the septal reset in creating a youthful eyelid-cheek complex in facial rejuvenation. *Plast Reconstr Surg* 2004; 113: 2124-44.
14. Moelleken B. The superficial subciliary cheek lift, a technique for rejuvenating the infraorbital region and nasojugal groove: a clinical series of 71 patients. *Plast Reconstr Surg* 1999; 104: 1863-74.
15. Mendelson BC, Muzaffar AR, Adams WP, Jr. Surgical anatomy of the midcheek and malar mounds. *Plast Reconstr Surg* 2002; 110: 905-11.
16. Muzaffar AR, Mendelson BC, Adams WP, Jr. Surgical anatomy of the ligamentous attachments of the lower lid and lateral canthus. *Plast Reconstr Surg* 2002; 110: 873-84.

17. Mitz V, Peyronie M. The superficial musculoaponeurotic system (SMAS) in the parotid and cheek area. *Plast Reconstr Surg* 1976; 58: 80-8.

18. De Cordier BC, de la Torre JI, Al-Hakeem MS, *et al*. Rejuvenation of the midface by elevating the malar fat pad: review of technique, cases, and complications. *Plast Reconstr Surg* 2002; 110: 1526-36.

19. Bourget J. Les hernies graisseuses de l'orbite: notre traitement chirurgical. *Bull Acad Med* (Paris) 1924; 92: 1270.

20. Castanares S. Blepharoplasty for herniated intraorbital fat: anatomical basis for a new approach. *Plast Reconstr Surg* 1951; 8: 46-58.

21. Manson PN, Clifford CM, Su CT, *et al*. Mechanisms of global support and post-traumatic enophthalmos: I. The anatomy of the ligament sling and its relation to intramuscular cone orbital fat. *Plast Reconstr Surg* 1986; 77: 193-202.

22. Camirand A, Doucet J, Harris J. Anatomy, pathophysiology, and prevention of senile enophthalmia and associated herniated lower eyelids. *Plast Reconstr Surg* 1997; 100: 1535-46.

23. de la Plaza R, Arroyo JM. A new technique for the treatment of palpebral bags. *Plast Reconstr Surg* 1988; 81: 677-87.

24. Adamson JE, McCraw JB, Carraway JH. Use of a muscle flap in lower blepharoplasty. *Plast Reconstr Surg* 1979; 63: 359-63.

25. Courtiss EH. Selection of alternatives in esthetic blepharoplasty. *Clin Plast Surg* 1981; 8: 739-55.

26. Furnas DW. The orbicularis oculi muscle. Management in blepharoplasty. *Clin Plast Surg* 1981; 8: 687-715.

27. Tessier P. Le lifting faciale sousperioste. *Ann Chir Plast Esthet* 1989; 34: 193-7.

28. Hester TR, Codner MA, McCord CD. The 'centrofacial' approach for correction of facial aging using the transblepharoplasty subperiosteal cheeklift. *Aesthetic Surg J* 1996; 16: 51-8.

29. Loeb R, Ed. *Aesthetic Surgery of the Eyelids*. New York: Springer-Verlag, 1989.

30. Loeb R. Nasojugal groove leveling with fat tissue. *Clin Plast Surg* 1993; 20: 393-400.

31. Loeb R. Fat pad sliding and fat grafting for leveling lid depressions. *Clin Plast Surg* 1981; 8: 757-76.

32. Hester TR, McCord CD, Nahai F, *et al*. Expanded applications for transconjunctival lower lid blepharoplasty. *Plast Reconstr Surg* 2001; 108: 271-2.

33. Lowry JC, Bartley GB, Litchy WJ. Results of levator-advancement blepharoptosis repair using a standard protocol: effect of epinephrine-induced eyelid position change. *Trans Am Ophthalmol Soc* 1996; 94: 165-73.

34. McCord CD Jr, Shore J, Putnam JR. Treatment of essential blepharospasm. II. A modification of exposure for the muscle stripping technique. *Arch Ophthalmol* 1984; 102: 269-73.

35. Honrado CP, Pastorek NJ. Long-term results of lower-lid suspension blepharoplasty: a 30-year experience. *Arch Facial Plast Surg* 2004; 6: 150-4.

36. Rizk SS, Matarasso A. Lower eyelid blepharoplasty: analysis of indications and the treatment of 100 patients. *Plast Reconstr Surg* 2003; 111: 1299-306.

37. Patipa M. Transblepharoplasty lower eyelid and midface rejuvenation: part I. Avoiding complications by utilizing lessons learned from the treatment of complications. *Plast Reconstr Surg* 2004; 113: 1459-68.

38. Patipa M Transblepharoplasty lower eyelid and midface rejuvenation: part II. Functional applications of midface elevation. *Plast Reconstr Surg* 2004; 113: 1469-74.

39. Zarem HA, Resnick JI. Expanded applications for transconjunctival lower lid blepharoplasty. *Plast Reconstr Surg* 1999; 103: 1041-3.

40. Seckel BR, Kovanda CJ, Cetrulo CL Jr, Passmore AK, Meneses PG, White T. Laser blepharoplasty with transconjunctival orbicularis muscle/septum tightening and periocular skin resurfacing: a safe and advantageous technique. *Plast Reconstr Surg* 2000; 106: 1127-41.

41. Barton FE, Ha R, Awada M. Fat extrusion and septal reset in patients with the tear trough triad: a critical appraisal. *Plast Reconstr Surg* 2004; 113: 2115-21.

42. Hester TR, Codner MA, McCord CD, *et al*. Evolution of technique of the direct transblepharoplasty approach for the correction of lower lid and midfacial aging: maximizing results and minimizing complications in a 5-year experience. *Plast Reconstr Surg* 2000; 105: 393-406.

43. Hamra ST. Evolution of technique of the direct transblepharoplasty approach for the correction of lower lid and midfacial aging: maximizing results and minimizing complications in a 5-year experience. *Plast Reconstr Surg* 2000; 105: 407-8.

44 Labandter HP. Use of the orbicularis muscle flap for complex lower lid problems: a 6-year analysis. *Plast Reconstr Surg* 1995; 96: 346-53.

45. Goldberg RA. Transconjunctival orbital fat repositioning: transposition of orbital fat pedicles into a subperiosteal pocket. *Plast Reconstr Surg* 2000; 105: 743-8.

46. Rohrich RJ. The superficial subciliary cheek lift, a technique for rejuvenating the infraorbital region and nasojugal groove: a clinical series of 71 patients. *Plast Reconstr Surg* 1999; 104: 1875-6.

Chapter 26

Chapter 27

Fibrin sealant in plastic surgery

David W Oliver BSc MB ChB FRCS FRCS (Plast.) 1
Consultant Plastic Surgeon
Iain S Whitaker BA (Hons) MA MB BChir MRCS 2
Specialist Registrar, Plastic Surgery

1 ROYAL DEVON AND EXETER HOSPITAL, EXETER, UK
2 THE WELSH CENTRE FOR BURNS AND PLASTIC SURGERY
MORRISTON HOSPITAL, SWANSEA, UK

Introduction

Fibrin sealants imitate the final phase of the blood coagulation process. On the tissue surface, fibrinogen is converted into a soluble fibrin monomer by the action of thrombin. Factor XIIIa (which is activated by calcium and thrombin) then acts to allow crosslinking of the fibrin monomer to create an insoluble high-molecular-weight fibrin polymer and a mechanically stable fibrin clot. Commercially available fibrin sealants mimic this phase of wound healing and are usually applied as a spray after re-constitution from their components in the operating theatre (Figure 1). Generally, two reconstituted vials (one containing fibrinogen, factor XIIIa and aprotinin, and the other, thrombin and calcium chloride) are sprayed together and this mixing forms the sealant as it reaches the wound surface. This mechanically stable fibrin clot has haemostatic and adhesive properties identical to the endogenous fibrin clot formed during the first phase of wound healing. Aprotinin is added in order to prevent the proteolytic degradation of fibrin by endogenous plasmin and prolong its presence in the wound.

This fibrin network is thought to reduce the amount of postoperative bleeding by sealing capillary vessels and allowing raw operative surfaces to adhere. Depending upon the concentrations of the thrombin and calcium component, the setting process can be manipulated such that adhesion will occur between a few seconds and several minutes after application.

Methodology

A Medline search was performed using search terms 'fibrin glue', 'fibrin sealant', 'platelet gel' and 'autologous sealant'. Bibliographic linkage was also used to retrieve secondary references.

Background

Fibrin sealant has been used for many years and has a wide range of clinical applications for wound support, tissue adhesion and haemostasis. The physiological mechanism for the formation of fibrin sealant was first described by Morawitz in 1905. Since this time attempts have been made to

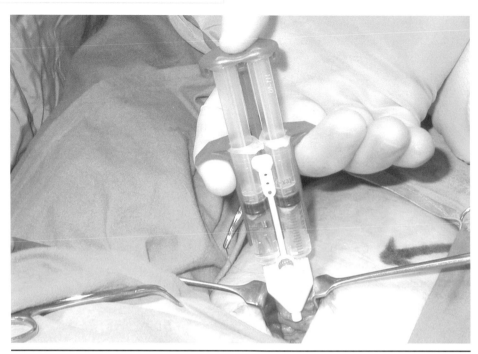

Figure 1. The application of fibrin sealant.

reproduce this mechanism for clinical use with varying success. In the 1940s a combination of thrombin (extrinsically added) and fibrinogen from the wound plasma was used in cataract operations [1]. Fibrin sealant was first marketed in 1983. It has now been used widely in both Europe and the US and many studies have shown fibrin sealant systems to be efficacious in controlling slow bleeding foci, diffuse oozing and lymphatic leaks in a wide range of applications [2] **(IV/C)**. The versatility is such that fibrin glue was used in up to 5% of all surgical procedures in a US hospital in 1995 [3] **(IV/C)**. For example, fibrin sealants have been used in liver resection and in cardiac surgery to aid haemostasis [4] **(IIa/B)**, to seal bronchial and alveolar leakages after pulmonary resections [5] **(Ib/A)** and in the treatment of bleeding gastroduodenal ulceration. These and other studies provide grade A and B evidence for the efficacy of these sealants [6] **(Ib/A)**. Because the exact composition and delivery system differ between products it may be difficult to draw parallels between them [7] **(IV/C)**.

Fibrin sealant incorporates human donor blood products making its use in elective cosmetic surgical procedures somewhat contentious on accord of a theoretical risk of transmission of hepatitis B and C virus (HBV, HCV), human immuno-deficiency virus (HIV) and human T cell leukaemia/lymphoma virus Type I or II (HTLV). A recent study into the risk of transmission of these infective agents, however, found no cases in over 20,000 blood transfusions [8] **(IIa/B)** and one commercially available fibrin sealant has now been used over 15 million times since 1991 without known transmission of pathogens.

It is possible to extract fibrinogen from the patient's own blood in the pre or peri-operative period. Concentrations of fibrinogen are lower than that produced from pre-prepared non-autologous products. Even commercially available fibrin sealants have been shown to contain basic fibroblast growth factor (bFGF), vascular endothelial growth factor (VEGF), transforming growth factor (TGF-ß1) and epidermal growth factor (EGF). However, if, in particular, platelets are included, the additional presence of growth factors in even higher concentrations (such as platelet-derived growth factor and transforming growth factor) may be beneficial for tissue repair and regeneration. The use of autologous platelet-rich plasma (platelet gel) and autologous platelet-poor plasma has also been advocated [9] (IIb/A) as an alternative to fibrin sealants. Some of these methods rely upon exogenous thrombin that may be of human or bovine origin. Thrombin and calcium chloride are combined with the autologous platelet-poor plasma to form fibrin glue. If larger volumes of this plasma are required it is possible to return the red blood cells to the patient using autologous blood salvage techniques. In the future techniques may become available that are cost-effective in preparing fibrin sealants by autologous plasma donation, carried out in the weeks prior to surgery to yield large volumes of concentrated fibrin sealants. Similarly, techniques using recombinant DNA technology to produce the components of fibrin sealant would avoid all risks associated with blood-derived products.

Evidence for use of fibrin sealants in plastic surgery

Face lifts

Fibrin sealant has been used extensively in face-lift surgery as a sizeable raw surface is created. Several non-randomised [10] (III/B), [11] (IIa/B), and randomised [12] (Ib/A) studies have shown that dressings and drains can be avoided using fibrin sealants and also platelet gel [13] (IIa/B). More recently, work by Marchac with improved levels of evidence has shown that the benefits of using fibrin sealants in face-lift surgery are not as great as previously suggested in reducing ecchymosis and oedema [14] (Ib/A). Other authors have applied the technique to the short scar face lift in large series but without randomisation [15] (III/B), and have also claimed benefits for the use of fibrin sealant in face-lift surgery [16] (Ib/A).

Blepharoplasty

There are two studies demonstrating advantages attributable to the use of fibrin sealant in lower blepharoplasties [17] (IIa/B), [18] (III/B), although in relatively low patient numbers and without randomisation.

Craniofacial surgery

Fibrin sealant has been used extensively in craniofacial surgery, including for tissue adhesion in endoscopic brow lifts [19] (III/B), where it has been shown to be less effective than bone anchored suture techniques in the long term [20] (IIa/B). This perhaps illustrates the predominant sealant rather than adhesive nature of fibrin glue. Sealants have also been used in large non-randomised case studies to seal dural tears, to secure bony fragments and to mix with powdered bone to form autologous bone graft during craniofacial surgery [21, 22] (III/B). The use of fibrin sealant in alveolar bone grafting has been found to significantly reduce bone resorption and improve graft integration and quality [23] (Ib/A).

Seroma formation

Two randomised trials have assessed the potential for fibrin sealant to reduce seroma formation after lymphadenectomy and cosmetic procedures such as abdominoplasty [24, 25] (Ib/A), the former finding no significant difference in seroma formation following lymphadenectomy beyond the first 24 hours but the latter demonstrating a statistically significant reduction in postoperative drainage and seroma formation following abdominoplasty (n=91). These findings have been corroborated in a series of patients undergoing abdominoplasty after massive weight loss [26] (III/B). Studies of fibrin sealant in axillary lymphadenectomy for breast cancer have not shown significant benefit [27] (Ib/A) and a meta-analysis [28] (Ia/A) on seroma formation in breast surgery concludes that the current evidence does not support the use of fibrin sealant following cancer resection to reduce postoperative drainage or seroma formation. However, there is evidence for a reduction in seroma formation following parotid surgery [29] (Ib/A), where it was able to significantly reduce postoperative drainage and seroma formation. Instillation of relatively large volumes of fibrin sealant into postoperative seromas has also been advocated [30] (III/C).

Skin grafting

Fibrin sealant is well suited to securing skin grafts, especially in areas where fixation is difficult; it reduces

Table 1. Level I and II evidence for the use of fibrin sealants.

	Levels	Grade	No studies	Recommendation
Face lift and blepharoplasty	Ib	A	2	+ benefit
	IIa	B	3	+ benefit
	Ib	A	1	No benefit shown
Craniofacial surgery	Ib	A	1	+ benefit
	IIa	B	1	No benefit shown
Prevention of seroma	Ib	A	2	+ benefit
	Ia	A	1	+ benefit
	Ia	A	1	No benefit shown
	Ib	A	1	No benefit shown
Skin grafting	Ib	A	3	+ benefit

seroma and haematoma formation between the graft and the bed due to the haemostatic and adhesive nature of the product. Studies in burns patients have demonstrated both a reduction in the incidence of sub-graft haematoma formation as well as improved graft take [31] **(Ib/A)**. Similarly improved graft take was observed in a series of complex genital reconstruction requiring skin grafting [32] **(III/B)**. The use of fibrin sealant with Integra™ in combination with negative-pressure therapy in the reconstruction of acute and chronic wounds [33] **(Ib/A)** has facilitated improved Integra take and a shorter time to second-stage skin grafting. Fibrin sealant has also been shown to be effective in reducing the blood loss from the donor site following skin grafting in burn patients, due to its haemostatic properties [34] **(Ib/A)**.

Other applications

Fibrin sealants have also been used for the non-suture repair of peripheral nerves; however, there is little clinical evidence to support this in comparison with conventional suture techniques. Animal studies have shown the benefits of fibrin sealant in reducing the number of sutures needed and reducing anastomotic bleeding time [35] **(IIa/B)** at microvascular anastomosis. *In vitro* studies have pointed towards a future use of fibrin products as a delivery system for the release of antibiotics [36] **(IIa/B)** or growth factors to a wound site. This has been exploited in follicular transplantation for male pattern baldness using autologous platelet growth factors [37] **(Ib/A)**.

Conclusions

Fibrin sealants have been shown to be efficacious in a variety of plastic surgical applications, summarised in Table 1. However, the available evidence for the use of fibrin sealants in plastic surgery is complicated by the number of different products available, their composition and mode of application.

For each clinical indication, the cost benefit of its use must be assessed in light of the evidence available.

Recommendations

<table>
<tr><td></td><td>Evidence level</td></tr>
</table>

Recommendations	Evidence level
◆ Fibrin sealant has a role in face lifting in selected patients.	Ib/A & IIa/B
◆ Fibrin sealant has no proven benefit in the reduction of seroma formation following lymphadenectomy.	Ib/A
◆ Fibrin sealant has been demonstrated to assist in stabilising split skin grafts.	Ib/A
◆ Cost-benefit implications for the use of fibrin sealant need to be assessed on an individual basis.	

References

1. Gareis-Helferich E, Decker W, Gross G, Dokter P, Geering H. Bindehautwundverschluss durch fibrinöse Verklebung (Closure of connective tissue wound). *Kiln Monatsbl Augenheilk* 1968; 153: 74-8.

2. Silver FH, Wang MC, Pins GD. Preparation and use of fibrin glue in surgery. *Biomaterials* 1995; 16: 891-903.

3. Spotnitz WD. Fibrin sealant in the United States: clinical use at the University of Virginia. *Thrombosis and Haemostasis* 1995; 74: 482-5.

4. Rousou J, Gonzalez-Lavin L, Cosgrove D, Weldon C, Hess P, Joyce L, *et al*. Randomized clinical trial of fibrin sealant in patients undergoing resternotomy or reoperation after cardiac operations. *J Thorac Cardiovasc Surg* 1989; 97: 194-203.

5. Mouritzen C, Dromer M, Keinecke HO. The effect of fibrin glueing to seal bronchial and alveolar leakages after pulmonary resections and decortications. *Eur J Cardiothorac Surg* 1993; 7: 75-80.

6. Rauws EM, Rutgeerts P, Wara P. Hoos A, Solleder E, Praus M, *et al*. Fibrin sealant (Beriplast R) vs Polidocanol 1% in the endoscopic treatment of bleeding gastroduodenal ulcers. *Endoscopy* 1996; 28: S19.

7. Martinowitz U, Spotnitz WD. Fibrin tissue adhesives. *Thrombosis and Haemostasis* 1997; 78: 661-6.

8. Regan FAM, Hewitt P, Barbara JAJ, Contreras M. Prospective investigation of transfusion transmitted infection in recipients of over 20,000 units of blood. *Br Med J* 2000; 320: 403-6.

9. Man D, Plosker H, Winland-Brown JE. The use of autologous platelet-rich plasma (platelet gel) and autologous platelet-poor plasma (fibrin glue) in cosmetic surgery. *Plast Reconstr Surg* 2001; 107: 229-39.

10. Marchac D, Pugash E, Gault D. The use of sprayed fibrin glue in facelifts. *Eur J Plast Surg* 1987; 10: 139-43.

11. Marchac D, Sandor G. Face lifts and sprayed fibrin glue: an outcome analysis of 200 patients. *Br J Plast Surg* 1994; 47: 306-9.

12. Oliver DW, Hamilton SA, Figle AA, Wood SH, Lamberty BGH. A prospective, randomized, double-blind trial of the use of fibrin sealant for face lifts. *Plast Reconstr Surg* 2001; 108: 2101-5.

13. Brown SA, Appelt EA, Lipschitz A, Sorokin ES, Rohrich RJ. Platelet gel sealant in rhytidectomy. *Plast Reconstr Surg* 2006; 118: 1019-25.

14. Marchac D, Greensmith AL. Early postoperative efficacy of fibrin glue in face lifts: a prospective randomized trial. *Plast Reconstr Surg* 2005; 115: 911-6.

15. Matarasso A, Rizk SS, Markowitz J. Short scar face-lift with the use of fibrin sealant. *Dematol Clin* 2005; 23: 495-504.

16. Fezza JP, Cartwright M, Mack W, Flaharty P. The use of aerosolized fibrin glue in face-lift surgery. *Plast Reconstr Surg* 2002; 110: 658-64.

17. Mommaerts MY, Beirne JC, Jacobs WI, Abeloos JS, De Clercq CA, Neyt LF. Use of fibrin glue in lower blepharoplasties. *J Craniomaxillofac Surg* 1996; 24: 78-82.

18. Mandel MA. Closure of blepharoplasty incisions with autologous fibrin glue. *Arch Ophthalmol* 1990; 108: 842-4.

19. Marchac D, Ascherman J, Arnaud A. Fibrin glue fixation in forehead endoscopy: evaluation of our experience with 206 cases. *Plast Reconstr Surg* 1997; 100: 704-12.

20. Jones BM, Grover R. Endoscopic brow lift: a personal review of 538 patients and comparison of fixation techniques. *Plast Reconstr Surg* 2004; 113: 1242-50.

21. Marchac D, Renier D. Fibrin glue in craniofacial surgery. *J Craniofac Surg* 1990; 11: 32-4.

22. Shaffrey CI, Spontnitz WD, Shaffrey ME, Jane JA. Neurosurgical applications of fibrin glue: augmentation of dural closure in 134 patients. *Neurosurgery* 1990; 26: 207-10.

23. Segura-Castillo JL, Aquirre-Camacho H, Gonzalez-Ojeda A, Michel-Perez J. Reduction of bone resorption by the application of fibrin glue in the reconstruction of the alveolar cleft. *J Craniofac Surg* 2005; 16: 105-12.

24. Oliver DW, Hamilton SA, Figle AA, Wood SH, Lamberty BGH. Can fibrin sealant be used to prevent post-operative drainage? A prospective randomised double blind trial. *Eur J Plast Surg* 2002; 24: 387-90.

25. Cruz-Korchin N, Korchin L. The use of fibrin sealant (Tisseel) in abdominoplasty. *Plast Reconstr Surg* 2005; 116: S23-4.

26. Downey SE. The use of fibrin sealant in prevention of seromas in the massive weight loss patients. *Plast Reconstr Surg* 2005; 116: S223-4.

27. Mustonen PK Harman MA Eskelinen MJ. The effect of fibrin sealant combined with fibrinolysis inhibitor on reducing the amount of lymphatic leakage after axillary evacuation in breast cancer. A prospective randomized clinical trial. *Scand J Surg* 2004; 93: 209-12.

28. Carless PA, Henry DA. Systematic review and meta-analysis of the use of fibrin sealant to prevent seroma formation after breast cancer surgery. *Br J Surg* 2006; 93: 810-9.

29. Mahara JM, Diamond C, Williams D, Seikaly H, Harris J. Tisseel to reduce postparotidectomy wound drainage: randomized, prospective, controlled trial. *J Otolaryngol* 2006; 35: 36-9.

30. Butler CE. Treatment of refractory donor-site seromas with percutaneous instillation of fibrin sealant. *Plast Reconstr Surg* 2006; 117: 976-85.

31. Mittermayer R, Wasserman E, Thurnher M, Simunek M, Redl H. Skin graft fixation by slow clotting fibrin sealant applied as a thin layer. *Burns* 2006; 32: 305-11.

32. Morris MS, Morley AF, Stackhouse DA, Santucci RA. Fibrin sealant as tissue glue: preliminary experience in complex genital reconstructive surgery. *Urology* 2006; 67: 688-91.

33. Jeschke MG Rose C, Angele P, Fuchtmeier B, Nerlich MN, Bolder U. Development of new reconstructive techniques: use of Integra in combination with fibrin glue and negative-pressure therapy for reconstruction of acute and chronic wounds. *Plast Reconstr Surg* 2004; 113: 525-30.

34. Nervi C, Gamelli RL, Greenhalagh DG, Luterman A, Hansbrough JF, Achauer BM, Gomperts ED, Lee M, Navalta L, Cruciani TR. A multicenter clinical trial to evaluate the topical hemostatic efficacy of fibrin sealant in burn patients. *J Burn Care Rehabil* 2001; 22: 99-103.

35. Cho AB, Jnr, Rames M. Effect of fibrin adhesive application in microvascular anastomosis: a comparative experimental study. *Plast Reconstr Surg* 2007; 119: 95-103.

36. Tredwell S, Jackson JK, Hamilton D, Lee V, Burt HM. Use of fibrin sealants for the localized, controlled release of cefazolin. *Can J Surg* 2006; 49: 347-52.

37. Uebel CO, da Silva JB, Cantarelli D, Martins P. The role of plasma growth factors in male pattern baldness surgery. *Plast Reconstr Surg* 2006; 118: 1458-67.

Chapter 28

Ablative and non-ablative techniques for rejuvenation of photo-aged skin

Nick Reynolds FRCS Ed
Specialist Registrar in Plastic Surgery
Kay Thomas MRCGP
Associate Clinical Specialist
John Kenealy FRACS
Consultant Plastic Surgeon

FRENCHAY HOSPITAL, BRISTOL, UK

Introduction

Whilst the aging process is an inescapable consequence of life, the retention of a youthful appearance for as long as possible has been the holy grail for many people. The increasing demand for surgical intervention through various face-lifting techniques has to some extent catered for this market. There are a number of issues with surgical face-lifting procedures, not only the side effects such as pain, infection, bleeding and scarring, but also the limitations, such as the difficulty in tightening the skin of the peri-oral and peri-orbital regions. With the introduction of ablative lasers, such as the CO_2 laser and Erbium YAG laser, it was hoped that some of these issues could be addressed.

Methodology

A Medline search was conducted using key words such as 'CO_2 laser', 'Erbium laser', 'ablative', 'non ablative', 'wrinkle reduction' and 'rhytid reduction'. A search was also made through our archive of the journal *Lasers in Surgery and Medicine* covering the past the past ten years.

Carbon dioxide lasers

The CO_2 laser first entered use in 1964 and has since become a cornerstone of laser therapy for a wide range of dermatological applications. However, the CO_2 laser has only been used in skin rejuvenation procedures since the early 1990s. This was initiated by the development of short pulsed CO_2 lasers and the introduction of the computer pattern generator (CPG), which enabled controlled bursts of laser energy to be given over a comparatively wide field. The CO_2 laser emits an invisible beam in the infrared spectrum at a wavelength of 10,600nm, with its target chromophore being water. The light energy is absorbed by the water in the tissue and the tissue is literally vapourised, leaving a zone of coagulative necrosis and a plume of cellular debris. The effect of this process on the skin is to remove the epidermis and a variable depth of the underlying dermis, usually down to the mid-level of the papillary dermis.

Regeneration of the skin takes place mainly from hair follicles, as well as from other skin appendages such as sweat glands. Remodelling of the dermis occurs at the same time, resulting in new collagen formation. Orringer et al demonstrated that connective tissue remodelling, induced by CO_2 laser resurfacing of photodamaged human skin [1] **(IIb/B)**, results in tightening of the skin.

This efficacy of the CO_2 laser has been corroborated by a number of clinical studies. Fitzpatrick et al [2] **(Ib/A)** assessed both peri-oral and peri-orbital wrinkles using a clinical scoring system for grading wrinkling and photodamage. Patients were observed post-treatment for one to 12 months and adverse events were recorded. The results showed an improvement in wrinkle scores for all types of wrinkling from mild to moderate to severe. Side effects included transient erythema and post-inflammatory hyperpigmentation, and one instance of an isolated hypertrophic scar.

Schwartz et al [3] **(Ib/A)** assessed the long-term efficacy and safety of the CO_2 laser. Facial wrinkles were almost completely ablated at the three and six-month follow-up. Some relapse was seen at one year, but the overall aesthetic result remained very good. Regions with dynamic wrinkles (e.g. the peri-oral region) showed more recurrence. The best and most durable results were seen in the cheeks.

The side effects of the CO_2 laser can be categorised into early, intermediate and late. The potential early side effects are infection, bleeding, pain, oedema and erythema. Infection as a result of the treatment can be severe and it is recommended that all patients are treated with prophylactic antibiotics. The risk of treating patients with a current herpes simplex virus infection as well as a latent infection has also been reported. Pain normally settles within 24 hours of treatment. Erythema can be very obvious and also persistent, sometimes taking several months to settle.

Intermediate complications include hyperpigmentation and hypopigmentation. Both these effects are well recognised, but whereas hyperpigmentation invariably settles with time, hypopigmentation can be persistent and occasionally permanent.

Late complications include scarring and late onset hypopigmentation. Laws [4] **(IV/C)** reported delayed hypopigmentation six months after a full facial CO_2 laser resurfacing procedure for widespread actinic keratoses. Histological examination revealed a normal number of melanocytes but a decrease in epidermal melanin. A similar finding has been reported after phenol chemical peels.

The Schwartz study [3] **(Ib/A)** examined the complications seen in over 200 patients: infection occurred in 13 patients (6%); 45 patients (21%) developed post-procedure hyperpigmentation; hypopigmentation was noted in 17 patients; and two patients (1%) developed postoperative scarring.

Fitzpatrick [2] **(Ib/A)** observed transient erythema and post-inflammatory hyperpigmentation, and one isolated hypertrophic scar in his study.

Nanni and Alster [5] **(IIa/B)** reported the complications that occurred after cutaneous CO_2 laser resurfacing using a retrospective analysis and chart review in 500 consecutive patients. The most common complication observed was postoperative erythema, which occurred in all patients, lasting an average of 4.5 months. Hyperpigmentation was seen in 37% of patients with a higher rate in darker skin phototypes. Acne flares, milia formation, and dermatitis occurred in 10-15% of patients. Postoperative infection with herpes simplex virus (HSV) was observed in 7.4%, regardless of prior HSV history. Hypopigmentation, scarring, and other local or disseminated infections occurred in less than 1%.

Hence, the CO_2 laser has been found to be an effective method of resurfacing but it is not without side effects. While its effectiveness stimulated a rapid uptake of this treatment, enthusiasm waned more as a result of prolonged recovery times, than a fear of side effects, as other laser and non-laser systems were aggressively marketed as showing equivalent results without the 'downtime'.

Erbium YAG laser

The Erbium laser has been marketed as an alternative to the CO_2 laser. The Erbium YAG laser uses a yttrium aluminium garnet crystal doped with the element Erbium. This produces upon excitation a laser beam of 2094nm, compared with a wavelength of 10,600nm for the CO_2 laser. At this wavelength the target chromophore, which as with the CO_2 laser is water, is up to 16 times more light-sensitive than at 10,600nm. The CO_2 laser is a photothermal laser with a marked coagulative effect. The Erbium laser is a photomechanical laser and for this reason has a very limited coagulative effect on the target tissue. Because the beam produced has such a strong affinity for its target chromophore, it only penetrates a short distance into the skin before its energy is fully absorbed. The water is rapidly converted to steam and expands, literally causing a micro-explosion in the target tissue. In doing so, a stream of tissue debris is ejected at rapid velocity with a resultant audible 'pop'. The ejected fragments carry most of the energy away with them so there is little heat energy remaining *in situ* to bring about a coagulative effect as occurs with the CO_2 laser. Because of these differences the Erbium laser will penetrate less deeply into the target tissue, producing only a shallow zone of ablation with minimal thermal injury.

The Erbium YAG laser is widely used in cosmetic resurfacing. However, in use on healthy tissue, once one passes beyond the papillary dermis there is profuse punctate bleeding, which hampers visibility, and reduces further absorption by the tissue. Consequently, this laser has been confined to roles where more precise and often localised resurfacing is required. There is a marked plume associated with this laser and it must be used in conjunction with a smoke extraction device.

A number of trials have reported the efficacy of the Er:YAG laser system in resurfacing. Teikemeier and Goldberg conducted a study on 20 patients with peri-oral, peri-orbital, and forehead wrinkles who were treated with the Er:YAG laser [6] **(Ib/A)**. Patients were evaluated at two days, one month, and two months for erythema, time of healing, degree of improvement, and pigment changes. All 20 patients showed improvement of their wrinkles, but the two-month follow-up period was probably not long enough for treatment oedema to subside and the true effect of treatment to be evident.

Perez [7] **(IIa/B)** evaluated the Er:YAG laser treatment of wrinkles clinically and histologically. The study involved 15 patients. Peri-oral, peri-orbital, and total face wrinkles were treated. After treatment, patients were evaluated daily for seven days and weekly for two months for erythema, healing time, improvement, and pigment changes. All patients showed some degree of improvement of their wrinkles. Histological examination showed tissue ablation down to the level of the granular layer after one pass; to the basal cell layer after two passes; to the papillary dermis after three to four passes; and deeper into the papillary and superficial reticular dermis after five to six passes.

Not surprisingly the Er:YAG laser has been the subject of comparative studies with the CO_2 laser (Figure 1). Ross compared one-pass CO_2 versus

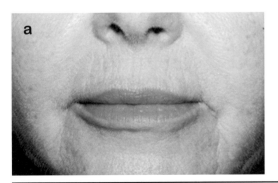
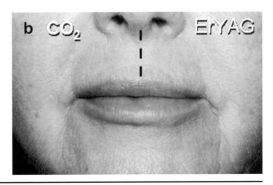

Figure 1. CO_2 and Er:YAG laser treatment of peri-oral wrinkles. a) Pre-treatment. b) Two months post-treatment. *Reproduced with permission from Cynosure Inc.*

multiple-pass Er:YAG laser resurfacing in the treatment of wrinkles [8] **(Ib/A)**. Thirteen patients with facial wrinkles underwent a side-by-side comparison using peri-orbital and peri-oral regions as treatment sites. One side was treated with a pulsed CO_2 laser and the other with an Er:YAG laser. Post-auricular skin was treated in an identical fashion to the study sites and biopsied for microscopic analysis. Their results showed no statistically significant differences between the lasers with respect to hyperpigmentation and wrinkle reduction. There was less erythema at the CO_2 laser-treated sites two weeks after treatment, but the differences had resolved by six weeks after treatment. Histological examination demonstrated equivalent dermal thermal injury on immediate postoperative biopsies and equivalent fibroplasia on subsequent biopsies. Both CO_2 and Er:YAG laser-treated sites showed overall modest wrinkle improvement compared with the pre-treatment photographs. Their conclusion was that CO_2 and Er:YAG lasers provides equivalent healing and cosmetic improvement, when used in a way that yields equivalent immediate postoperative histological results.

A randomised prospective study by Newman et al [9] **(Ib/A)** looked at the clinical effects on upper lip wrinkles of a variable pulse Er:YAG laser compared with pulsed CO_2 laser resurfacing. Twenty-one patients were treated and the results proved the Er:YAG laser to be just as safe and effective as a resurfacing tool.

The side effect profile of the Er:YAG laser is similar to that of the CO_2 laser, as shown in a study by Tanzi and Alster [10] **(IIa/A)**. This evaluated postoperative wound healing and short- and long-term side effects of single-pass CO_2 and multiple-pass, long-pulsed Er:YAG laser skin resurfacing for the treatment of facial photodamage and atrophic scars. The average time to re-epithelialisation was 5.5 days with the CO_2 laser and 5.1 days with the Erbium laser. All patients experienced postoperative erythema, lasting an average of 4.5 weeks after single-pass CO_2 laser treatment and 3.6 weeks after multiple-pass long-pulsed Er:YAG laser treatment. Hyperpigmentation was seen in 46% of patients treated with the CO_2 laser and 42% of the patients treated with the long-pulsed Er:YAG laser, but this settled within three months. There were no reports of hypopigmentation or scarring.

Non-ablative resurfacing with lasers and other light systems

The issue of side effects and subsequent downtime for the patient following treatment with ablative resurfacing has led to the development of non-ablative laser treatments. Several different lasers have been used along with non-laser intense pulsed light treatments.

Pulsed dye laser

The pulsed dye laser generally works at wavelengths between 570 and 590nm. At this range it is an effective vascular laser and is able to selectively heat haemoglobin within the dermal plexus. The basis of pulsed dye laser wrinkle reduction lies in the photothermal induction of pro-collagen III expression resulting in subsequent collagen remodelling [11] **(IIb/B)**. Anderson and Parrish's principle of selective photothermolysis [12] **(IIb/B)** shows that this is achieved through the heating of the subdermal plexus. A paper by Bjerring [13] **(IIb/B)** points out that the pulsed dye laser is selectively targeting the subdermal plexus using oxyhaemoglobin and, to a lesser extent, deoxyhaemoglobin, as its target chromophores. By selectively heating but not disrupting the subdermal plexus, there is induction of the procollagen and hence collagen remodelling. Some studies have shown little or no improvement after treatment [14] **(IIa/B)**. Nevertheless, there is enough evidence to suggest that it can work in selected patients [13, 15-19] **(IIa/B)**. Zelickson [16] **(IIa/B)** et al showed in 1999 that new collagen formation occurred 12 weeks post-treatment with a 585nm pulsed dye laser using a pulse width of 0.45ms and fluences of up to 6.5J/cm². Bjerring [13] **(IIa/B)** demonstrated an increase in procollagen type III, using sub-purpuric thresholds and Omi et al [20] also detected new collagen formation, again at low fluences. Omi states: "new collagen formation was readily observed within four weeks of the laser therapy. Clinically, wrinkle improvement is also observed from four weeks after the therapy."

Sadick [11] **(IIa/B)**, however, argues that improvement in the appearance of wrinkles may not occur for up to 18 months post-treatment.

In our own randomised controlled clinical trial [21] **(Ib/A)**, 26 volunteers (25 female and one male) received one treatment to the peri-orbital wrinkles around one eye, using the other as the control. They were then observed at three and six months post-treatment. They then received three treatments spaced four weeks apart and were again observed at three and six months. At the end of the trial a panel of three blinded assessors scored photographs of the subjects independently using the Fitzpatrick wrinkle scoring system. All data were subjected to statistical analysis using non-parametric t-tests. The results revealed no significant differences in the wrinkle scores of the patients upon completion of the trial protocols.

Nd:YAG and KTP lasers

The long-pulsed Nd:YAG laser uses a neodymium yttrium aluminum garnet crystal to produce laser light at a wavelength of 1064nm. The KTP laser uses a potassium titanyl phosphate crystal to produce light at 532nm. This is achieved by employing the crystal as a frequency doubler with the Nd:YAG crystal, thus halving the wavelength to 532nm. It is for this reason that a number of trials tend to compare these lasers side by side.

In a paper titled "Combination 532nm and 1064nm lasers for non-invasive skin rejuvenation and toning" [22] **(IIa/B)**, Lee employed a long-pulsed, 532nm potassium titanyl phosphate (KTP) laser and a long-pulsed 1064nm Nd:YAG laser, both separately and combined, in a prospective non-randomised study. A total of 150 patients were treated. All subjects were treated at least three times and at most six times, at monthly intervals, and were observed for up to 18 months after the last treatment. All 150 patients were reported to have exhibited mild to moderate improvement in the appearance of wrinkles, moderate improvement in skin toning and texture, and great improvement in the reduction of redness and pigmentation. The KTP laser used alone produced results superior to those of the Nd:YAG laser. Results from combination treatment with both KTP and Nd:YAG lasers were slightly superior to those achieved with either laser alone.

Another study by Tan et al [23] **(IIa/B)** assessed patients who underwent two treatments with the 532nm laser to one side of the face and with both lasers to the other side, followed by three treatments with the 1,064nm laser to both sides. The patients were evaluated before, during, and up to four months after treatment. The author's conclusions were simply that the 532nm KTP and 1,064nm Nd:YAG lasers can be effectively and safely used for non-invasive skin rejuvenation.

The effectiveness of the Nd:YAG laser was further assessed by Trelles et al [24] **(IIa/B)**. This study used the long-pulsed Nd:YAG laser in the non-ablative treatment of peri-ocular and peri-oral wrinkles. Ten patients with facial wrinkles were treated with the long-pulsed 1064nm Nd:YAG laser. All patients had a total of three treatments, once every two weeks. Improvements in the appearance of wrinkles was noted. The greatest level of effect was seen two months after the final treatment and effects were still visible at the six-month period, but showed a tendency to decrease.

Woo and Handley compared the pulsed dye and Nd:YAG lasers [25] **(IIa/B)**. In their study, seven subjects had one side of their peri-orbital wrinkles treated with pulsed dye laser. The second part of the study involved using the long-pulsed Nd:YAG laser 532nm to treat the contralateral wrinkles in five subjects. Pre-treatment and post-treatment photographs were taken and blinded assessors were asked to choose the better of the two unlabelled photographs. Neither the pulsed dye laser nor the long-pulsed Nd:YAG laser appeared to produce any improvement in moderate to severe facial wrinkles. The difficulty with this study was that it did not evaluate the 1064nm wavelength and so it is not directly comparable with other papers mentioned.

Diode lasers

These lasers emit infrared light at 1450nm using solid state diodes. Not surprisingly they have also been evaluated in the non-ablative treatment of wrinkles. The results have been varied.

Chapter 28

all degrees of wrinkling, be they mild, moderate or severe. As a trade off these ablative devices also have the greatest side effect profile, but low long-term complication rates.

Some studies have shown that non-ablative devices are effective in treating mild to moderate wrinkles, but not consistently in all patients, and the results have not always been reproducible by other practitioners. Much of the observed effects may be due to tissue oedema and hence are not long-lasting. Many studies are compromised by short follow-up.

Dermal remodelling and new collagen formation following ablative resurfacing is similar to that which occurs in the formation of scar tissue. It may, therefore, be the case, that dermal scarring and subsequent contracture are key to later rejuvenation. Paradoxically, non-ablative systems, which heat the deeper dermis, if effective, may cause more widespread dermal fibrosis than ablative systems. The long-term consequence of this is yet to be seen.

Recommendations	Evidence level
◆ CO_2 and Erbium YAG lasers are effective in improving the appearance of facial wrinkling.	Ib/A
◆ The side effect profile of these two systems is both well understood and well documented.	Ib/A
◆ There is sufficient evidence to suggest that non-ablative systems and, in particular, pulsed dye laser systems may have little or no long-term benefits in improving the appearance of wrinkles.	Ib/A
◆ The side effect profile of these systems, however, is relatively low.	Ib/B
◆ Currently, there are no sufficient robust data to suggest that radiofrequency sytems have any effect on improving the appearance of facial wrinkles.	IIb/B
◆ Based on the above evidence the only reliable systems currently on the market are the ablative CO_2 and Er YAG lasers.	Ib/A

References

1. Orringer JS, Kang S, Johnson TM, Karimipour DJ, Hamilton T, Hammerberg C, Voorhees JJ, Fisher GJ. Connective tissue remodeling induced by carbon dioxide laser resurfacing of photodamaged human skin. *Arch Dermatol* 2004; 140(11): 1326-32.

2. Fitzpatrick RE, Goldman MP, Satur NM, Tope WD. Pulsed carbon dioxide laser resurfacing of photo-aged facial skin. *Arch Dermatol* 1996; 132(4): 395-402.

3. Schwartz RJ, Burns AJ, Rohrich RJ, Barton FE Jr, Byrd HS. Long-term assessment of CO_2 facial laser resurfacing: aesthetic results and complications. *Plast Reconstr Surg* 1999; 103(2): 592-601.

4. Laws RA, Finley EM, McCollough ML, Grabski WJ. Alabaster skin after carbon dioxide laser resurfacing with histologic correlation. *Dermatol Surg* 1998; 24(6): 633-6.

5. Nanni C, Alster TS. Complications of carbon dioxide laser resurfacing. An evaluation of 500 patients. *Dermatol Surg* 1998; 24(6): 633-6.

6. Teikemeier G, Goldberg DJ. Skin resurfacing with the erbium: YAG laser. *Dermatol Surg* 1997; 23(8): 685-7.

7. Perez MI, Bank DE, Silvers D. Skin resurfacing of the face with the Erbium:YAG laser. *Dermatol Surg* 1998; 24(6): 653-8; discussion 658-9.

8. Ross EV, Miller C, Meehan K, McKinlay J, Sajben P, Trafeli JP, Barnette DJ. One-pass CO_2 versus multiple-pass Er:YAG laser resurfacing in the treatment of rhytides: a comparison side-by-side study of pulsed CO_2 and Er:YAG lasers. *Dermatol Surg* 2001; 27(8): 709-15.

9. Newman JB, Lord JL, Ash K, McDaniel DH. Variable pulse erbium:YAG laser skin resurfacing of perioral rhytides and side-by-side comparison with carbon dioxide laser. *Lasers Surg Med* 2000; 26(2): 208-14.

10. Tanzi EL, Alster TS. Single-pass carbon dioxide versus multiple-pass Er:YAG laser skin resurfacing: a comparison of postoperative wound healing and side-effect rates. *Dermatol Surg* 2003; 29(1): 80-4.

11. Sadick NS. Update on non-ablative light therapy for rejuvenation: a review. *Lasers Surg Med* 2003; 32: 120-8.

12. Anderson RR, Parrish JA. Microvasculature can be selectively damaged using dye lasers: a basic theory and experimental evidence in human skin. *Lasers Surg Med* 1981; 1: 263-76.

13. Bjerring P, Clement M, Heickendorff L. Egevist H, Kiernan M. Selective non-ablative wrinkle reduction by laser. *Jr Cutaneous Laser Therapy* 2000; 2: 9-15.

14. Menaker G, Wrone D, Williams R, Moy R. Treatment of facial rhytids with a non-ablative laser: a clinical and histological study. *Dermatol Surg* 1999; 25: 440-4.

15. Fitzpatrick R, Goldman M, Satur N, Tope W. Pulsed carbon dioxide laser resurfacing of photoaged facial skin. *Arch Dermatol* 1996; 132: 395-402.

16. Zelickson B, Kilmer S, Bernstein E, Chotzen V, Dock J, Mehregan D, Coles C. Pulsed dye laser therapy for sun damaged skin. *Lasers Surg Med* 1999; 25: 229-36.

17. Goldberg D. Non-ablative subsurface remodelling: clinical and histologic evaluation of a 1320nm Nd:YAG laser. *Jr Cutaneous Laser Therapy* 1999; 1: 153-7.

18. Goldberg D. Cutler K. Non-ablative treatment of rhytids with intense pulsed light. *Lasers Surg Med* 2000; 26: 196-200.

19. Goldberg D, Metzler C. Skin resurfacing utilising a low fluence Nd:YAG laser. *Jr Cutaneous Laser Therapy* 1999; 1: 23-7.

20. Omi T, Kawana S, Sato S, Honda M. Ultrastructural changes elicited by a non-ablative wrinkle reduction laser. *Lasers Surg Med* 2003; 32: 46-9.

21. Reynolds N, Thomas K, Baker L, Adams C, Kenealy J. Pulsed dye laser and non-ablative wrinkle reduction. *Lasers Surg Med* 2004; 34(2): 109-13.

22. Lee MW. Combination 532-nm and 1064-nm lasers for noninvasive skin rejuvenation and toning. *Arch Dermatol* 2003; 139(10): 1265-76. Erratum in: *Arch Dermatol* 2004; 140(5): 625.

23. Tan MH, Dover JS, Hsu TS, Arndt KA, Stewart B. Clinical evaluation of enhanced nonablative skin rejuvenation using a combination of a 532 and a 1,064nm laser. *Lasers Surg Med* 2004; 34(5): 439-45.

24. Trelles MA, Alvarez X, Martin-Vazquez MJ, Trelles O, Velez M, Levy JL, Allones I. Assessment of the efficacy of nonablative long-pulsed 1064-nm Nd:YAG laser treatment of wrinkles compared at 2, 4, and 6 months. *Facial Plast Surg* 2005; 21(2): 145-53.

25. Woo WK, Handley JM. A pilot study on the treatment of facial rhytids using nonablative 585-nm pulsed dye and 532-nm Nd:YAG lasers. *Dermatol Surg* 2003; 29(12): 1192-5; discussion 1195.

26. Hohenleutner S, Koellner K, Lorenz S, Landthaler M, Hohenleutner U. Results of nonablative wrinkle reduction with a 1,450-nm diode laser: difficulties in the assessment of 'subtle changes'. *Lasers Surg Med* 2005; 37(1): 14-8.

27. Goldberg DJ, Rogachefsky AS, Silapunt S. Non-ablative laser treatment of facial rhytides: a comparison of 1450-nm diode laser treatment with dynamic cooling as opposed to treatment with dynamic cooling alone. *Lasers Surg Med* 2002; 30(2): 79-81.

28. Tanzi EL, Williams CM, Alster TS. Treatment of facial rhytides with a nonablative 1,450-nm diode laser: a controlled clinical and histologic study. *Dermatol Surg* 2003; 29(2): 124-8.

29. Kopera D, Smolle J, Kaddu S, Kerl H. Nonablative laser treatment of wrinkles: meeting the objective? Assessment by 25 dermatologists. *Br J Dermatol* 2004; 150(5): 936-9.

30. Raulin C, Greve B, Grema H. IPL technology: a review. *Lasers Surg Med* 2003; 32: 78-87.

31. Katugampola GA, Lanigan SW. Five years experience of treating port wine stains with the flashlamp pumped pulsed dye laser. *Br J Dermatol* 1997; 137: 750-4.

32. Bitter PH. Noninvasive rejuvenation of photodamaged skin using serial, full-face intense pulsed light treatments. *Dermatol Surg* 2000; 26(9): 835-42; discussion 843.

33. Kligman DE, Zhen Y. Intense pulsed light treatment of photoaged facial skin. *Dermatol Surg* 2004; 30(8): 1085-90.

34. Hedelund L, Due E, Bjerring P, Wulf HC, Haedersdal M. Skin rejuvenation using intense pulsed light: a randomized controlled split-face trial with blinded response evaluation. *Arch Dermatol* 2006; 142(8): 985-90.

35. Hammes S, Greve B, Raulin C. Electro-optical synergy (ELOS) technology for nonablative skin rejuvenation: a preliminary prospective study. *J Eur Acad Dermatol Venereol* 2006; 20(9): 1070-5.

36. Fitzpatrick R, Geronemus R, Goldberg D, Kaminer M, Kilmer S, Ruiz-Esparza J. Multicenter study of noninvasive radiofrequency for periorbital tissue tightening. *Lasers Surg Med* 2003; 33(4): 232-42.

37. Weiss RA, Weiss MA, Munavalli G, Beasley KL. Monopolar radiofrequency facial tightening: a retrospective analysis of efficacy and safety in over 600 treatments. *J Drugs Dermatol* 2006; 5(8): 707-12.

Chapter 28

Chapter 29

Hand and facial composite tissue allotransplantation

Iain S Whitaker BA (Hons) MA MB BChir MRCS
Research Fellow, Plastic Surgery
John H Barker MD PhD
Professor of Surgery

Plastic Surgery Research Laboratory
University of Louisville, Kentucky, USA

Introduction

Composite tissue allotransplantation of hand and facial tissues is now a clinical reality. To date, 20 individuals have received seven double hand, 12 single hand and one thumb transplant worldwide. Several of these cases are more than eight years post-transplant and only two graft failures have been reported, one due to non-compliance [1] and the other, due to unclear aetiology [2, 3] (Table 1). Overall, the functional outcomes and patient satisfaction have been reported to be good [2, 3]. In addition, four cases of head and neck allotransplantation have been reported, two in China [4, 5] and two in France [6, 7].

The microsurgical techniques required to successfully transplant hand and facial tissues are well established and are used in daily practice by the plastic surgery community worldwide. In composite tissue allotransplantation (CTA), however, the immunological principles of graft rejection and failure, as well as the mechanism of action, routine regimens, dosages and toxicities of the drugs used to manipulate the immune system, are far removed from the knowledge base of the general plastic surgeon. In order to give patients the possibility of this new treatment option, it is important that plastic surgeons have a working knowledge of the relevant scientific and technical principles. In this chapter, we provide the reader with a very brief history of CTA, the hand and facial CTAs performed to date with medium and short-term results, the 'real risks' associated with immunotherapy and the 'risk acceptances' of different groups of individuals. A time-line with the history of CTA, and a complete listing of hand and face transplants performed to date are also provided. It is important to note that the complex psychosocial and ethical issues associated with these new procedures are being developed as new clinical cases are being performed and followed up.

Methodology

Sources for this chapter include a comprehensive literature search using the PubMed and EMBASE databases, along with personal experiences of composite tissue allotransplantion and personal communication with pioneers in the field.

Table 1. Chronology of human allotransplantation.

Type of CTA	Date performed	Location	Institution	Recipient age & gender	Immunotherapy	Graft survival	Patient survival	Acute rejection	Chronic rejection
				HAND TRANSPLANTS					
Single hand transplant	Feb-1963	Guayaquil, Ecuador	(*)	28 y/o male	Cortisone /6-mercaptopurine/ azathioprine (AZA) & hydrocortisone	(-) Rejection & removal 3 wks post-transplant; due to insufficient immunosuppression	(+)	(+)	(-)
Single hand transplant	Sep-1998	Lyon, France	Hopital Edouard Herriot	48 y/o male	FK506/MMF/ Prednisone	(-) Rejection & removal of hand 2yrs 4mo post-transplant; due to non-compliance	(+)	(+)	(+)
Single hand transplant	Jan-1999	Louisville, USA	Jewish Hospital	37 y/o male	FK506/MMF/ Prednisone	(+)	(+)	(+)	(-)
Single hand transplant	Sep-1999	Guangzhou, China	Nanfang Hospital	39 y/o male	FK506/MMF/ Prednisone	(-) Rejection & removal of hand 1yr 8mo post-transplant; Unknown cause	(+)	(+)	(-)
Single hand transplant	Jan-2000	Guangxi, China	1st Affiliated Hospital, Guangxi Univ.	27 y/o male	FK506/MMF/ Prednisone	(+)	(+)	(*)	(-)
Double hand transplant	Jan-2000	Lyon, France	Hopital Edouard Herriot	33 y/o male	FK506/MMF/ Prednisone	(+)	(+)	(+)	(-)
Digital transplant	Jan-2000	Yantai, China	Shandong Provincial Hospital	18 y/o male	(*)	(+)	(+)	(*)	(-)
Double hand transplant	Mar-2000	Innsbruch, Austria	Universitats klinik fur Chirurgie	45 y/o male	(*)	(+)	(+)	(+)	(-)
Single hand transplant	May-2000	Kuala-Lumpur Malaysia	Selayang Hospital	1 m/o female	None (identical twin)	(+)	(+)	(-)	(-)
Double hand transplant	Sep-2000	Guangzhou, China	Nanfang Hospital	(*)	(*)	(+)	(+)	(*)	(-)
Single hand transplant	Oct-2000	Milano, Italy	Milano-Bicocca University	35 y/o male	(*)	(+)	(+)	(+)	(-)

Table 1. Chronology of human allotransplantation *continued*.

Type of CTA	Date performed	Location	Institution	Recipient age & gender	Immunotherapy	Graft survival	Patient survival	Acute rejection	Chronic rejection
Double hand transplant	Jan-2001	Harbin, China	1st Affiliated Hospital, Harbin Medical Univ.	(*)	(*)	(+)	(+)	(*)	(-)
Single hand transplant	Feb-2001	Louisville, USA	Jewish Hospital	36 y/o male	FK506/MMF/ Prednisone	(+)	(+)	(+)	(-)
Single hand transplant	Oct-2001	Milano, Italy	Milano-Bicocca University	(*)	FK506/MMF/ Prednisone	(+)	(+)	(*)	(-)
Single hand transplant	Jun-2002	Brussels, Belgium	Erasme Univ. Hospital	(*)	(*)	(+)	(+)	(*)	(-)
Single hand transplant	Nov-2002	Milan, Italy	Milano-Bicocca University	(*)	FK506/MMF/ Prednisone	(+)	(+)	(*)	(-)
Double hand transplant	Feb-2003	Innsbruch, Austria	Universitats- klinik fur Chirurgie	(*)	(*)	(+)	(+)	(*)	(-)
Double hand transplant	May-2003	Lyon, France	Hopital Edouard Herriot	(*)	FK506/MMF/ Prednisone	(+)	(+)	(*)	(-)
Single hand transplant	Nov-2006	Louisville, USA	Jewish Hospital	58 y/o male	FK506/MMF/ Prednisone	(+)	(+)	(*)	(-)
Double hand transplant	Nov-2006	Valencia, Spain	Hospital La Fe	47 y/o female	FK506/MMF/ Prednisone	(+)	(+)	(*)	(-)

FACIAL TISSUE TRANSPLANTS

Type of CTA	Date performed	Location	Institution	Recipient age & gender	Immunotherapy	Graft survival	Patient survival	Acute rejection	Chronic rejection
Cephalo- cervical skin flap & 2 ears	Sep-2003	Nanjing, China	Jinling Hospital	72 y/o female	FK506/MMF/ Prednisone/Zenapax	(+)	(+)	(-)	(-)
Face transplant	Nov-2005	Amiens, France	Hopital Edouard Herriot	38 y/o female	FK506/MMF/ Prednisone	(+)	(+)	(+)	(-)
Face transplant	Apr-2006	Xi'an, China	Xijing Hospital	30 y/o male	FK506/MMF/ Prednisone	(+)	(+)	(*)	(-)
Face transplant	Jan-2007	Paris France	Henri-Mondor Hospital	29 y/o male	FK506/MMF/ Prednisone	(+)	(+)	(*)	(-)

*Data unavailable

Chapter 29

The history of hand and facial composite tissue allotransplantation

"The more sand that has escaped from the hourglass of our life, the clearer we should see through it." (Table 1) [8]

Jean Paul

Hand transplantation

In November 1997, the 1st International Symposium on CTA was held in Louisville, Kentucky, to discuss "the barriers standing in the way of performing human hand transplants". The meeting brought together leading experts in the fields of reconstructive surgery, transplant immunology, and medical ethics. The two days of discussions focused primarily on immunological and ethical barriers and while many opinions were aired, the overall consensus of those present at the meeting was that sufficient research had been done and the time had come to move hand transplantation research into the clinical arena.

The same year, at the Plastic Surgery Research Laboratory at the University of Louisville, animal experiments showed that the immunosuppressive regimen (tacrolimus/MMF/corticosteroid) effectively suppressed CTA 'skin' rejection for the duration of the experiment with relatively low toxicity. Based on these findings the University of Louisville team immediately applied to the hospital's institutional review board for approval to perform ten human hand transplants and at the same time presented their findings at an international hand surgery meeting in Vancouver, subsequently published in a landmark paper [9].

Based on these results, between 1998 and 1999, teams in Lyon (France) [10, 11], Louisville (USA) [9] and Guangzhou (China) performed the first successful human hand transplants using a tacrolimus/MMF and corticosteroid combination therapy [12]. At the time of writing this chapter, 20 individuals have received seven double hand, 12 single hand and one thumb transplant worldwide. Seven of these are more than eight years post-transplant and only two graft failures have been reported, one due to non-compliance [1] and the other

performed in China, due to unclear aetiology [3]. Overall, the functional outcomes and patient satisfaction have been reported to be good [3] **(IIb/B)** (see Table 1).

Face transplantation

To date, four cases of head and neck allotransplantation have been reported, two in China [4, 5] and two in France [6, 7] (Table 1). Facial transplantation has captured the interest and imagination of the media, scientists, and the lay public. Our face is much more than the anatomical location where our olfactory, auditory and visual organs are situated. We use facial expressions to communicate with the world around us and our face is the window through which others see and come to know us. It is this great importance we attach to our face that makes facial disfigurement such a devastating condition. Perception of the face dominates peoples' views of disfigured individuals, and their facial appearance becomes their defining feature. Stevenage and McKay found in their research that job recruiters had a negative perception of facially disfigured applicants, which was associated with an adverse bias of work-related skills [13]. Facially disfigured individuals are frequently reclusive, hiding from social relationships that others take for granted. Of all the physical handicaps, none is as socially devastating as facial disfigurement. In a large number of cases, facial disfigurement leads to depression, social isolation, and increased risk of suicide [14, 15].

The first suggestion to the public that face transplantation was actually being considered as a clinical possibility in the UK stemmed from a presentation made by surgeons at London's Royal Free Hospital in the UK, at the December 2002 meeting of the British Association of Plastic Surgeons [16]. Members of the media were in attendance, reporting on the event, and began to speculate that a face transplant was indeed a clinical reality and this sparked media frenzy. This frenzy reached its height in Britain in December 2002 when the media singled out a young lady with facial disfigurement and reported that she had been selected as the first face transplant recipient [17]. In response to this, the Royal College of Surgeons (RCS) formed a "Working Party on Facial Transplantation" consisting of experts in the fields of ethics, reconstructive surgery, psychology and transplantation to assess the current scientific merits of face transplantation. Sir Peter Morris, the Head of the RCS and Chair of the Working Party recommended "...that until there is further research and the prospect of better control of complications it would be unwise to proceed with human facial transplantation" [18]. The report ended welcoming comments on their findings. In response to the RCS report, the University of Louisville team, who presented their position at the Public Debate at the London Museum, published their response. They concluded that "the major technical, immunological and ethical barriers standing in the way of performing human facial transplantation have been overcome" and that "in a select population of severely disfigured individuals, facial transplantation, despite its recognised risks, could provide a better treatment option than current methods" and thus "should move into its clinical research phase" [19]. Immediately following this, the same team in Louisville published their ethical guidelines for performing facial transplantation in the *American Journal of Bioethics* [19]. A key component of this set of ethical guidelines was "Open Display and Public and Professional Discussion and Evaluation", and opinions were invited from several related fields, including the surgical teams in the UK, France and the Cleveland Clinic in the US. Fifteen commentaries [20-34] were published alongside the Louisville teams' ethical guidelines and their response to the commentaries [35].

In 2004, in preparation to perform clinical face transplants, a team in Paris, France, led by Professor Laurent Lantieri submitted a proposal to the French government's advisory council on bioethics (Comité Consultatif National d'Ethique; CCNE). The Council responded in a report entitled "Composite tissue allotransplantation (CTA) of the face; full or partial facial transplant". The report concluded that while it was not 'ethical' to perform a full face transplant at the time, a partial face transplant (a triangle-shaped part of the face including the nose and mouth) could be performed [36].

Later, in October 2005, an institutional review board at the Cleveland Clinic in Cleveland, USA, approved a proposal submitted by a team at their hospital, led by Dr. Maria Siemionow, to proceed with human face transplants [37], at which time the team began to screen potential patients. Also in 2005, in the US, the American Society for Plastic Surgery (ASPS) and the American Society of Reconstructive Microsurgery (ASRM) issued their 'guiding principles' recommending "that due to the unknown risks and benefits, those involved in this important work move forward in incremental steps" [38, 39].

In November, 2005, in Amiens, France, a surgical team led by Dr. Bernard Devauchelle and Jean-Michel Dubernard announced that they had performed a partial face transplant on a 38-year-old female, whose face had been disfigured by a dog bite (Table 1). The surgery involved transplanting a triangular graft of tissue extending from the nose to the chin including the lips. Initial reports indicate that the recipient is doing well and both the medical community and the lay public have reacted favourably to the procedure [40, 41] **(IV/C)**. Immediately following this, an ethics committee in the UK granted permission to the Royal Free Hospital in London to perform a facial transplant [37].

In April 2006, a team in Xi'an, capital of Shaanxi Province in northwest China, performed a face transplant on a 30-year-old male with facial disfigurement resulting from a bear bite. Initial reports indicate that the patient is doing well [42] **(IV/C)**.

Risk acceptance

To investigate risk versus benefit issues in CTA, the University of Louisville gathered a multi-disciplinary team, led by the senior author, including respected scientists and clinicians in the fields of psychology (body image), psychiatry, bioethics, sociology and plastic, head and neck, ophthalmologic and transplant surgery. This team expanded the risk versus benefit research they had begun with hand transplantation [43] to questions relevant to face transplantation. A questionnaire-based instrument (Louisville Instrument for Transplantation; LIFT) was developed and validated [44] to assess the amount of risk individuals would be willing to accept to receive different types of non-life-saving transplant procedures (foot, single and double hand, larynx, hemi- and full-face CTAs and kidney transplants). Using the LIFT they questioned over 300 individuals with real life experiences in the risks of immunosuppression (kidney transplant recipients) [45] and individuals who could benefit from one of these procedures (limb amputees [46], laryngectomy patients [47]), and individuals who had suffered facial disfigurement [48]. Of all those questioned in this series of studies, regardless of their individual life experience, there was unanimous acceptance of the risks involved to receive a face transplant **(IIb/B)**. Of particular interest was the fact that they would risk even more to receive a face than a kidney transplant which is considered standard care and for which there is no risk versus benefit debate. It was based on these findings that the University of Louisville team considered that the time had come to move facial transplantation research into a clinical phase [19, 49].

Real risks of immunosuppression

Critics of CTA contend that the risks posed by life-long immunosuppression required to prevent rejection do not justify the benefits of this novel treatment. Their argument is based mainly on the Royal College of Surgeons' Report on facial transplantation in 2003 [18], which states that the risk of graft loss is 10% from acute rejection in the first year, the risk of chronic rejection is around 30-50% of patients in the first 2-5 years, and the risks of drug toxicity are hypertension, renal toxicity, diabetes, dyslipidaemia, infection, non-compliance and malignancy.

Although there are undeniable risks of life-long immunosuppression, these particular estimates are inaccurate and misleading, as these data are derived from solid organ transplant studies, often employing drugs other than those used in face/hand transplantation (tacrolimus/mycophenolate mofetil/corticosteroids). In addition to this, there is also a substantial difference between the initial health status of face versus solid organ transplant recipients. Combine this with the composition, function and antigenicity of facial tissue being highly distinct from solid organs, and the 'real risks' are arguably very different.

When the clinical data from studies of human hand transplants using tacrolimus/mycophenolate mofetil/

corticosteroids (>43-month follow-up), with comparable health status, tissue composition and antigenicity are considered, we find human hand transplant studies report a 0% graft loss at one year [2, 3] **(IIb/B)** and a chronic rejection rate of 0% at two years [2, 3] **(IIb/B)**. The studies report non-compliance, acute rejection episodes (treated) and infection up to 43 months post-transplant, but as yet we have not seen other systemic toxic effects or malignancies [2, 3] **(IIb/B)**.

The low incidence of graft loss observed in human hand transplants is possibly due to the early detection of acute rejection episodes and early treatment. The low incidence of chronic rejection could be explained by the relatively short-term follow-up (43 months) in addition to early detection and treatment of acute rejection episodes. The low incidence (in the medium term) of drug toxicity in human hand transplants is perhaps due to the stronger initial health status of hand versus solid organ transplant recipients. Undeniably, these are medium-term results, and with longer-term follow-up the results may change, and systemic toxic effects and malignancies may occur.

Conclusions

Hand and facial transplantations are now a clinical reality. As has been the case in so many advances in medicine, while these new treatments seem like an enormous leap forward, in reality the individual components necessary to accomplish these advancements are well established and have been routinely used in clinical practice for some time. The microsurgical techniques used to transplant a hand or facial tissue, while complex, are commonly practised by reconstructive plastic surgeons. The immuno-suppression medications used to prevent rejection have been used in thousands of organ transplant recipients. All of the logistics used to identify, select, harvest and transport the donor tissue have been developed and are used routinely in solid organ procurement.

As scientists and physicians it is now our duty to ensure that hand and facial transplantation moves into the clinical research phase in a thoughtful and well planned manner. To achieve this, it is essential that teams proposing to perform these new procedures have the necessary technical and immunological expertise, but more importantly, that they develop and adhere to well defined ethical guidelines. These guidelines should include open display and public and professional discussion and evaluation. By openly sharing and discussing our successes as well as our

failures we will assure that this new and exciting medical frontier will reach mainstream medicine as quickly as possible and thus be made available to so many who suffer with these disfiguring deformities.

Recommendations

Recommendation	Evidence level
◆ To date, 20 individuals have received seven double hand, 12 single hand and one thumb transplant worldwide and, overall, the functional outcomes and patient satisfaction have been reported to be good.	IIb/B
◆ Three successful face transplants have been performed worldwide	IV/C
◆ Using the LIFT questionnaire, there is evidence to demonstrate that patients are willing to accept the consequences of life-long immunosuppression for the opportunity to receive a face transplant.	IIb/B
◆ Human hand transplant studies report a 0% graft loss at one year, and a chronic rejection rate of 0% at two years.	IIb/B
◆ Non-compliance, acute rejection episodes (treated) and infection have been observed, but as yet, there have been no reports of other systemic toxic effects or malignancies following human allotransplantation.	IIb/B

References

1. Kanitakis J, Petruzzo P, Jullien D, *et al*. Pathological score for the evaluation of allograft rejection in human hand (composite tissue) allotransplantation. *Eur J Dermatol* 2005; 15: 235-8.
2. Lanzetta M, Petruzzo P, Vitale, G, *et al*. Human hand transplantation: what have we learned? *Transplant Proc* 2004; 36: 664-8.
3. Lanzetta M, Petruzzo P, Margreiter R, *et al*. The International Registry on Hand and Composite Tissue Transplantation. *Transplantation* 2005; 79: 1210-4.
4. China's 1st face transplant successful, 2006 (cited April 15, 2006); available from: http://news.xinhuanet.com/english/2006-04/14/content_4425653.htm.
5. Jiang HQ, Wang Y, Hu XB, *et al*. Composite tissue allograft transplantation of cephalocervical skin flap and two ears. *Plast Reconstr Surg* 2005; 115: 31e-5; discussion 36e-7.
6. Man gets world's third partial face transplant. French doctors give 27-year-old with disfiguring disease a new nose, chin. (cited January 23, 2007); available from: http://www.msnbc.msn.com/id/16767785/.
7. Devauchelle B, Badet L, Lengelé B, Morelon E, Testelin S, Michallet M, D'Hauthuille C, Dubernard JM. First human face allograft: early report. *Lancet* 2006; 368(9531): 203-9.
8. Wigmore SJ. Face transplantation: the view from Birmingham, England. *South Med J* 2006; 99: 424-6.
9. Jones JW, Gruber SA, Barker JH, *et al*. Successful hand transplantation. One-year follow-up. Louisville Hand Transplant Team. *N Engl J Med* 2000; 343: 468-73.
10. Dubernard JM, Owen E, Herzberg G, *et al*. Human hand allograft: report on first 6 months. *Lancet* 1999; 353: 1315-20.
11. Dubernard JM, Owen E, Lefrancois N, *et al*. First human hand transplantation. Case report. *Transpl Int* 2000; 13 Suppl 1: S521-4.
12. Francois CG, Breidenbach WC, Maldonado C, *et al*. Hand transplantation: comparisons and observations of the first four clinical cases. *Microsurgery* 2000; 20: 360-71.
13. Stevenage S, McKay Y. Model applicants: the effect of facial appearance on recruitment decisions. *British Journal of Psychology* 1999; 90: 221-34.
14. Robinson E, Rumsey N, Partridge J. An evaluation of the impact of social interaction skills training for facially disfigured people. *Br J Plast Surg* 1996; 49: 281-9.
15. Ye EM. Psychological morbidity in patients with facial and neck burns. *Burns* 1998; 24: 646-8.
16. The UK Face Transplant Information Website, 2006 (cited March 15, 2006); available from: http://www.facialtransplantation.org.uk/content/info2.asp.

17. Dougherty H. Burns girl to have first face transplant, 2003 (cited April 26, 2006); available from: http://www.thisislondon.com/news/articles/3609267?source= Evening%20Standard.

18. Morris P, Bradley A, Doyal L, *et al*. Facial Transplantation: Working Party report, 2003 (cited April 30, 2006); available from: http://www.rcseng.ac.uk/rcseng/content/publications/docs/facial_transplantation.html.

19. Wiggins OP, Barker JH, Martinez S, *et al*. On the ethics of facial transplantation research. *Am J Bioeth* 2004; 4: 1-12.

20. Strong, C. Should we be putting a good face on facial transplantation? *Am J Bioeth* 2004; 4: 13-4; discussion W23-31.

21. Petit F, Paraskevas A, Lantieri L. A surgeon's perspective on the ethics of face transplantation. *Am J Bioeth* 2004; 4: 14-6; discussion W23-31.

22. Butler PE, Clarke A, Ashcroft RE. Face transplantation: when and for whom? *Am J Bioeth* 2004; 4: 16-7; discussion W23-31.

23. Caplan, A. Facing ourselves. *Am J Bioeth* 2004; 4: 18-20; discussion W23-31.

24. Rumsey N. Psychological aspects of face transplantation: read the small print carefully. *Am J Bioeth* 2004; 4: 22-5; discussion W23-31.

25. Agich GJ, Siemionow M. Facing the ethical questions in facial transplantation. *Am J Bioeth* 2004; 4: 25-7; discussion W23-31.

26. Morreim EH. About face: downplaying the role of the press in facial transplantation research. *Am J Bioeth* 2004; 4: 27-9; discussion W23-31.

27. Baylis F. A face is not just like a hand: pace Barker. *Am J Bioeth* 2004; 4: 30-2; discussion W23-31.

28. Robertson JA. Face transplants: enriching the debate. *Am J Bioeth* 2004; 4: 32-3; discussion W23-31.

29. Maschke KJ, Trump E. Facial transplantation research: a need for additional deliberation. *Am J Bioeth* 2004; 4: 33-5; discussion W23-31.

30. Ankeny RA, Kerridge I. On not taking objective risk assessments at face value. *Am J Bioeth* 2004; 4: 35-7; discussion W23-31.

31. Goering S. Facing the consequences of facial transplantation: individual choices, social effects. *Am J Bioeth* 2004; 4: 37-9; discussion W23-31.

32. Miles SH. Medical ethicists, human curiosities, and the new media midway. *Am J Bioeth* 2004; 4: 39-43.

33. Chambers T. How to do things with AJOB: the case of facial transplantation. *Am J Bioeth* 2004; 4: 20-1.

34. Trachtman H. Facing the truth: a response to "On the ethics of facial transplantation research" by Wiggins, *et al*. *Am J Bioeth* 2004; 4: W33-4.

35. Banis J, Barker J, Cunningham M, *et al*. Response to selected commentaries on the AJOB target article "On the Ethics of Facial Transplantation Research". *Am J Bioeth* 2004; 4: W23-W31.

36. Working Group-Comité Consultatif National d'Ethique (CCNE): Composite Tissue Allotransplantation of The Face (Full or Partial Facial Transplant), 2004 (cited April 30, 2006); available from: http://www.ccne-ethique.fr/english/start.htm.

37. Okie S. Facial transplantation: brave new face. *N Engl J Med* 2006; 354: 889-94.

38. Position of the American Society for Reconstructive Microsurgery on Facial Transplantation, 2006 (cited March 15, 2005); available from: http://www.microsurg.org/asrmFTP.pdf.

39. Facial Transplantation ASRM/ASPS Guiding Principles, 2006; available from: http://www.microsurg.org/ftGuidelines.pdf.

40. Dubernard JM, Lengelé B, Morelon E, *et al*. Outcomes 18 months after the first human partial face transplantation. *N Engl J Med* 2007; 357(24): 2451-60.

41. Butler PE, Hettiaratchy S, Clarke A. Facial transplantation: a new gold standard in facial reconstruction? *J Plast Reconstr Aesthet Surg* 2006; 59: 211-2.

42. Chinese face op man 'doing well' 2006 (cited May 6, 2006); available from: http://news.bbc.co.uk/1/hi/world/asia-pacific/4915290.stm.

43. McCabe S, Rodocker G, Julliard K, *et al*. Using decision analysis to aid in the introduction of upper extremity transplantation. *Transplant Proc* 1998; 30: 2783-6.

44. Cunningham M, Majzoub R, Brouha PCR, *et al*. Risk acceptance in composite tissue allotransplantation reconstructive procedures. Instrument design and validation. *Eur J Trauma* 2004; 30: 12-6.

45. Brouha P, Naidu D, Cunningham M, *et al*. Risk acceptance in composite-tissue allotransplantation reconstructive procedures. *Microsurgery* 2006; 26: 144-9.

46. Majzoub RK, Cunningham M, Grossi F, *et al*. Investigation of risk acceptance in hand transplantation. *J Hand Surg* (Am) 2006; 31: 295-302.

47. Reynolds CC, Martinez SA, Furr A, *et al*. Risk acceptance in laryngeal transplantation. *Laryngoscope* 2006; 116(10): 1770-5.

48. Barker JH, Furr A, Cunningham M, *et al*. Investigation of risk acceptance in facial transplantation. *Plast Reconstr Surg* 2006; 118(3): 663-70.

49. Barker J, Vossen M, Banis J. The technical, immunological and ethical feasibility of face transplantation. *Int J Surg* 2004; 2: 8-12.

Chapter 30

Hyperbaric oxygen therapy in plastic surgery

Christian Mills MRCS CHT
Registrar, Plastic and Reconstructive Surgery

ROYAL DEVON AND EXETER HOSPITAL, EXETER, UK
HYPERBARIC MEDICINE PHYSICIAN, DIVING DISEASES RESEARCH CENTRE, PLYMOUTH, UK

Introduction

Hyperbaric oxygen therapy (HBO) is the intermittent inhalation of 100% oxygen at pressures greater than that at sea level. It is widely recognised as the primary treatment for decompression illness, although only around 5% of treatments carried out by large hyperbaric centres are for this indication. In total there are 13 clinical conditions for which HBO has been advocated (Table 1). Of these, four are commonly encountered by plastic and reconstructive surgeons. The evidence supporting the use of HBO for these conditions is considered in this chapter.

History

Medical treatment using supra-atmospheric pressures predates the discovery of oxygen. As early as 1662, compressed air was used as a treatment for a wide variety of conditions including heart disease, respiratory failure, uraemia, diabetes and cancer.

The use of 100% oxygen at greater than atmospheric pressure was introduced around the turn of the 20th century for the treatment of caisson disease (decompression sickness) and later refinements to treatment protocols were made by the US Navy in support of military diving operations. In the 1950s, Boerema, a Dutch cardiovascular surgeon, investigated the use of HBO and hypothermia to facilitate surgery for congenital cardiac defects [1]. At around the same time, advances in cardiopulmonary bypass made the use of these techniques obsolete.

In 1967 the Undersea Medical Society, founded by US Navy Diving and Submarine Medical Officers, began regulation of the emerging new specialty of hyperbaric medicine and a report detailing the indications for hyperbaric therapy was issued in 1977 [2].

Practicalities

HBO is delivered by means of a hyperbaric chamber. There are two general chamber designs, mono-place and multi-place (Figure 1). Although less readily available, multi-place chambers allow direct access to the patient during treatment but require a greater support infrastructure and a larger number of trained staff. In the UK there are, at present, approximately 20 hyperbaric units divided into classes

Table 1. Recognised indications for hyperbaric oxygen therapy.

- Air or gas embolism
- Carbon monoxide poisoning
- Clostridial myonecrosis
- Crush injury, compartment syndrome and other acute traumatic ischaemias
- Decompression sickness
- Enhancement of healing of selected problem wounds
- Exceptional blood loss anaemia
- Necrotising soft tissue infection
- Refractory osteomyelitis
- Radiation tissue damage
- Compromised skin grafts and flaps
- Thermal burns
- Intracranial abscess

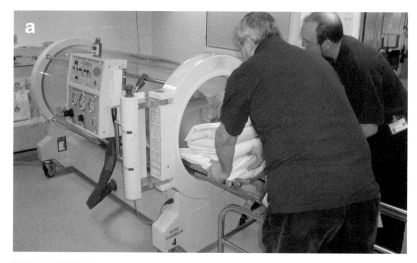

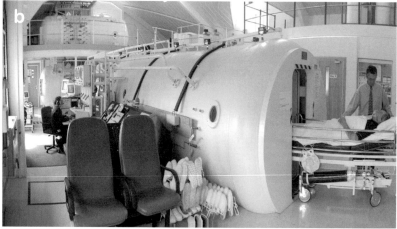

Figure 1. Hyperbaric chambers. a) Mono-place. b) Multi-place.

Chapter 30

depending on chamber type and the level of medical and hospital support available. Standard HBO treatments are delivered at the highest partial pressure of oxygen that can be tolerated without the induction of oxygen toxicity. A typical treatment schedule would involve breathing 100% oxygen at 2.2-2.4 Atmospheres Absolute (ATA) (222.9-243.2 kPa) for a total of 90 minutes (Figure 2). Brief air breaks are introduced during the treatment to minimise the risk of oxygen toxicity.

Complications

The potential complications of HBO therapy include barotrauma, oxygen toxicity (affecting the lungs, central nervous system and optic lens) and confinement anxiety. Most adverse events are self-limiting and resolve when treatment is discontinued. Barotraumatic otitis can be managed with temporary tympanostomy tubes and some centres use these prophylactically.

Mechanisms of action

HBO exerts its effects through two broad mechanisms. Firstly, there is the physical effect of raised ambient pressure on gas bubbles and gas-filled spaces, such as the lungs, as described by Boyle's Law. In the context of decompression sickness gas bubbles lodged in the vascular tree are thus reduced in size. It is the pharmacological effects of HBO, however, that are of most relevance to this chapter.

Increased tissue oxygen delivery

Breathing 100% oxygen at raised pressures markedly increases the amount of oxygen dissolved in plasma. For typical HBO treatment pressures the increase in oxygen carriage is approximately 10-15-fold. Arterial blood oxygen content is calculated using the following formula:

$$O_2 \text{ (ml/dl blood)} =$$
$$[Hb(g/dl) \times SaO_2(\%) \times 1.34(Hb\ O_2\ capacity)]$$
$$+ 0.003PO_2(mmHg)$$

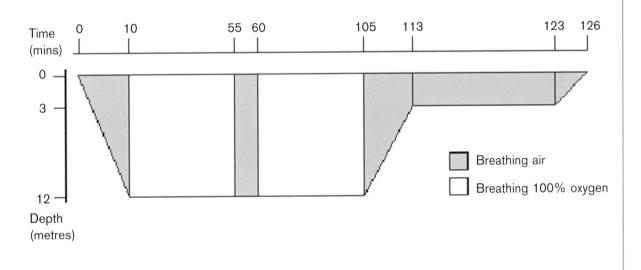

Figure 2. A typical HBO treatment profile.

Tissue oxygen concentration gradients are steeper and the distance over which oxygen can diffuse from the capillary bed into tissues increases. This may be sufficient to restore normal function to cells which are suffering cellular hypoxia. Such high concentrations of oxygen also have a range of dose-dependent pharmacological effects.

Leukocyte microbial killing

HBO has been shown to have both bactericidal and bacteristatic effects. At oxygen concentrations below 30mmHg, leukocytes are unable to generate an oxidative burst and are unable to effectively kill microbes. By increasing tissue oxygen tensions, HBO can restore the killing abilities of polymorphonuclear leukocytes.

Enhanced fibroblast proliferation

Fibroblasts synthesise the extracellular matrix of many tissues and provide a structural framework for the inward migration of re-populating cells. They are the most common connective tissue cell and are critical to the wound healing process. HBO has been shown experimentally to enhance fibroblastic proliferation [3, 4].

Increased collagen formation

The collagen that is synthesised by fibroblasts restores the extracellular structure and strength to healing wounds. The hydroxylation of collagen is an important step in formation of the collagen triple helix and this process is directly dependent upon the presence of oxygen. HBO has been shown to facilitate the post-translational modification of collagen in hypoxic tissues.

Neoangiogenesis in ischaemic tissues

Neoangiogenesis is the growth *de novo* of a micro-vascular system. It involves budding from local capillaries and is an essential part of the wound repair and regeneration process. HBO has been shown in animal and human studies to increase capillary density in healing tissues and also in tissues damaged by therapeutic irradiation [5].

Neutrophil adhesion

Neutrophil adhesion to the vascular endothelium is recognised as a major component in the pathophysiology of ischaemia-reperfusion injury. HBO has been documented to reduce neutrophil adhesion and to attenuate ischaemia-reperfusion injury in a number of experimental models [6-8].

Stem cell mobilisation

Most recently it has been demonstrated that a single exposure to HBO causes a doubling in the number of stem cells present in the peripheral circulation of humans, and after 20 treatments the increase is up to eight-fold [9]. The full role of these progenitor cells in the pharmacological effects of HBO has yet to be established but a role in neovascularisation has been proposed.

Methodology

PubMed was searched using combinations of the following terms 'hyperbaric oxygenation'[MeSH], 'burns', 'fasciitis', 'necroti*', 'graft', 'flap', 'wound' and 'healing'. In addition, the reference lists of review articles were examined for other relevant literature.

Necrotising soft tissue infections

Necrotising fasciitis (NF) is a rapidly progressing infection of the subcutaneous tissues and fascia. It is frequently life or limb-threatening. The mainstays of treatment have been examined elsewhere in this text, but essentially remain early surgery and broad-spectrum antibiotics. Intravenous immunoglobulin, recombinant Protein C and HBO have all been used in attempts to improve survival.

Experimental studies

The effectiveness of HBO in combination with penicillin in the management of NF has been established in a murine model of streptococcal myositis [10]. Both penicillin alone and penicillin plus HBO significantly reduced the number of colony forming units in specimens, but significantly longer survival was associated with combined therapy.

Tissue oxygen tensions have been measured in healthy volunteers and patients with NF undergoing HBO [11]. Six patients and three volunteers had tissue gas tensions measured using silastic tube tonometry in the subcutaneous tissues of the upper arm. Arterial gases were also measured. HBO raised blood oxygen concentration seven-fold and tissue oxygen tension four-fold in the NF group. These changes were not significantly different from the healthy volunteers.

Clinical studies

The earliest clinical analysis was a retrospective study to compare standard therapy alone and in combination with HBO [12]. Twenty-nine cases were examined with 17 receiving HBO. Despite the HBO group having been considered to have had worse prognostic indicators for the disease, mortality was significantly less in this group compared with the non-HBO group (23% vs 66%). In addition, the HBO group required fewer debridements as part of their treatment **(III/B)**.

A multi-centre retrospective analysis subsequently considered 54 cases of NF [13]. Thirty patients received HBO in this study. No significant difference in either duration of ICU/hospital stay or in the duration of antibiotic treatment was observed, and although there was a trend towards lower mortality in the HBO group this similarly failed to reach statistical significance. Interestingly, in this study the patients in the HBO group underwent more operations compared with those receiving standard treatment alone. It should be noted, however, that once again those patients in the HBO group tended to have poorer prognosis disease **(III/B)**.

Another later retrospective study [14] further challenged the role of HBO in the management of NF

with mortality rates of 36% in the HBO group compared with 25% amongst controls receiving standard treatment, although owing to small numbers of patients this difference was not statistically significant. The mean number of debridements was also higher in the HBO group (3.3 vs. 1.5) **(III/B)**.

In a small series of six cases of cervical NF, all of which were considered to have been odontogenic in origin, no deaths were reported following treatment with immediate broad-spectrum antibiotics and surgical debridement followed by HBO [15]. In three cases, HBO was commenced within 24 hours of diagnosis and in one case on the 19th postoperative day. The authors suggest that HBO may have a role in the management of NF but should be considered only after surgical debridement and intravenous antibiotic therapy have been initiated **(III/B)**.

The most recent retrospective analysis was reported in 2005 [16]. Forty-two consecutive patients with NF were treated with HBO in addition to aggressive surgery, antibiotics and critical care. No controls were included in the study. Mortality was 11.9% and only two amputations were carried out, both before transfer to the reporting facility. The average number of surgical debridements was 2.8 and the average number of HBO treatments was seven. Barotrauma and confinement anxiety were reported as complications of HBO but none were severe enough to prevent treatment. These results compare favourably with published mortality rates for the disease **(III/B)**.

Reviews

A thorough review of the role of HBO in the management of NF was published in 2005 but conclusions were guarded owing to the paucity of clinical studies and low case numbers available for comparison [17] **(IV/C)**.

Summary

HBO has been widely discussed as a potential adjunctive measure in the treatment of severe soft tissue infections such as NF and gas gangrene. Certainly there is considerable work investigating the mechanisms through which HBO exerts its pharmacological effects, and although the rationale for the use of HBO in the management of NF would appear to be sound, there is little evidence to support its efficacy in the literature. In the meantime, surgical debridement and intravenous high-dose antibiotic treatment should be instigated without delay, and the role for HBO remains to be fully elucidated in the context of a well conducted, prospectively randomised controlled clinical trial.

Failing skin grafts and flaps

Skin grafts

HBO can be used to prepare an ischaemic wound bed for skin grafting through the stimulation of neoangiogenesis and granulation tissue formation. In addition, it may have some influence on reducing the bacterial load within the wound. Several studies have also examined a role for HBO in assisting graft take postoperatively.

Experimental studies

An accelerated time to healing has been demonstrated in a rat wound healing model following the use of HBO in combination with skin grafting compared with grafting alone [18]. Time to full re-epithelialisation at partial and full-thickness wound sites reduced from 14 and 25.6 days, respectively, in the standard treatment group to 8.8 and 18.7 days in the HBO treatment group.

Full-thickness skin grafts have also been studied in a canine model [19]. In this study, HBO combined with hydroxyl-ethyl pentafraction starch (HEPFS) and deferoxamine was shown to improve graft survival in comparison with historical control data.

Clinical studies

Only one clinical study, from 1967, of 48 patients has compared split skin graft take with and without HBO [20]. A 29% improvement in the area of successful graft take was observed in the HBO treatment group. However, 'complete' take (defined

as >95%) was only achieved in 64% of HBO patients and 17% of non-HBO patients, and clearly the findings of this study may bear little relevance to the modern era **(IIb/B)**.

Composite grafts

Composite grafts are made up of several tissue types, the most common of which are skin, fat and cartilage. It is generally recognised that the majority of composite grafts will take if no part is more that 5mm from a vascularised tissue bed. HBO has been used to extend this distance and facilitate the grafting of ever larger composites.

Experimental studies

Using a rabbit ear model, Rubin showed that 46.9% of a 4x2cm side cut-out composite graft survived nine days when supported by HBO, compared with 16.2% of the control group [21].

An additional rabbit ear model, involving amputation of the distal 2cm and immediate reattachment [22], compared graft take when treated with HBO, dimethylthiourea, or melatonin, with untreated controls. Graft survival was assessed at one, two and three weeks. The authors were unable to demonstrate a clear benefit to HBO treatment compared with the control group at any stage. They did, however, point out some inconsistency between their chosen methods of assessing graft survival.

In a further study, incorporating both of the above models, HBO was administered for ten days and assessment of graft survival made at day 18 [23]. By this stage no tip grafts survived in either HBO or control group. In the side cut out group, however, only one of the ten HBO rabbits showed complete loss of the graft, compared with seven out of eight in the control group.

Clinical studies

One small series in the literature describes the treatment of six peri-orbital reconstructions with 'larger than normal' composite grafts. All six grafts survived in this series [24] (III/B).

Case reports also document successful replantation of a traumatically amputated nose [25] and the transfer of a large composite graft from the ear to the nasal tip [26], both supported with adjuvant HBO and both successful (III/B).

Finally, a series of five patients underwent nasal reconstruction using an ear lobule composite graft, treated with adjunctive HBO [27] (III/B). All patients experienced complete graft take. Interestingly, a further patient underwent the same procedure without HBO and the graft failed. The procedure was repeated using adjuvant HBO and was successful on the second attempt.

Local flaps

Experimental studies

An early study from 1965 showed a significant reduction in the degree of tip necrosis in random pattern flaps raised on the dorsum of a rat when HBO was administered at 2 ATA for three to four hours per day for four days [28]. Unfortunately, however, mortality was high due to oxygen toxicity.

A similar study using a guinea pig dorsal flap demonstrated a 22% increase in viable flap length in the HBO-treated group [29]. Histological examination of the flap was also carried out and increased capillary ingrowth and epithelial regeneration in the treatment group was observed.

HBO has also been investigated for its synergistic effect with other treatments [30]. When combined with allopurinol and topical silver sulphadiazine, HBO failed to improve flap survival, although combining HBO with tocopherol or superoxide dismutase and catalase was shown to be beneficial.

The effect of HBO on an inferiorly-based transverse rectus abdominis muscle (TRAM) flap in the rat has also been examined [31]. The HBO group demonstrated a 52.5% survival of the skin paddle, compared with 38.5% in the control group. Angiography revealed an increased capillary network in the flaps receiving HBO.

These results concur with those obtained in a random pattern flap model in pigs, in which HBO significantly increased the percentage area of the surviving flap between 12 and 26% [32, 33].

Clinical studies

There are little data regarding the use and effectiveness of HBO in improving flap viability clinically.

One prospective non-randomised trial of HBO treatment for ischaemic random pattern flaps has been reported [34]. Over the course of a one-year period, 11 episodes of flap necrosis were reported and only one of these failed to respond to HBO treatment. A retrospective analysis revealed a flap failure rate of 8.5-11.8% without HBO, compared with 4.5% for the year under investigation (IIb/B).

A retrospective review has also reported on 65 patients who received HBO to support flap survival [35]. HBO was indicated where there appeared to be incipient flap necrosis or pre-identified risk factors. Of these patients, 55% healed completely with a further 34% showing marked improvement in flap viability (III/B).

Free flaps

The only evidence in support of HBO treatment in the context of free tissue transfer comes from animal models. These have largely concentrated upon prolonging ischaemic time with the use of HBO and have yielded encouraging results [36-38].

Summary

While in animal models at least, HBO does seem to extend the viability of local random pattern flaps, there is little good evidence regarding the effectiveness of HBO in the salvage of compromised flaps in clinical practice.

As suggested by Friedman [39], multi-centre prospective clinical studies to compare HBO with other mechanical and pharmacological interventions are needed to evidence the effectiveness of this treatment modality for incipient flap failure in patients.

Thermal burns

Burn wound pathophysiology is well described elsewhere in this text, and it is an understanding of the metabolic responses to a major burn injury that provides us with the rationale for HBO treatment.

The use of HBO therapy in the management of thermal burns has been documented in published literature as early as 1965. It has been hypothesised that HBO exerts its effects through several mechanisms. In animal models, HBO has consistently been shown to reduce oedema formation [40], to restore normal tissue oxygen levels [41] and to attenuate the systemic inflammatory response in a variety of conditions [42]. HBO causes a profound inhibition of neutrophil activation thus minimising the associated endothelial injury [43].

Experimental studies

An early study of HBO in a rat full-thickness burn wound model demonstrated the restoration of normal tissue oxygen tension, although the effects of HBO wound healing were less clear [44].

More rapid epithelialisation of the burn wound and an earlier return of capillary patency (by India ink perfusion) have also been illustrated in a guinea pig model of partial-thickness burns [45]. A generalised reduction in post-burn oedema attributable to HBO treatment has been observed in a murine scalded ear model [40].

HBO and piracetam have together been shown to decrease the early extension of deep partial-thickness burns [46]. In a rat model of 5% TBSA partial-thickness burns, HBO was administered 12-hourly until day three. Small but statistically significant reductions in skin appendage destruction, epidermal basal layer destruction and dermal/epidermal leukocyte infiltration were noted in the HBO treated group.

The effects of HBO on a burn wound model in human volunteers have also been studied [47]. Twelve volunteers received a standardised UV burn to the forearm and were randomised to receive HBO at 2.4 ATA twice daily for three days, or a surface equivalent oxygen concentration at the same pressure. Wound size, hyperaemia and exudation significantly favoured the HBO-treated group, but there was no significant difference in surface re-epithelialisation. Furthermore, a similar burn study in a guinea pig model, which compared HBO with normobaric 100% oxygen (NBO) and silver sulphadiazine, demonstrated significantly increased re-epithelialisation in the NBO group [48].

Most recently a rat model of deep partial-thickness burns was used to compare silver sulphadiazine in combination with either HBO or a sham HBO [49]. HBO treatment resulted in a significant reduction in local tissue oedema, an increase in neoangiogenesis, an increased number of regeneratory active follicles and more rapid re-epithelialisation. In contrast with other studies, there was no difference in leukocyte margination or necrosis staging.

Investigators have also examined the role of HBO in the prevention of bacterial translocation following burns [50]. A study using a 30% burn rat model has shown how thermal injury causes both bacterial proliferation within the gut lumen and transmural translocation. Amongst rats receiving HBO, both proliferation and translocation were significantly reduced at day three and eight.

Clinical studies

One double-blind randomised controlled trial of 16 burns patients has investigated mean healing times following HBO compared with a sham treatment [51] **(Ib/A)**. Time to healing was significantly shorter in patients exposed to HBO (19.7 days versus 43.8 days; p<0.01). Fluid requirements were small and the risk of graft failure was less with HBO. Other outcome measures, such as mortality and morbidity rate, were not recorded.

In a later paired case-control study, 36 burns patients receiving HBO were compared with 36 age- and % BSA-matched controls [52]. With respect to wound healing the two groups were broadly similar, but there was a worrying prevalence of renal toxicity and bacterial sepsis in the HBO group **(IIa/B)**.

Finally, a further randomised controlled trial has been conducted randomising 121 burns patients to standard treatment with or without HBO [53]. No statistically significant differences in length of stay, mortality, acute fluid requirements and number of operations were identified **(Ib/A)**.

Reviews

A comprehensive but non-systematic review in 1994 considered the evidence for the role of HBO in burns management [54]. The findings of this review suggested that HBO was able to facilitate a significant reduction in morbidity, mortality, length of hospital stay and the need for surgery **(IV/C)**.

Ten years on, the use of HBO in the management of thermal burns was the subject of a Cochrane systematic review [55]. Only two randomised controlled trials were identified, conducted 23 years apart, which met their inclusion criteria [51, 53]. These two studies were felt to be too dissimilar and of insufficient quality to allow them to be combined in a meta-analysis. Encouraging results were acknowledged from one of the studies but the overall conclusion was that there was insufficient evidence to support the routine use of HBO in the management of severe burns **(Ia/A)**.

Summary

It seems logical that HBO should ameliorate the production of inflammatory mediators at burn wound sites through a reduction in tissue hypoxia. Despite this there remains a lack of evidence from well conducted clinical trials to support its use. Clearly this remains a potential area for further research and HBO may yet find a role in the management of severe burns.

Problem wounds

Problem wounds are generally recognised by clinicians as those that fail to heal despite treatment with standard recognised medical and surgical techniques. The most common chronic wounds encountered in western medical practice are due to diabetes, vascular disease (arterial or venous), sustained pressure or therapeutic irradiation. Common to all these conditions is tissue hypoxia at the wound site:

- Diabetic foot ulcers are usually the result of a combination of peripheral neuropathy and/or peripheral vascular disease. The annual incidence of foot ulcers in diabetics may be as high as 10% and around 12% of diabetics with foot ulcers progress to amputation [56].
- Venous ulcers are due to raised venous pressure secondary either to reflux or obstruction. The prevalence of venous ulcers has been estimated at 20/1000 people aged over 80 years [57].
- Arterial ulcers are due to impaired perfusion to the feet or legs. They generally represent the end stages of lower limb atherosclerosis and are the peripheral manifestation of a generalised disease process.
- Pressure ulcers are often deep, extending down to underlying muscle or bone. They are due to unrelieved pressure in the immobile patient and have a prevalence of 6-10% in UK NHS hospitals [58].

HBO has been used for the treatment of chronic wounds since the 1960s [59].

Diabetic ulcers (Figure 3)

Unlike much of hyperbaric medicine, there are several randomised controlled trials that examine the efficacy of HBO in the treatment of diabetic wounds and the prevention of distal amputation.

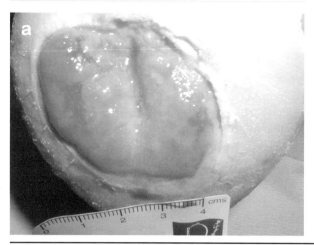 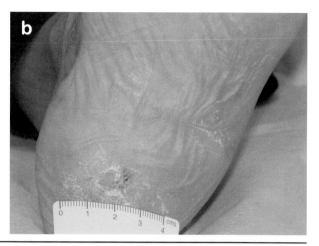

Figure 3. A diabetic ulcer treated with hyperbaric oxygen therapy. a) Pre-treatment. b) Post-treatment.

Randomised controlled trials

The earliest randomised controlled trial recruited 30 patients to treatment by either standard care alone or standard care plus HBO using 3 ATA on four occasions over four weeks [60]. Patients were not blinded. The endpoints of the study were major and minor distal amputation. Two major amputations were required in the HBO group, compared with seven amongst controls. This difference just failed to reach statistical significance **(Ib/A)**.

A further randomised controlled trial, again non-blinded, included 70 patients in similar treatment arms with HBO delivered at 2.2-2.5 ATA daily for 20-40 treatments [61]. Once again, there was an observed reduction in major amputations in the HBO group **(Ib/A)**.

The most recent double-blinded randomised controlled trial to address this issue randomised 18 patients to wound care plus sham HBO or wound care with HBO [62]. The study reported a significantly higher rate of wound healing and a significantly lower rate of amputations in the HBO group compared with the sham group **(Ib/A)**.

Reviews

A systematic review of the literature in 2003 considered all published trials and case series with more than five cases of problematic diabetic wounds treated by HBO [63]. While these studies overall suggested that HBO might be of some benefit to non-healing diabetic ulcers, in general the quality of studies was poor and there was insufficient evidence to recommend HBO as an adjunctive therapy **(Ia/A)**.

In 2004, a Cochrane systematic review was undertaken [64]. Five trials met eligibility criteria for inclusion, enabling the evaluation of a total of 163 patients in a single meta-analysis. The relative risk of major amputation with HBO was found to be 0.31 (p=0.0006), with four patients needing to be treated to avoid one amputation. Given the small number of studies available for scrutiny and the modest number of patients, and methodological and reporting inadequacies of those studies, the guarded conclusion of the meta-analysis was that large randomised controlled trials of high methodological rigour are required to determine the true benefit of HBO therapy for diabetic ulceration **(Ia/A)**.

Venous ulceration

Randomised controlled trials

One double-blind trial has explored the use of HBO in the management of venous ulceration. Sixteen non-diabetic patients in whom large vessel disease had been excluded were randomised to receive either air or 100% oxygen at 2.5 ATA [65]. The residual wound area was assessed after two, four and six weeks. After four weeks there was a significant difference in the mean reduction in wound area in favour of the HBO-treated group (22% vs. 3.7%; p<0.05), and at six weeks the difference was even greater (2.7% vs. 35.7%; p<0.001) **(Ib/A)**.

Reviews

Venous ulcers were also included in the Cochrane review of HBO therapy [64]. Only one trial was cited in which there was no significant difference in healing between HBO and sham treatment groups. Overall there appears to be less evidence for the efficacy of HBO in the management of venous ulceration compared with diabetic ulceration and any true benefit remains to be proven in the context of a large well conducted randomised controlled trial **(Ia/A)**.

Arterial ulcers

The primary treatment for ulceration due to arterial insufficiency is revascularisation of the affected limb. Once this is achieved, then ulcers generally heal rapidly. There is no evidence to support the use of HBO in the treatment of arterial ulcers [66] **(Ia/A)**.

Radiation ulceration

Radiation-induced ulceration, including osteoradionecrosis, has long been thought of as a prime indication for HBO therapy, and has similarly been the subject of a Cochrane review [67]. This review pointed towards a potential benefit from HBO in the management of late radiation tissue injury involving the head and neck and the perineum following abdomino-perineal resection and radiotherapy for low anorectal carcinoma. In addition, the risk of osteoradionecrosis developing in the mandible following dental extraction in the radiotherapy field appears to be reduced by prophylactic HBO. As before, more study is warranted **(Ia/A)**.

Summary

The evidence in support of HBO is perhaps strongest when addressing tissue hypoxia at chronic wound sites. In this context, as in others, HBO remains a perfectly logical and tantalising solution to poor wound healing but there is a lack of level I and II evidence precluding its widespread clinical development. In addition, there will always be financial and logistical barriers to development of HBO as a treatment modality, but there is now the beginnings of an evidence base upon which future studies can build.

Conclusions

The use of HBO has been advocated in the management of a range of conditions. Several of these fall within the scope of plastic surgical practice. There is evidence to support the use of HBO in the treatment of necrotising soft tissue infections although this does not reach a high level. The case for the use of HBO in chronic diabetic foot ulcers is stronger, with randomised controlled trials and systematic reviews supporting its selective use. There is some low level evidence to suggest that HBO may be of help in salvaging compromised skin flaps. Despite being a recognised indication for HBO, a systematic review of the literature does not support its use in this context. In all these areas, there is clear scope for further, more rigorous trials to be carried out. Where any evidence of efficacy is conclusively demonstrated, this will need to be backed up by favourable economic analysis before HBO can receive widespread acceptance.

Acknowledgement

The author would like to thank the Diving Diseases Research Centre in Plymouth, UK, for their help in the preparation of this chapter and also for providing the illustrations.

Chapter 30

Chapter 30

Recommendations

	Evidence level
◆ Where HBO is readily available, its use, in addition to surgery, antibiotics and critical care, may reduce mortality in necrotising fasciitis.	IIb/B
◆ Compromised skin flaps can sometimes be salvaged by using HBO.	III/C
◆ The currently available evidence does not support the use of HBO in the management of thermal burns.	Ia/A
◆ HBO can help prevent major amputations in diabetic patients with foot ulcers.	Ia/A
◆ When added to standard wound care, HBO can help chronic diabetic ulcers heal.	Ia/A

References

1. Boerema I, Huiskes JW, Kroll JA, Kroon B, Lokin E, Meyne NG. High atmospheric pressure as an aid to cardiac surgery. *Arch Chir Neerl* 1956; 8(3): 193-211.

2. Kindwall EP. Hyperbaric Oxygen Therapy: A Committee Report. Bethesda, Md: UMS; 1977. Report No.: Undersea Medical Society Report 5-23-77.

3. Kang TS, Gorti GK, Quan SY, Ho M, Koch RJ. Effect of hyperbaric oxygen on the growth factor profile of fibroblasts. *Arch Facial Plast Surg* 2004; 6(1): 31-5.

4. Kunnavatana SS, Quan SY, Koch RJ. Combined effect of hyberbaric oxygen and N-acetylcysteine on fibroblast proliferation. *Arch Otolaryngol Head Neck Surg* 2005; 131(9): 809-14.

5. Marx RE, Ames JR. The use of hyperbaric oxygen therapy in bony reconstruction of the irradiated and tissue-deficient patient. *J Oral Maxillofac Surg* 1982; 40(7): 412-20.

6. Bouachour G, Cronier P, Gouello JP, Toulemonde JL, Talha A, Alquier P. Hyperbaric oxygen therapy in the management of crush injuries: a randomized double-blind placebo-controlled clinical trial. *J Trauma* 1996; 41(2): 333-9.

7. Buras J. Basic mechanisms of hyperbaric oxygen in the treatment of ischemia-reperfusion injury. *Int Anesthesiol Clin* 2000; 38(1): 91-109.

8. Buras JA, Reenstra WR. Endothelial-neutrophil interactions during ischemia and reperfusion injury: basic mechanisms of hyperbaric oxygen. *Neurol Res* 2007; 29(2): 127-31.

9. Thom SR, Bhopale VM, Velazquez OC, Goldstein LJ, Thom LH, Buerk DG. Stem cell mobilization by hyperbaric oxygen. *Am J Physiol Heart Circ Physiol* 2006; 290(4): H1378-86.

10. Zamboni WA, Mazolewski PJ, Erdmann D, Bergman BA, Hussman J, Cooper MD, *et al*. Evaluation of penicillin and hyperbaric oxygen in the treatment of streptococcal myositis. *Ann Plast Surg* 1997; 39(2): 131-6.

11. Korhonen K, Kuttila K, Niinikoski J. Tissue gas tensions in patients with necrotising fasciitis and healthy controls during treatment with hyperbaric oxygen: a clinical study. *Eur J Surg* 2000; 166(7): 530-4.

12. Riseman JA, Zamboni WA, Curtis A, Graham DR, Konrad HR, Ross DS. Hyperbaric oxygen therapy for necrotizing fasciitis reduces mortality and the need for debridements. *Surgery* 1990; 108(5): 847-50.

13. Brown DR, Davis NL, Lepawsky M, Cunningham J, Kortbeek J. A multicenter review of the treatment of major truncal necrotizing infections with and without hyperbaric oxygen therapy. *Am J Surg* 1994; 167(5): 485-9.

14. Shupak A, Shoshani O, Goldenberg I, Barzilai A, Moskuna R, Bursztein S. Necrotizing fasciitis: an indication for hyperbaric oxygenation therapy? *Surgery* 1995; 118(5): 873-8.

15. Langford FP, Moon RE, Stolp BW, Scher RL. Treatment of cervical necrotizing fasciitis with hyperbaric oxygen therapy. *Otolaryngol Head Neck Surg* 1995; 112(2): 274-8.

16. Escobar SJ, Slade JB, Jr., Hunt TK, Cianci P. Adjuvant hyperbaric oxygen therapy (HBO_2) for treatment of necrotizing fasciitis reduces mortality and amputation rate. *Undersea Hyperb Med* 2005; 32(6): 437-43.

17. Jallali N, Withey S, Butler PE. Hyperbaric oxygen as adjuvant therapy in the management of necrotizing fasciitis. *Am J Surg* 2005; 189(4): 462-6.

18. Shulman AG, Krohn HL. Influence of hyperbaric oxygen and multiple skin allografts of the healing of skin wounds. *Surgery* 1967; 62: 1051.

19. Hosgood G, Hodgin EC, Strain GM, Lopez MK, Lewis DD. Effect of deferoxamine and hyperbaric oxygen on free, autogenous, full-thickness skin grafts in dogs. *Am J Vet Res* 1995; 56(2): 241-7.

20. Perrins DJ. Influence of hyperbaric oxygen on the survival of split skin grafts. *Lancet* 1967; 1(7495): 868-71.

21. Rubin JS, Marzella L, Myers RA, Suter C, Eddy H, Kleiman L. Effect of hyperbaric oxygen on the take of composite skin grafts in rabbit ears. *J Hyperbaric Med* 1988; 3: 79.

22. Lim AA, Wall MP, Greinwald JH, Jr. Effects of dimethylthiourea, melatonin, and hyperbaric oxygen therapy on the survival of reimplanted rabbit auricular composite grafts. *Otolaryngol Head Neck Surg* 1999; 121(3): 231-7.

23. McClane S, Renner G, Bell PL, Early EK, Shaw B. Pilot study to evaluate the efficacy of hyperbaric oxygen therapy in improving the survival of reattached auricular composite grafts in the New Zealand White rabbit. *Otolaryngol Head Neck Surg* 2000; 123(5): 539-42.

24. Gonnering RS, Kindwall EP, Goldmann RW. Adjunct hyperbaric oxygen therapy in periorbital reconstruction. *Arch Ophthalmol* 1986; 104(3): 439-43.

25. Nichter LS, Morwood DT, Williams GS, Spence RJ. Expanding the limits of composite grafting: a case report of successful nose replantation assisted by hyperbaric oxygen therapy. *Plast Reconstr Surg* 1991; 87(2): 337-40.

26. Rapley JH, Lawrence WT, Witt PD. Composite grafting and hyperbaric oxygen therapy in pediatric nasal tip reconstruction after avulsive dog-bite injury. *Ann Plast Surg* 2001; 46(4): 434-8.

27. Friedman HI, Stonerock C, Brill A. Composite earlobe grafts to reconstruct the lateral nasal ala and sill. *Ann Plast Surg* 2003; 50(3): 275-81.

28. McFarlane RM, DeYoung G, Henry RA. Prevention of necrosis in experimental pedicle flaps with hyperbaric oxygen. *Surg Forum* 1965; 16: 481-2.

29. Manson PN, Im IJ, Myers RA, Hoopes JE. Improved capillaries by hyperbaric oxygen in skin flaps. *Surg Forum* 1980; 31: 564.

30. Stewart RJ, Moore T, Bennett B, Easton M, Newton GW, Yamaguchi KT. Effect of free-radical scavengers and hyperbaric oxygen on random-pattern skin flaps. *Arch Surg* 1994; 129(9): 982-7.

31. Ramon Y, Abramovich A, Shupak A, Ullmann Y, Moscona RA, Shoshani O, et al. Effect of hyperbaric oxygen on a rat transverse rectus abdominis myocutaneous flap model. *Plast Reconstr Surg* 1998; 102(2): 416-22.

32. Kernahan DA, Zingg W, Kay CW. The effect of hyperbaric oxygen on the survival of experimental skin flaps. *Plast Reconstr Surg* 1965; 36: 19-25.

33. Pellitteri PK, Kennedy TL, Youn BA. The influence of intensive hyperbaric oxygen therapy on skin flap survival in a swine model. *Arch Otolaryngol Head Neck Surg* 1992; 118(10): 1050-4.

34. Perrins DJ. The effect of hyperbaric oxygen on ischemic skin flaps. In: *Skin Flaps*. Grabb WC, Myers MB, Eds. Boston: Little Brown; 1975: 53.

35. Bowersox JC, Strauss MB, Hart GB. Clinical experience with hyperbaric oxygen therapy in the salvage of ischemic skin flaps and grafts. *J Hyperbaric Med* 1986; 1: 141.

36. Angel MF, Im MJ, Chung HK, Vander Kolk CA, Manson PN. Effects of combined cold and hyperbaric oxygen storage on free flap survival. *Microsurgery* 1994; 15(9): 648-51.

37. Kaelin CM, Im MJ, Myers RA, Manson PN, Hoopes JE. The effects of hyperbaric oxygen on free flaps in rats. *Arch Surg* 1990; 125(5): 607-9.

38. Edwards RJ, Im MJ, Hoopes JE. Effects of hyperbaric oxygen preservation on rat limb replantation: a preliminary report. *Ann Plast Surg* 1991; 27(1): 31-5.

39. Friedman HI, Fitzmaurice M, Lefaivre JF, Vecchiolla T, Clarke D. An evidence-based appraisal of the use of hyperbaric oxygen on flaps and grafts. *Plast Reconstr Surg* 2006; 117(7 Suppl): 175S-90.

40. Nylander G, Nordstrom H, Eriksson E. Effects of hyperbaric oxygen on oedema formation after a scald burn. *Burns Incl Therm Inj* 1984; 10(3): 193-6.

41. Korhonen K, Kuttila K, Niinikoski J. Subcutaneous tissue oxygen and carbon dioxide tensions during hyperbaric oxygenation: an experimental study in rats. *Eur J Surg* 1999; 165(9): 885.

42. Imperatore F, Cuzzocrea S, Luongo C, Liguori G, Scafuro A, De AA, et al. Hyperbaric oxygen therapy prevents vascular derangement during zymosan-induced multiple-organ-failure syndrome. *Intensive Care Med* 2004; 30(6): 1175-81.

43. Thom SR, Mendiguren I, Hardy K, Bolotin T, Fisher D, Nebolon M, et al. Inhibition of human neutrophil beta2-integrin-dependent adherence by hyperbaric O_2. *Am J Physiol* 1997; 272(3 Pt 1): C770-7.

44. Gruber RP, Brinkley FB, Amato JJ, Mendelson JA. Hyperbaric oxygen and pedicle flaps, skin grafts, and burns. *Plast Reconstr Surg* 1970; 45(1): 24-30.

45. Korn HN, Wheeler ES, Miller TA. Effect of hyperbaric oxygen on second-degree burn wound healing. *Arch Surg* 1977; 112(6): 732-7.

46. Germonpre P, Reper P, Vanderkelen A. Hyperbaric oxygen therapy and piracetam decrease the early extension of deep partial-thickness burns. *Burns* 1996; 22(6): 468-73.

47. Niezgoda JA, Cianci P, Folden BW, Ortega RL, Slade JB, Storrow AB. The effect of hyperbaric oxygen therapy on a burn wound model in human volunteers. *Plast Reconstr Surg* 1997; 99(6): 1620-5.

48. Shoshani O, Shupak A, Barak A, Ullman Y, Ramon Y, Lindenbaum E, et al. Hyperbaric oxygen therapy for deep second degree burns: an experimental study in the guinea pig. *Br J Plast Surg* 1998; 51(1): 67-73.

49. Bilic I, Petri NM, Bezic J, Alfirevic D, Modun D, Capkun V, et al. Effects of hyperbaric oxygen therapy on experimental burn wound healing in rats: a randomized controlled study. *Undersea Hyperb Med* 2005; 32(1): 1-9.

50. Akin ML, Gulluoglu BM, Erenoglu C, Dundar K, Terzi K, Erdemoglu A, et al. Hyperbaric oxygen prevents bacterial translocation in thermally injured rats. *J Invest Surg* 2002; 15(6): 303-10.

51. Hart GB, O'Reilly RR, Broussard ND, Cave RH, Goodman DB, Yanda RL. Treatment of burns with hyperbaric oxygen. *Surg Gynecol Obstet* 1974; 139(5): 693-6.

52. Waisbren BA, Schutz D, Collentine G, Banaszak E, Stern M. Hyperbaric oxygen in severe burns. *Burns Incl Therm Inj* 1982; 8(3): 176-9.

53. Brannen AL, Still J, Haynes M, Orlet H, Rosenblum F, Law E, et al. A randomized prospective trial of hyperbaric oxygen in a referral burn center population. *Am Surg* 1997; 63(3): 205-8.

54. Cianci P, Sato R. Adjunctive hyperbaric oxygen therapy in the treatment of thermal burns: a review. *Burns* 1994; 20(1): 5-14.

55. Villanueva E, Bennett MH, Wasiak J, Lehm JP. Hyperbaric oxygen therapy for thermal burns. *Cochrane Database Syst Rev* 2004; 3: CD004727.

56. Apelqvist J, Larsson J, Agardh CD. Long-term prognosis for diabetic patients with foot ulcers. *J Intern Med* 1993; 233(6): 485-91.

57. Callam MJ, Ruckley CV, Harper DR, Dale JJ. Chronic ulceration of the leg: extent of the problem and provision of care. *Br Med J* (Clin Res Ed) 1985; 290(6485): 1855-6.

Chapter 30

58. O'Dea K. The prevalence of pressure damage in acute care hospital patients in the UK. *J Wound Care* 1999; 8(4): 192-4.

59. Kulonen E, Niinikoski J. Effect of hyperbaric oxygenation on wound healing and experimental granuloma. *Acta Physiol Scand* 1968; 73(3): 383-4.

60. Doctor N, Pandya S, Supe A. Hyperbaric oxygen therapy in diabetic foot. *J Postgrad Med* 1992; 38(3): 112-4, 111.

61. Faglia E, Favales F, Aldeghi A, Calia P, Quarantiello A, Oriani G, *et al.* Adjunctive systemic hyperbaric oxygen therapy in treatment of severe prevalently ischemic diabetic foot ulcer. A randomized study. *Diabetes Care* 1996; 19(12): 1338-43.

62. Abidia A, Laden G, Kuhan G, Johnson BF, Wilkinson AR, Renwick PM, *et al.* The role of hyperbaric oxygen therapy in ischaemic diabetic lower extremity ulcers: a double-blind randomised-controlled trial. *Eur J Vasc Endovasc Surg* 2003; 25(6): 513-8.

63. Wang C, Schwaitzberg S, Berliner E, Zarin DA, Lau J. Hyperbaric oxygen for treating wounds: a systematic review of the literature. *Arch Surg* 2003; 138(3): 272-9.

64. Kranke P, Bennett M, Roeckl-Wiedmann I, Debus S. Hyperbaric oxygen therapy for chronic wounds. *Cochrane Database Syst Rev* 2004; (2): CD004123.

65. Hammarlund C, Sundberg T. Hyperbaric oxygen reduced size of chronic leg ulcers: a randomized double-blind study. *Plast Reconstr Surg* 1994; 93(4): 829-33.

66. Roeckl-Wiedmann I, Bennett M, Kranke P. Systematic review of hyperbaric oxygen in the management of chronic wounds. *Br J Surg* 2005; 92(1): 24-32.

67. Bennett MH, Feldmeier J, Hampson N, Smee R, Milross C. Hyperbaric oxygen therapy for late radiation tissue injury. *Cochrane Database Syst Rev* 2005; 20(3): CD005005.

Chapter 30